the Unofficial Guide™ to Living with Diabetes

by Maria Thomas
with
Dr. Loren W. Greene

Hungry Minds, Inc.

Hungry Minds, Inc.
909 Third Avenue
New York, NY 10022
www.hungryminds.com

This publication contains the opinions and ideas of its authors and is designed to provide useful advice to the reader on the subject matter covered. Any references to any products or services do not constitute or imply an endorsement or recommendation. The publisher and the authors specifically disclaim any responsibility for any liability, loss, or risk (financial, personal, or otherwise) that may be claimed or incurred as a consequence, directly or indirectly, of the use and/or application of any of the contents of this publication. All matters regarding your health require medical supervision. Consult your physician before adopting any suggestions in this publication, as well as about any condition that may require medical attention.

Certain terms mentioned in this book that are known or claimed to be trademarks or service marks have been capitalized. Hungry Minds does not attest to the validity, accuracy, or completeness of this information. Use of a term in this book should not be regarded as affecting the validity of any trademark or service mark.

ISBN: 0-02-862919-1

Manufactured in the United States of America

10 9 8 7 6 5 4

First edition

Acknowledgments

I want to thank the friends, family members, and colleagues who provided invaluable help along the way:

Many thanks to my co-author, Loren Wissner Greene, M.D., without whom this project could not have succeeded. Loren brought an encyclopedic knowledge of diabetes, unflagging energy, and much good humor to our work together, which has been a pleasure.

Many thanks, too, to my superb editor at Macmillan, Jennifer Williams. Jennifer has great taste and great tact, and I profited greatly from both while writing this book. The reader will profit, too. I also want to thank Jennifer very much for her kindness and patience throughout.

Thanks to Nancy Mikhail and Jennifer Perillo at Macmillan for getting us started and seeing us through.

The following people offered their knowledge, advice, and encouragement at many times and in many ways: Susan Filkins; Damienne Real; Louise, Francesca, and Benedette Palazzola; Barbara Winkelman; Eric Zorn; Rachael Williams; Michael Osheowitz; Ruth Taubman; Clare Johnson; Dino Valouritis; David Abramis; and especially Clayton Thomas, M.D. and Peggy Thomas. I am very grateful to you all.

Thank you from the bottom of my heart to Jeanne Levy-Hinte.

Finally, I want to thank my big-hearted husband, Clayton, who keeps me laughing, no matter what. Thank you, dear!

—Maria Thomas

My co-author, Maria Thomas, made this whole project possible. She had an amazing ability to absorb information and translate it into the most user-friendly language and synthesize loads of information into a coherent book. It was always fun to work with her and even to struggle together. Our editor at Macmillan, Jennifer Williams, was always a pleasure to work with too with her gentle care, encouragement and ability to negotiate the difficult waters. Joy Bauer and Nancy Mikhail were kind enough to invite me to participate in this project and Jennifer Perillo helped tremendously to direct and encourage us as we went along.

I want to thank my parents, Aileen and Irwin Wissner; my parents-in-law, Vera and Martin Greene, and my husband, Norman, for encouraging me along my journey in medicine. My particularly inspiring teachers and professors and inspiring colleagues along the way (in chronological order), included Mrs. Lillian Silverman, Dr. David Ehrenfeld, Dr. Eric Holtzman, Dr. Charles Hollander, Dr. Norton Spritz, Dr. Lawrence Rosman, Dr. Marie Pulini, Dr. Ira Laufer, and Dr. Herbert Samuels. Drs. Claresa Levetan and Richard Hellman have shown how good control in diabetes improves outcome. Dr. Valerie Peck deserves special thanks for "covering" me through my times off working on this book. Joy McKnight has helped me with endless faxing and mailings. Other uncited and insightful contributors have included: Scott Blum, Barbara Bove, Mario Ehrlach, Gregory Gallaro, Howard Gladstone, Carrie Greco, Christine Hart, Brian Hearn, Colette Kramer, Elaine Kubiak, Carol Mazin, Anu Menen, Eleanor O'Rangers, Jane Sealy, Kathleen Tregnaghi, Michael Verga, Richard Weil, Kathleen Wessels, and Marilyn Zayfert.

I would also like to thank my daughters, Alison and Becky and our sitter, Ruth Oliver, for putting up with a mother who was often absent in her devotion to keyboard medicine. Most importantly, I would again like to thank Norman for helping me make the big leap into human computerdom.

—Dr. Loren W. Greene

Contents

The *Unofficial Guide* Reader's Bill of Rights

We Give You More Than the Official Line

Welcome to the *Unofficial Guide* series of Lifestyles titles—books that deliver critical, unbiased information that other books can't or won't reveal—*the inside scoop*. Our goal is to provide you with the *most accessible,useful* information and advice possible. The recommendations we offer in these pages are not influenced by the corporate line of any organization or industry; we give you the hard facts, whether those institutions like them or not. If something is ill-advised or will cause a loss of time and/or money, we'll give you ample warning. And if it is a worthwhile option, we'll let you know that, too.

Armed and Ready

Our hand-picked authors confidently and critically report on a wide range of topics that matter to smart readers like you. Our authors are passionate about their subjects, but have distanced themselves enough from them to help you be armed and protected, and help you make educated decisions as you go through your process. It is our intent that, from having read this book, you will avoid the pitfalls everyone else falls into and get it right the first time.

Don't be fooled by cheap imitations; this is the *genuine article Unofficial Guide* series from Macmillan Publishing. You may be familiar with the proven track record of the travel *Unofficial Guides*, which have more than 3 million copies in print. Each year thousands of travelers—new and old—are armed with a brand new, fully updated edition of the flagship *Unofficial Guide to Walt Disney World*, by Bob Sehlinger. It is our intention here to provide you with the same level of objective authority that Mr. Sehlinger does in his brainchild.

The Unofficial Panel of Experts

Every work in the Lifestyle *Unofficial Guides* is intensively inspected by a team of three top professionals in their fields. These experts review the manuscript for factual accuracy, comprehensiveness, and an insider's determination as to whether the manuscript fulfills the credo in this Reader's Bill of Rights. In other words, our Panel ensures that you are, in fact, getting "the inside scoop."

Our Pledge

The authors, the editorial staff, and the Unofficial Panel of Experts assembled for *Unofficial Guides* are determined to lay out the most valuable alternatives available for our readers. This dictum means that our writers must be explicit, prescriptive, and, above all, direct. We strive to be thorough and complete, but our goal is not necessarily to have the "most" or "all" of the information on a topic; this is not, after all, an encyclopedia. Our objective is to help you narrow down your options to the best of what is available, unbiased by affiliation with any industry or organization.

In each *Unofficial Guide* we give you:

- Comprehensive coverage of necessary and vital information
- Authoritative, rigorously fact-checked data
- The most up-to-date insights into trends
- Savvy, sophisticated writing that's also readable
- Sensible, applicable facts and secrets that only an insider knows

Special Features

Every book in our series offers the following six special sidebars in the margins that were devised to help you get things done cheaply, efficiently, and smartly.

1. "Timesaver"—tips and shortcuts that save you time.

2. "Moneysaver"—tips and shortcuts that save you money.

3. "Watch Out!"—more serious cautions and warnings.

4. "Bright Idea"—general tips and shortcuts to help you find an easier or smarter way to do something.

5. "Quote"—statements from real people that are intended to be prescriptive and valuable to you.

6. "Unofficially..."—an insider's fact or anecdote.

We also recognize your need to have quick information at your fingertips, and have thus provided the following comprehensive sections at the back of the book:

1. **Glossary:** Definitions of complicated terminology and jargon.

2. **Resource Guide:** Lists of relevant agencies, associations, institutions, Web sites, etc.

3. **Recommended Reading List:** Suggested titles that can help you get more in-depth information on related topics.

4. **Important Documents:** "Official" pieces of information you need to refer to, such as government forms.

5. **Important Statistics:** Facts and numbers presented at a glance for easy reference.

6. **Index.**

Letters, Comments, and Questions from Readers

We strive to continually improve the *Unofficial* series, and input from our readers is a valuable way for us to do that. Many of those who have used the *Unofficial Guide* travel books write to the authors to ask questions, make comments, or share their own discoveries and lessons. For Lifestyle *Unofficial Guides*, we would also appreciate all such correspondence, both positive and critical, and we will make best efforts to incorporate appropriate readers' feedback and comments in revised editions of this work.

How to write to us:

Unofficial Guides
Macmillan Lifestyle Guides
Macmillan Publishing
1633 Broadway
New York, NY 10019
Attention: Reader's Comments

The Unofficial Guide
Panel of Experts

The *Unofficial* editorial team recognizes that you've purchased this book with the expectation of getting the most authoritative, carefully inspected information currently available. Toward that end, on each and every title in this series, we have selected a minimum of three "official" experts comprising the "Unofficial Panel," who painstakingly review the manuscripts to ensure: factual accuracy of all data; inclusion of the most up-to-date and relevant information; and that, from an insider's perspective, the authors have armed you with all the necessary facts you need—but the institutions don't want you to know.

For *The Unofficial Guide to Living with Diabetes,* we are proud to introduce the following panel of experts:

Dr. William A. Petit, Jr, M.D., F.A.C.P., F.A.C.E. Dr. Petit is the Medical Director of the Joslin Center for Diabetes at New Britain General Hospital. He is also an Assistant Professor of Clinical Medicine at Yale. Dr. Petit is board certified in Endocrinology, Diabetes and Metabolism.

Dr. Petit received his medical degree from the University of Pittsburgh School of Medicine. He completed an internship and residency at Strong Memorial Hospital, Rochester, New York. His post-doctoral fellowship was in Endocrinology and Metabolism at Yale University School of Medicine.

Dr. Petit is the Past President of the American Diabetes Association-Connecticut Affiliate. He was a member of the ADA Board of Directors and was elected to the ADA Hall of Merit.

Karen H. McAvoy, R.N., M.S.N., C.D.E. Karen McAvoy has been the Education Coordinator at the Joslin Center for Diabetes at New Britain General Hospital since 1996. Previously, she was a Diabetes Clinical Nurse Specialist at Yale-New Haven Hospital from 1993 through 1996. She is a Certified Diabetes Educator. She received her B.S.N. at St. Anslem College, Manchester, New Hampshire, and her M.S.N. at Yale University, New Haven, Connecticut.

Dessa Hartz, R.D., C.D.E. Dessa Hartz is a Clinical Dietitian at the Division of Endocrinology and the Diabetes Center for Children at the Children's Hospital of Philadelphia.

Introduction

I t's tempting to begin with the statistics: An estimated 20 million Americans have diabetes, and the number is rising. The United States spends close to $130 *billion* per year on diabetes health-care costs and time lost from work due to diabetes, which amount to almost 15 percent of total health-care expenditures. Diabetes is the leading cause of adult blindness, lower-limb amputations, and end-stage kidney failure in the United States; and it is a major contributor to the incidence of heart disease, nerve damage, and stroke.

The Rest of the Story

As sweeping and dramatic as these figures are, they tell only a part of the story. Diabetes places unique and recurring daily demands on each person affected by it. The treatment of most other serious diseases is in the hands of health-care professionals. But diabetes treatment is conducted largely by the "patient," who shoulders the primary responsibility for managing the disease. If you have diabetes, you—and only you—can take the steps that will help you to achieve the fundamental goal of diabetes management: keeping your blood-sugar levels from soaring too high or plummeting too low.

Yet successful diabetes treatment also means working with a team of health-care professionals— endocrinologists, diabetes educators, dietitians, ophthalmologists, podiatrists, and sometimes additional professionals. This is because diabetes affects and can damage virtually every part of the body. Poorly controlled diabetes can lead to the devastating, even deadly complications we mentioned above. The person with diabetes must have a team of practitioners who will help him or her to detect complications in the earliest stages, when they are most treatable.

Diabetes: Daily Demands

Assembling your diabetes treatment team is one of the first, and sometimes one of the most challenging, steps you must take to get your diabetes under control. But we repeat: It is the person who has diabetes who must work to keep his or her blood-sugar levels under control, each and every day, in order to feel good and to prevent or delay the development of diabetic complications.

Your team of professionals can't do this for you. Proper blood-sugar control means being aware of and controlling the interaction between the many factors that affect blood-sugar levels—factors that people who do not have diabetes rarely give much thought to. The person with diabetes must monitor the effects of eating, exercise, stress levels, and medications on her blood-sugar levels. She must frequently check her blood for the amount of sugar in it, and must adjust her food intake, food choices, medication dose and schedule, and the duration and intensity of exercise, all depending upon her blood-sugar readings. These are the daily "nuts and bolts" of diabetes self-care. When you add to this the emotional demands of coping with diabetes, and the impact it can have on families, friends, and loved ones, the day-to-day, individual picture can seem more overwhelming than all the national statistics combined.

How This Book Can Help

That's where this book comes in. If you or someone close to you has diabetes, you're probably feeling somewhat daunted by all that there is to know about the disease, about managing it, and about avoiding frightening complications. But think about this: You're not so overwhelmed that you're not seeking to educate yourself; after all, you've picked up this book. Your strength is showing! You're on the right track, and you've come to the right place.

The objective of *The Unofficial Guide to Living with Diabetes* is straightforward: to provide essential, complex medical information about all aspects of diabetes in the most organized and clear manner possible. We want you to grasp the technical facts about diabetes, but our bent is firmly practical, not academic. You won't be overwhelmed by too much medical information, nor disappointed by too little down-to-earth advice about *what to do*. You'll gain a basic understanding of the latest medical information on diabetes, but you'll also be armed with an arsenal of practical tips for coping with diabetes every day—from how to contain treatment costs and make the best dietary choices to how to respond to the emotional and family upheavals that can accompany diabetes.

Speak Up!

Another primary goal of this book is to prepare you to deal effectively with the health-care system and professionals with whom you will be interacting. Many of us feel a certain amount of awe and intimidation in the presence of those white coats. Our goal is to foster a little healthy independence, to promote your ability to speak up and advocate for yourself, despite the fear or helplessness you may understandably feel. In this day of impersonal, profit-oriented health care, self-advocacy is an essential skill for all patients. It is especially important, though, for people with diabetes, who must interact frequently with an array of caregivers and may need to fight to receive the full benefit of their insurance coverage. We tell you what you need to know to get your needs across to your doctor without working against him or her; how to find and select highly qualified professionals (and how to check up on their credentials); and how to evaluate new or alternative treatments *for yourself.*

The Psychological Side

Having diabetes, or any chronic disease, is an emotional as well as a physical experience. We've worked hard not to neglect the psychological side of living with diabetes. We explain what the major emotional impacts of diabetes can be—how to recognize the emotional "complications" of diabetes, how to address them effectively on your own, and when and how to seek professional help. We've made sure to include hard-to-find advice and information for friends and family members of people with diabetes: What is your role? How can you be most helpful? What is *not* helpful? And we haven't forgotten essential tips for parents of children and teenagers with diabetes, as well as special sections focusing on women, men, diabetes and sexuality, diabetes and pregnancy, and living alone with diabetes.

You'll also find here all the information you need to protect yourself against employment discrimination (yes, it happens), as well as information on traveling with diabetes, dining out, and how to gracefully navigate those food-laden office parties and other social functions.

Finding the Information You Need

Finally, we've packed our appendices with information on invaluable resources for people with diabetes: the best diabetes books and magazines, and how to find them; the leading diabetes organizations, and how to contact them; and other diabetes-related organizations and professional groups. We're especially proud of our comprehensive guide to Internet resources for people with diabetes. If you're worried about missing any of the many (and growing) resources out there that can help you to cope with diabetes, relax; we've done the research for you.

Looking Ahead

Yes, the statistics on diabetes are scary. But those same numbers have sparked new interest in finding better treatments, even a cure, for diabetes. Respect for the seriousness of diabetes is growing: In 1998, President Clinton earmarked $300 million for diabetes research over the next five years. The budget passed by Congress for 1999 includes another $1.9 billion for the National Institutes of Health, part of which will fund diabetes research. That money will be put to good use: In the mid-1990s, the National Institutes of Health launched two first-of-their-kind major diabetes studies. One is the Diabetes Prevention Trial-Type 1, which will examine the genetic roots and means of prevention of type 1 diabetes (formerly called *juvenile diabetes*). The other is the Diabetes Prevention Program, which will help to determine the best ways to prevent type 2 diabetes in people at risk for developing this disease (formerly called *adult-onset diabetes*). In the meantime, scientists are beginning to unlock the mysteries behind insulin resistance, a primary factor in type 2 diabetes, and the role of the immune system in causing type 1 diabetes. And new technology for transplanting healthy pancreas cells into people with diabetes is being developed, offering hope of a cure for diabetes that doesn't rely on difficult and costly whole-pancreas transplants.

Corporate America is also putting money into diabetes research. As the number of people with diabetes increases with increases in our population's age, obesity, and lack of physical activity, major drug and medical supply companies are investing in improving diabetes medications and tools. They're making rapid headway on advances such as the insulin pump, microfine syringes, "bloodless" blood-sugar monitoring, and "needleless" insulin.

It's an exciting time in diabetes research. Some people, like Dr. Lois Jovanovic of the Sansum Medical Research Foundation, believe that we will have a cure for diabetes by the year 2000. Dr. Jovanovic, who happens to have diabetes, is the director of the Santa Barbara Diabetes Project, an international research effort that has pledged to meet this millennial goal. Headquartered at Sansum, the Santa Barbara Project is bringing together the hard work, enthusiasm, and ambition of diabetes experts around the world, in hopes of accelerating the growing pace of diabetes research. You can read more about this fascinating project in Chapter 17.

Whether or not a cure for diabetes is found by the end of this century, today people can face the challenge of diabetes with confidence. After all, diabetes is a *manageable* disease. And our understanding of what diabetes is; how to treat it; and how to delay, prevent, and treat complications is steadily improving. With the spread of knowledge has come the emergence of a well-informed, supportive diabetes community, as a look at the number of publications and Internet sites devoted to diabetes will tell you. Education and support are your strongest allies. You are not alone, and you needn't be uninformed. It is our hope that this book will help to educate and support you, and will become one of your keys to a healthier life with diabetes.

A Word on the Term "Diabetic"

The authors of this book respect the important distinction between the terms "people with diabetes" and "diabetes". A conscious effort has been made, therefore, to use "people with diabetes" wherever possible. The distinction in terms is meant, also, as a reminder that no one should ever be defined solely by the condition of his or her health.

The Essentials

PART I

GET THE SCOOP ON...
What diabetes really is ▪ The roles of glucose
and insulin ▪ The liver and diabetes ▪ The
basics of daily treatment ▪ The difference
between insulin and oral medications ▪
The scope of diabetes

Defining Diabetes

Y ou've just been diagnosed with diabetes, or someone you know has. Funny how a word you've long had a passing familiarity with can suddenly become so compelling, so confusing, and so scary. What is diabetes, really? What is actually happening in your body?

Learning that you have a serious disease can make you feel more alone than you have ever felt before. That's a normal reaction. But did you know that diabetes is one of the most common chronic diseases of adults and children in the United States? An estimated 20 million Americans have diabetes. That's about 6 percent of the population, or one in seventeen people. Each day brings about 1,800 new diagnoses; each year over 650,000 new cases are diagnosed.

There are two types of diabetes, types 1 and 2, which we discuss at length in the next chapter. Either type can occur in people of any age, but, in general, type 1 occurs more often in children and type 2 in adults. Here are some more diabetes facts:

3

- About 90 to 95 percent of all cases are type 2 diabetes.

- Nearly 11 percent of Americans age sixty-five to seventy-four have type 2 diabetes.

- Among Americans ages forty-five to seventy-four, 6 percent of Caucasians, 10 percent of African Americans, and 14 percent of Mexican Americans and Puerto Ricans have type 2 diabetes.

- Among some Native American groups, fully half of adults have type 2 diabetes.

Type 1 diabetes, formerly called *juvenile-onset* or *insulin-dependent* diabetes, affects close to 130,000 children and teenagers in the United States.

Given these numbers, and the fact that diabetes can damage the heart, kidneys, eyes, and nervous system, it's no wonder that diabetes exacts a huge toll on the nation's health-care budget. Diabetes costs the United States approximately $130 billion per year, or close to 15 percent of total health-care expenditures. About half of diabetes-related costs are indirect, involving time lost from work, disability payments, or premature deaths. The other half consists of direct medical costs, such as doctors' fees, treatment supplies, and hospitalizations. Diabetes hospitalizations add up to about $6 million in-hospital days per year.

Sadly, diabetes is the leading cause of blindness in adults, end-stage kidney disease, and amputations in the United States. It is also the sixth leading cause of death by disease.

Keep in mind that the prevalence of diabetes is likely to increase as our population ages, becomes more obese and more sedentary, and as the Latino,

Native American, and African American populations grow.

So much for the entire United States of America. Let's get back to you: what diabetes means for you, and what is happening in your body.

Wasted energy

Here's what's happening: Your body cells are failing to absorb the sugar that is circulating in your bloodstream, with the result that far too much sugar is accumulating in your blood instead of entering cells and providing them with essential energy. Blood sugar, or *glucose* (the terms are interchangeable), derives from the foods we eat and is meant to enter cells and provide essential energy for their normal functioning. The body is not designed to cope with large amounts of sugar that stay in the blood, and serious complications develop from this. Untreated or poorly managed diabetes can lead to kidney damage, heart disease, coma, stroke, blindness, nerve damage, sores that won't heal, amputation, and infections throughout the body. Adults who have diabetes have four times the risk of developing heart disease as nondiabetic adults. (See Chapter 4.)

Sugar and symptoms

Diabetes's toll on the body is evident in its most common diagnostic symptoms: powerful thirst, frequent urination, and weight loss. As blood sugar reaches "overflow" proportions, the kidneys begin a heroic effort to flush excess sugar from the body through the urine. The body becomes dehydrated and a driving thirst results. The kidneys, of course, are seriously taxed by this burden; high levels of glucose are abnormal, and the body will do what it can

> 66
> When my sister was diagnosed with type 2 diabetes, I was really scared for her. Even though she's forty-three, she'll always be my 'little sister.' But now, I see her exercising, and eating right. Her lifestyle is healthier than it's ever been!
> —Anna, age forty-six
> 99

to correct the problem. Another response from the body is that cells, starved for glucose, begin burning fat and protein for energy. This breakdown of fat creates chemical by-products called *ketones*, which disturb the crucial and delicate alkaline/acidity balance of the blood. The blood becomes dangerously acidic, a condition called *diabetic ketoacidosis*, which can end in coma and death if unchecked. This rarely happens today, but prior to the 1920s, when pharmaceutical insulin became available, all people with type 1 diabetes eventually died from diabetic ketoacidosis. Today, diabetic ketoacidosis is fatal in 2 to 9 percent of cases.

It's not always obvious

Dramatic as these symptoms are, it's important to note that many people who have one type of diabetes, type 2, exhibit no symptoms or only mild symptoms, at least in the early stages of the disease. Their blood-sugar levels, nonetheless, are excessively high.

The hormone *insulin*, produced by the pancreas, controls the amount of sugar in the bloodstream. People with type 1 diabetes produce little or no insulin; people with type 2 diabetes do produce insulin, but for various reasons their bodies cannot make full use of the insulin produced. (There will be more on this in Chapter 2.) Due to their complete lack of insulin (which must be supplied by injection), type 1 diabetics experience more volatile ups and downs in blood-sugar levels, and the early symptoms of their disorder—before treatment with insulin injections is started—are more dramatic and dangerous.

Bright Idea
If you've recently learned you have diabetes, you may feel like there is too much to know about this complex disease. Give yourself time to take information in. It's not necessary, or possible, to understand everything all at once.

When blood sugar stays high

Rampant blood-sugar levels, whether obvious or not, wreak havoc on the body. It's extremely important to your health that glucose leaves the bloodstream and enters your cells to nourish them. Glucose is the end result of the digestion of carbohydrates. During digestion, what you eat is broken down into simple components that enter the bloodstream. Fats become fatty acids (typically stored); proteins become amino acids (typically used to build and repair tissue); and carbohydrates become glucose. All of these can be used as fuel for cells, but normally glucose is the body's primary, most "user-friendly" energy source.

After digestion, glucose passes through the walls of the small intestine into the bloodstream and on to all parts of the body. Again, glucose is not supposed to linger in the blood, circulating aimlessly. This is what happens, however, in diabetics. Their cells do not absorb glucose, and their blood becomes saturated with unhealthy amounts of unused, wasted glucose. Imagine holding a gas nozzle three feet away from your open gas cap: Fuel gushes plentifully (as the glucose enters the bloodstream), but it never enters the engine (cells) that needs it in order to get you down the highway.

Normally, the body vigilantly orchestrates the transfer of glucose from the blood into body cells. In nondiabetics, glucose in the blood tends to remain at or around the same level most of the day, usually balanced somewhere between 60 to 140 milligrams (mg) of glucose per deciliter (dl) of blood. (60 mg/dl represents low glucose levels prior to eating; 140 mg/dl represents higher levels, following a meal.) In people with untreated or poorly managed

Watch Out!
Did you know that urine tests alone are not sufficient to diagnose diabetes? Your doctor must perform blood tests to be certain.

diabetes, however, the average level of sugar is much higher than normal, and glucose levels are far more prone to large swings up or down. (See Figures 1, 2, and 3.)

Note! ➜
1. This is the blood-sugar level of a person without diabetes. The blood-sugar level rises after meals but stays in the normal range of 70 to 126 mg/dl throughout the day.

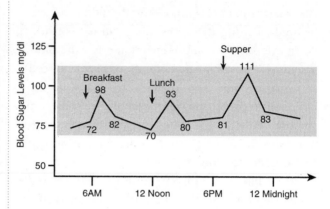

Note! ➜
2. Blood-sugar levels in people with well-controlled diabetes vary slightly before and after meals, but remain in the normal range most of the time. The average blood sugar in this case is 108 mg/dl.

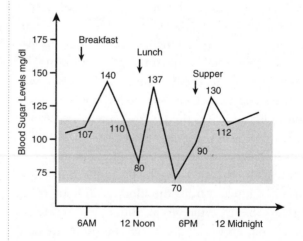

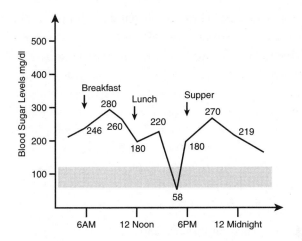

← Note!
3. Blood-sugar levels in people with poorly controlled diabetes are erratic, rising sharply after meals, then plummeting. Levels are high, on average. In this case the average blood sugar is 212 mg/dl.

Why does glucose remain in the blood of diabetics?

Insulin and blood-sugar control

Blood-sugar levels in people with diabetes are out of control; too much glucose remains in the blood and goes unused by cells. The key to understanding why this happens is insulin, which ensures that blood sugar goes from the bloodstream into the body's cells.

Insulin is not blood sugar and blood sugar is not insulin. Blood sugar comes from digested foods, while insulin is a hormone, one of many produced by the body. Hormones are chemicals produced by various glands or structures that travel through the bloodstream with vital "instructions" for other cells and organs. For instance, the female hormone *estrogen* is produced in the ovary; each month the ovary releases estrogen, which stimulates the uterine wall to begin the buildup of tissue that is shed in menstruation (unless pregnancy occurs). The hormone *melatonin* is produced by the pineal gland in the brain; when this gland secretes melatonin, it signals the brain to sleep and to wake up.

Insulin is made by a gland called the *pancreas*, a roughly banana-sized and -shaped organ that is found behind and somewhat below the stomach. The pancreas produces insulin in tiny multicellular structures called the *islets of Langerhans*, of which there are about 100,000 in a normal pancreas. One type of cell in the islets is the *beta cell*, which plays the most important role in producing insulin and also stores insulin for future use.

Beta cells: insulin powerhouses

It is the pancreatic beta cells that control the release of insulin, determining when and how much to release. When glucose begins entering the bloodstream following digestion, the beta cells respond to this and release the hound insulin. Here is where insulin's role in diabetes comes in: It is the hormone that tells body cell membranes to "open up" to sugar in the blood. Think of insulin as an escort to the blood sugar, one that has the power to open cell doors. Without insulin, cell membranes remain closed to glucose and, therefore, blood glucose levels remain high. (Conversely, when glucose is properly ushered into body cells, large amounts do not remain in the blood: If Macy's Department Store opens its doors at 8:00 a.m. to the customers thronging outside on a sale day, not many customers are left out on the street. Insulin is the Macy's doorman of glucose.)

Insulin must be present in the bloodstream in order for glucose to be absorbed into body cells where it belongs. The beta cells in the pancreas release insulin when blood-sugar levels rise. If insulin were not present to escort glucose into cells, too much sugar would stay in the blood.

The pancreas: insulin mastermind

The healthy pancreas performs a continuous and exquisite balancing act, managing to sustain smooth, stable blood-sugar levels by releasing just the right amount of insulin as glucose levels wax and wane throughout the day. The beta cells release stored insulin first, and then produce more if more is needed, say, after a carbohydrate-rich meal.

Once insulin has succeeded in getting the necessary amount of glucose into cells, the pancreas responds by tapering off the insulin release. This prevents blood-sugar levels from plummeting too low, which can lead to loss of consciousness. The brain requires large amounts of glucose to function. High blood-sugar levels, therefore, are not the pancreas's only concern. It works to prevent precipitous drops in blood sugar as well. Dangerously low blood sugar is called *hypoglycemia*, and it can be a life-threatening situation. (See Chapter 5.)

The liver: pancreatic helpmate

It may surprise you to know that the liver, too, plays an important role in blood-sugar control. Liver cells pick up and store glucose that is not immediately needed by the body for energy, thus removing excess sugar from the bloodstream. Unused glucose that is stored in the liver becomes a substance called *glycogen*, which can rapidly be converted back into glucose when energy needs are high (during exercise, for example) or when food intake is temporarily low, as during sleep.

The liver breaks down glycogen and releases it as glucose under orders from the pancreas, the glandular mastermind behind the regulation of blood-sugar levels. It is *glucagon*, another hormone produced by the pancreas, that stimulates the liver

Unofficially...
The word *diabetes* comes from the Greek word for "siphon." Ancient healers noticed that diabetics seemed caught up in an endless cycle of taking in water (extreme thirst) and eliminating it (frequent urination).

Bright Idea
Has someone close to you recently been diagnosed with diabetes? Your local American Diabetes Association can give you information about magazines and books published specifically for people with diabetes. A gift subscription or book might be just the thing. For more information, call the ADA at (800) 342-2383, or visit their Web site at: www. diabetes.org.

to release stored glucose. (Under stressful situations, especially if blood sugar drops very low, the stress hormone *adrenaline* will also trigger glycogen breakdown.) Thus the pancreas makes sure that adequate amounts of sugar are sent out to cells as necessary, and it can be responsible for raising blood-sugar levels as well as lowering them. In people who have had type 1 diabetes for years, glucagon stores in the liver may be low, hampering the body's swift correction of low blood sugar.

The healthy pancreas works to protect the body from the dangers of dramatic swings in blood-sugar levels. The pancreas releases finely calibrated amounts of insulin when blood-sugar levels rise; it pulls back on insulin secretion as blood sugar is absorbed from the bloodstream; and it releases glucagon (the liver-stimulating hormone) when blood-sugar levels begin to fall below healthy levels. Insulin acts on all cells, opening them up to absorb blood sugar; glucagon acts on the liver, stimulating it to release stored glucose back into the bloodstream.

It's a remarkable system, and if you're lucky enough not to have diabetes, you never give it a second thought. The person with diabetes, on the other hand, must think about blood-sugar control every day.

Health, quality of life, and, at times, life itself depend upon this conscious effort.

A day in the life of a person with type 1 diabetes

A person with diabetes faces the daily, even hourly, challenge of maintaining blood-sugar levels that are as close to normal as possible. A metabolic system that functions automatically in the nondiabetic body becomes the conscious task of the person with diabetes, who must in effect take on the job of the pancreas. The person with diabetes must try to balance the major factors affecting blood-sugar levels:

- Timing of meals
- Timing of snacks
- Choice of foods
- Timing and dosage of insulin or other medications
- Timing and intensity of exercise. (Exercise has an impact on glucose levels because it utilizes stored and available glucose, and for other reasons that are discussed in Chapter 9.)

Before breakfast

A routine day in the life of a person with type 1 diabetes begins before breakfast each morning with a blood test to check the glucose level. He or she must prick a finger in order to get a sizeable drop onto a chemically treated strip of paper. Taking the sample hurts a little, but not as much as it once did, when lancets—the small, sharp-pointed instruments used to get blood samples—were wider and less refined.

Getting a reading: the glucose meter

Once a drop of blood has been placed on the paper strip, most people with diabetes today use a specially designed blood glucose meter to read the strip. The meter is a highly accurate computerized device, small enough to fit in the palm of the hand, which gives a digital reading of the blood-sugar level "caught" on the strip.

Prior to the introduction of glucose meters, people with diabetes used color charts to check glucose levels. The chemically treated paper strip reacts with

Bright Idea
When taking a blood sample from your finger, prick the side, not the tip. There are fewer nerve endings on the sides, so it's less painful. Many people use a lancet device that allows them to administer the prick to just the right depth by pushing a button, just like using a ballpoint pen.

the blood sample to create a color. The strip is then matched with a color on the chart that represents that glucose level. A problem with the color chart method is that strips can develop colors that fall between colors on the chart, forcing people to estimate their glucose level.

Before blood testing became common, diabetics checked their urine for high blood sugar. This method for checking glucose levels is now obsolete. The limitations of urine testing are that

- Sugar does not begin to spill over into the urine until the amount in the blood is already very high.

- Urine testing reflects what was happening in the blood several hours ago, not what is happening now.

- Urine testing cannot tell you if your blood sugar is dropping too low (that is, if you are heading into hypoglycemia).

- In some cases, glucose is present in the urine of non-diabetic people, for example, pregnant women.

For the record: the blood-sugar log

Once the blood sample has been taken and read by the meter, the blood-sugar level must be recorded in a daily log. Your blood-sugar log is an indispensable tool in your diabetes treatment. Although most glucose meters will store a number of blood test results for recall, it is the daily log that gives a picture of your glucose patterns within each day and over time. It allows you to rapidly consider a lot of information. (See Appendix D for a sample blood-sugar log.)

How often a person with diabetes checks his or her blood-sugar level varies widely, based upon how difficult it is to control the blood sugar, whether or not the person injects insulin, how often it is injected, and other aspects of the treatment regimen. This is discussed in detail in Chapter 5. Typically, type 1 diabetics check their glucose level three to five times per day. Each time the blood sugar is checked, the finding is logged in the daily record. This usually includes a note on the dose and type of insulin injected following the check (if insulin is used), and any other factors that might be relevant to that reading, for instance, what was eaten at the last meal, or if exercise occurred.

Insulin injections: why?

All people with type 1 diabetes must take insulin to survive. Their bodies do not produce any insulin. A person with type 2 diabetes may or may not need to take insulin, depending upon how much insulin his or her pancreas produces.

Insulin can only be taken by injection; there is no such thing—yet—as "insulin pills" or "oral insulin." (But there are non-insulin oral medications for type 2 diabetes. See Chapter 6.)

Insulin is injected so that, ideally, there is always enough insulin present and active in the bloodstream to handle the rises in blood sugar that occur as food is digested.

Most people with type 1 diabetes, who want good control of their blood-sugar levels, inject themselves with insulin two to five times per day. Insulin injection schedules vary, based upon the individual's personal schedule and activity level, the need for flexibility at meal times, and personal goals for achieving blood-sugar control. Insulin regimens are discussed in more detail in Chapter 5.

> **66**
> I was amazed to discover how many books there are especially for kids with diabetes. I found them in our library, plus you can get some wonderful books from the American Diabetes Association.
> —Paula, mother of Ben, ten-year-old with type 1 diabetes
> **99**

The first injection

Before eating breakfast, the person using insulin has done a blood-sugar test and has recorded the results in her blood-sugar log. She must now prepare and inject her pre-breakfast dose of insulin.

There are different types of insulin, distinguished by how long it takes the insulin to become active in the body. One new form of insulin (called *lispro insulin*) is rapid-acting; it is active by about fifteen minutes after injection. Some insulin is short-acting; it is ready to work within thirty minutes of being injected, peaks rapidly, and leaves the body within three hours or so. Other insulins are intermediate-acting; it takes them forty-five to sixty minutes to become active, and their peak effectiveness occurs from two to eight hours after injection. Long-acting insulin starts working in two to four hours, with its peak effectiveness occurring at about sixteen hours following injection.

Each person injects the type or mixture of insulin that has been recommended by his or her health-care team. In the morning, it is common to inject a combination of short-acting and intermediate-acting insulins. That way, the short-acting insulin will handle the rise in blood glucose that follows breakfast, while the intermediate-acting insulin will be there for a midmorning snack or for lunch.

Some people may inject one shot of intermediate-acting insulin, or a mixture of intermediate- and long-acting insulin, in the morning.

The injection site

Diabetics who inject insulin do not use the same injection site every time. Repeated injections can cause skin reactions that can hamper the absorption of insulin. Instead, a general area of injection is chosen—frequently, the abdomen—and injection sites within that area are rotated. All injections must be made into the fat tissue lying just below the skin, the *subcutaneous* fat.

Waiting to eat

Once the injection has been made, it is necessary to give the insulin time to infuse itself into the bloodstream before eating. In the morning, this may mean a wait of fifteen to thirty minutes, if very short or short-acting insulin is used, or thirty to forty-five minutes, if only intermediate-acting insulin is used. The goal is to time meals and injections so that the post-meal rise in blood sugar will occur while there is active insulin in the bloodstream.

Off to work or school

People with diabetes need to think about the state of their blood sugar many times throughout the day. Whether you use insulin or not, it is often necessary to do blood glucose checks to see whether glucose has climbed too high or fallen too low, or to see how a certain meal or physical activity has affected your glucose level. If something's amiss, steps must be taken to get the glucose level back on track. If you take insulin, most regimens will require that you administer an injection or two during the day.

All of this means that people with diabetes must always have with them "the tools of the trade": a diabetes kit bag. Here's what you'll find in the average kit:

- One or two types of insulin (in small vials or in prefilled syringes)
- Syringes or insulin pen (holds premeasured insulin cartridge and includes needle)
- Antiseptic wipes, for cleaning injection sites

Watch Out!
There is no such thing as "a touch" of diabetes or "a little sugar." You either have diabetes or you don't. (See Chapter 3.)

- Blood glucose meter

- Glucose meter strips

- Lancet device for doing blood tests

- Extra lancets

- Blood-sugar log book and pens

- Tissues and cotton balls

- Snacks containing quickly digestible sugar in case blood sugar gets too low, such as raisins, hard candy, a container of orange juice, or specially prepared glucose tablets or gel.

The diabetes kit is essential to your health. Carrying it is no small effort if you already carry a briefcase, backpack, gym bag, or some combination of these!

Before lunch

Timesaver
Don't forget that most glucose meters can hold in memory a certain number of blood test readings. If you don't have time during the day to record a reading in your log book, hold it in the meter's memory and record that reading later when you have a moment to spare.

As a meal approaches, your question must be, "Will there be enough active insulin in my bloodstream to cover the glucose that will enter my bloodstream following this meal?" As lunchtime nears, you may inject a prelunch dose of rapid- or short-acting insulin, depending upon your insulin regimen. If you injected a dose of intermediate-acting insulin in the morning, it should be peaking in action right about lunchtime, so you might not administer insulin before lunch. Again, it depends upon the insulin regimen your doctor has prescribed for you.

In either case, it's necessary to check blood glucose levels again, and to record them. And type 2 diabetics who are not on insulin may also check their glucose levels before lunch.

An important task

The point of checking glucose levels is to see if your level is stable—not too high and not too low. If your glucose level is too low before a meal, it may be necessary to eat right away to avoid *hypoglycemia*. If it is too high, you may need to inject insulin and wait for it to enter your bloodstream before eating, in order to avoid an even higher glucose level after the meal. Or it may be necessary to make an adjustment in your insulin dose, based on recommendations you've already gone over with your health-care providers to prepare for "highs" and "lows." It all depends upon what types of insulin you use, how often you inject insulin, and what blood glucose levels are appropriate for you.

And another thing . . .
The daily effort to control blood glucose levels means that people with diabetes need to choose their foods carefully and to control their portion sizes.

Too many carbohydrates throughout the day mean higher glucose levels because carbohydrates are the main source of blood glucose. A meal that is overly rich in carbohydrates can cause a spike in blood sugar that may be too much for the amount of insulin in the bloodstream to handle. An overly large meal or snack can do the same thing, throwing the most conscientiously applied insulin regimen temporarily off the track.

People with diabetes must learn to eat with their blood-sugar levels in mind. Food is primarily a source of sustenance and enjoyment for all of us, diabetic or not, but diabetics must also look at each meal and snack in terms of its potential effect on the next glucose reading. It's another of the daily tasks of managing diabetes.

Bright Idea
Eating five or six small meals a day, instead of three larger meals, can help to keep blood-sugar levels more stable while also providing a more even flow of energy.

Adding in exercise

Exercise, too, is something that people with diabetes must plan for rather carefully. This is because exercise lowers blood-sugar levels by burning up glucose. The body needs the additional energy during exercise.

This glucose-lowering effect is a good thing, and doctors generally advise diabetic patients to exercise regularly as a part of their management program (and because of the many other health benefits of exercise!). But since exercise affects glucose levels for six to eight hours, and with regular exercise, for as long as thirty-six hours after the fact, people with diabetes need to factor it in to their daily treatment plan.

The main objective is to avoid hypoglycemia induced by exercise. Before engaging in exercise, by which we mean moderately intense aerobic activity lasting twenty to thirty minutes or more, the person with diabetes must

- Do a blood glucose test
- Eat a snack if blood glucose is low, or
- Eat a snack to keep blood sugar stable during exercise
- Make sure a snack is on hand during exercise, just in case blood sugar drops
- Make sure that someone exercising with him or her knows the signs of hypoglycemia
- Do another blood glucose test during the exercise period, if exercise lasts an hour or longer (hiking or biking, for example)
- Test blood glucose after exercise
- Adjust insulin dosages before or after exercise, or both, according to doctor's instructions

It's a lot to think about! The good news is that most people with diabetes can and should exercise (with their doctor's approval). The downside is that this requires adjustments in the overall daily plan. Fortunately, juggling all of these factors becomes second nature over time.

Dinner and bedtime

As at lunchtime, the approach of dinner calls for another glucose test and (if prescribed) a predinner insulin injection, which may combine rapid- or short-acting insulin (to handle the postmeal glucose rise) with long-acting insulin (to last throughout the night). The glucose test result and insulin type and dose should be logged in the logbook.

Before bed, it's a good idea to examine your bare feet for any trouble spots that could develop into foot ulcers (wounds that don't heal easily, if at all). Your health-care team will teach you to look for areas of redness, pain, numbness, coldness, and irritation—all possible warning signs of underlying circulation or nerve problems that could predispose you to foot ulcers.

Another bedtime consideration is the bedtime snack. During the night, your predinner or bedtime injection of long-acting insulin is at work in your bloodstream, but (normally) you do not get up to eat. This means that if you go to bed on an empty stomach, there may be too much insulin and too little glucose by midnight or later, in the hours before dawn. You could become hypoglycemic while you sleep.

To avoid this, your doctor may recommend that you eat a snack before bed. Typically, the bedtime snack includes a specific amount of carbohydrate and protein—milk and crackers, for example—

Watch Out!
If you have diabetes and are physically active, it is especially important that you check your bare feet daily for signs of potential foot sores.

which tends to promote a slow, steady rise in glucose through the night while the insulin is acting.

Prescribed snacks are a regular feature of diabetes management.

Other considerations

We've given a basic overview of the daily diabetes tasks that the person with type 1 diabetes must balance in order to keep blood-sugar levels as stable as possible. Note, however, that we've described a routine schedule. We haven't yet touched on the challenges of coping with real-life difficulties, such as:

- Managing food intake and keeping glucose levels stable when you have a stomach flu and nothing you eat stays down
- Ordering food at a restaurant
- The goodies-packed office or classroom party
- The colleague or peer who asks you if "you really ought to be eating that"

We'll do our best to address these topics, and more, in the pages to come. Here, our intention has been to introduce you to the basic concepts and tasks involved in the daily management of type 1 diabetes.

The diabetic person lives with the fact that poorly controlled blood-sugar levels lead to very serious health problems. None of us can take our future health for granted, but on a day-to-day basis, many of us do. The diabetic person doesn't have this luxury.

Daily management of type 2 diabetes

It's far more difficult to describe the average day of a person with type 2 diabetes, even though 90 to 95

Unofficially...
Diabetes has been diagnosed in almost every breed of cat and dog in America. It usually appears in older, overweight animals, and in most cases can be controlled through proper diet and exercise. Sometimes, though, insulin injections are necessary.

percent of diabetics have this type of diabetes. The severity of type 2 diabetes varies among individuals, and within individuals over time, and there are more treatment options and philosophies.

Most people with type 2 diabetes do not require insulin, although some do. Sometimes type 2 diabetes can progress or worsen to the point that external insulin is required. (Please be aware that this does not mean the type 2 diabetic has developed type 1 diabetes! Other features distinguish the disorders, and they cannot "change into" one another. See Chapter 2.) People with type 2 diabetes, however, generally are not dependent upon insulin injections because their pancreases do produce some insulin. They have an internal source of insulin; the problem is that their bodies don't do a good job of using the insulin to get glucose out of the blood and into the cells. Their livers supply sugar to the bloodstream, even when blood-sugar levels are high. This causes their blood-sugar levels to be too high, despite the presence of natural insulin.

People with type 2 diabetes, therefore, must also monitor and control their blood-sugar levels. While they may not be tied to an injection schedule, they too must perform a balancing act among diet, exercise, and (in most cases) the effects of oral medication taken in order to keep blood sugar stable. Oral medications are taken anywhere from once to three times a day. The daily life of people with type 2 diabetics is certainly affected by the disease, and if they do not control their blood sugar, people with type 2 diabetes are at risk for developing the same serious complications as type 1 diabetics. Whether diabetes is type 1 or type 2, high blood-sugar levels are extremely unhealthy! And with both types of diabetes, it is equally important to control blood sugar levels in order to decrease the risk of complications.

Diet, exercise, and weight loss

Some people with type 2 diabetes find that they can keep blood-sugar levels in the healthy range by

- Limiting the portion sizes of all foods, especially carbohydrates
- Increasing exercise, and
- Changing their eating pattern from three large meals a day to smaller, more frequent meals (which tends to reduce large rises or spikes in blood sugar)

Although this is simpler, perhaps, than adhering to a strict self-injection program, it can still mean making fundamental, permanent lifestyle changes.

The majority of people with type 2 diabetes are overweight—obesity is a risk factor for type 2 diabetes—and the type 2 diabetic may face the task of losing weight as part of a disease management regimen. It's not always easy. Like people with type 1 diabetes, people with type 2 diabetes who want the best health possible must give a lot of thought to diet and physical activity. It's a commitment.

Blood glucose monitoring and type 2 diabetes

What about blood checks? We've seen that insulin-dependent diabetics must check their blood-sugar levels several times during the day. In people with type 2 diabetes, these levels tend to be less volatile and it is usually not necessary to check them as often. Medical opinion on this can vary, however. Doctors used to think that glucose monitoring was not as important for type 2 diabetics, but recent

Bright Idea
Exercise doesn't just lower blood glucose levels; it also reduces insulin resistance. Some research indicates that people at high risk for type 2 diabetes can lower their risk through exercising regularly.

research has clarified the importance of good blood-sugar control for all diabetics.

A lot depends on the specific person, especially on how well blood sugar is controlled by diet and exercise and whether oral medication is taken to enhance insulin's action in the body. A person with type 2 diabetes may check his or her blood sugar from as infrequently as once every other day to as often as four times each day. (See Chapter 6.) It's important to remember that, regardless of their prescribed frequency, blood-sugar checks are an indispensable part of regular treatment for every person with diabetes.

Oral medications for type 2 diabetes

Doctors may prescribe certain medications for people who have type 2 diabetes. Contrary to popular belief, these medications are not oral insulin or insulin in pill form. (Insulin cannot be swallowed because it is destroyed by enzymes in the stomach. Scientists are working on a solution to this problem; see Chapter 16.) Medications prescribed for type 2 management are discussed in detail in Chapter 6. These drugs help to keep blood-sugar levels lower, typically, depending upon the medication used, by stimulating the pancreas to release insulin, by helping insulin to get glucose into cells, by helping the liver to control its release of stored glucose, or by slowing down the intestinal absorption of carbohydrates.

Oral medications and hypoglycemia

People with type 2 diabetes who take oral medications need to guard against glucose levels dropping too low, which can happen because these medicines may enhance insulin secretion or the body's

Watch Out!
Complications of diabetes, like vision damage, kidney disease, and nerve damage, can occur before you know you have type 2 diabetes. In order to detect diabetes sooner, The American Diabetes Association has lowered the diagnostic blood glucose level for diabetes from 140 mg/dl to 125 md/dl.

sensitivity to insulin, or may decrease the availability of glucose. People with type 2 diabetes who take medication therefore need to be careful not to delay or skip meals, and to eat enough food (within the caloric and portion limits established in their meal plans). They also need to keep in mind exercise's lowering effects on blood sugar, which can mean a lot of juggling if they are trying to lose weight as well. All of this requires more frequent blood tests to track the effects of the medications.

Checking for diabetes complications

Finally, type 2 diabetics must monitor themselves for signs of diabetes complications just as type 1 diabetics do. Proper foot care, for example, is just as necessary for type 2 diabetics as for type 1 diabetics.

The growing impact of diabetes

The figures given at the beginning of this chapter tell the story: The number of people affected by diabetes is large and growing. It may be scant comfort to know that a serious disease afflicting you or a loved one is so widespread. But the upside of diabetes's growing impact is that it spurs public and medical commitment to researching the disease and improving treatment. And if you have received a diagnosis of diabetes, you can count yourself lucky in one respect: An estimated half of all people who have type 2 diabetes are unaware of it and are not under treatment. Obviously, these people are at grave risk for serious complications.

Diabetes can have a devastating impact. But it is a treatable, manageable disease. The management of diabetes is ultimately in the hands of the person who has it. Responsibility for the treatment of diabetes cannot be handed over to health-care

> **"**
> I decided I could live a long and healthy life with diabetes—but not if I kept ignoring it!
> —Barry, age twenty-four, with type 1 diabetes
> **"**

professionals. With diabetes, the patient's under-standing of and response to the disease—not just the doctor's—can make a real difference in the effectiveness of treatment.

Knowledge is power. Read on!

Just the facts

- If diabetes is untreated or poorly controlled, levels of sugar (glucose) in the bloodstream are chronically and dangerously high.

- Each day, people with diabetes strive to control blood-sugar levels through a delicate balancing of diet, exercise, and any medications (insulin or oral medications) prescribed.

- The challenge of daily treatment is to mimic as closely as possible the functioning of a healthy pancreas.

- This includes preventing sugar "lows" as well as "highs."

- People with type 2 diabetes are at risk for the same serious complications that can develop in type 1 (insulin-dependent) diabetics.

- Whether or not you take insulin, diabetes is a self-managed disease that demands daily attention.

GET THE SCOOP ON...
The basic differences between types 1 and 2 ▪
What puts you at risk for having either type? ▪
The "pregnancy" diabetes ▪ Cow's milk and
diabetes ▪ Can diabetes be prevented or cured?

One Name, Two Diseases: Types 1 and 2 Explained

Chapter 2

Y ou don't have a solid working knowledge of diabetes if you don't understand the differences between types 1 and 2. That's what we'll focus on in this chapter: essential information, concepts, and terms that are basic to understanding diabetes.

Let's begin with some fundamental, perhaps surprising, similarities between these two forms of diabetes:

- Both types can occur in people of any age.

- Both types may require the use of pharmaceutical insulin.

- Both types cause high blood-sugar levels, which will lead to serious long-term complications if not controlled.

- Type 2 is not less serious than type 1! They are equally serious diseases.

No doubt you recall hearing about "juvenile" and "adult-onset" diabetes. These terms are dated and do not accurately correspond to type 1 and type 2, respectively. However, it is true that most diabetes occurring in children is type 1 diabetes, while diabetes occurring in people over forty is usually type 2 diabetes. But only about half of type 1, "juvenile" diabetes cases appear in children and teens; usually the rest occur in adults under the age of thirty. And among some ethnic groups that are highly predisposed to type 2 diabetes, such as certain Native American families, children as young as ten may have the so-called "adult-onset" type. The terms *type 1* and *type 2* have replaced the older terms now that we know that adults and young people can develop either type.

Whether type 1 or type 2, we know that diabetes results from a failure of the body to control the amount of sugar circulating in the bloodstream. We know also that insulin is the key to healthy absorption of blood sugar by the body's cells. Let's look at the way problems with insulin and blood sugar occur in the two forms of diabetes.

Type 1 diabetes: you're not making insulin

If you have type 1 diabetes, your pancreas (the large, insulin-producing gland behind the stomach) cannot do its job because it is under attack by your immune system. Type 1 diabetes begins as an autoimmune disease that targets the pancreas. For reasons that aren't clear, the body's immune system begins to destroy the highly specialized, insulin-producing beta cells in the pancreas. Research suggests that certain genetic factors, viruses, and other environmental forces may be at the root of this destructive process; see the discussion below on risk factors.

As the beta cells are destroyed, insulin production is greatly diminished and may stop completely. This usually occurs within a short time period, especially in children, but it can also take months or as many as ten or more years for full-blown diabetes to develop.

The person with type 1 diabetes has an ill, damaged pancreas with a very small internal source of insulin, or none at all. This is why people with type 1 diabetes are always dependent upon an external source of insulin for blood-sugar control. Type 1 diabetes represents a shutting down of insulin production at its very source, the pancreas. Because the pancreas has stopped producing insulin, the type 1 diabetic has no choice but to take over the job of the pancreas for life. He or she must learn to supply the appropriate amounts of insulin to the body whenever it is needed in order to maintain healthy blood-sugar levels. It's an exacting task, usually requiring two to three doses of insulin per day and perhaps more, thoughtful meal planning, and blood-sugar readings (see Chapter 5).

Type 2 diabetes: you are making insulin, but . . .

While type 1 diabetes is caused by a clear-cut lack of insulin production, the causes of type 2 diabetes are more complex and less well understood. Type 2 diabetes is not triggered by the autoimmune destruction of pancreatic cells and a cessation of insulin production. Some people with type 2 diabetes may, in fact, produce excess amounts of insulin. However, they become as seriously diabetic as those with type 1 disease for one, or a combination of, the following reasons:

Unofficially...
Frederick Banting, the young Canadian physician who discovered insulin, was driven to become a doctor and find a cure for diabetes because his childhood sweetheart died of diabetes when Banting was fifteen years old.

■ Their bodies cannot make full use of the available insulin (that is, they are *insulin resistant*).

■ Their pancreatic beta cells, while not under autoimmune attack, are sluggish and don't produce enough insulin to keep their blood-sugar levels normal.

■ They have fewer beta cells than is normal, and therefore don't produce enough insulin. (This is more likely in long-standing type 2 diabetes.)

■ They have one or several problems with the hormonal signaling system underlying blood-sugar control (for example, their livers may release glucose even when the blood-sugar level is high).

■ Their *need* for insulin has increased due to obesity, and the pancreas cannot keep up with the increased demand.

Understanding type 2 diabetes, then, takes us from the focus on the damaged pancreas in type 1 diabetes to looking at the way the body uses (or doesn't use) insulin that has been produced. In type 2 diabetes, the pancreas is producing at least some insulin, yet glucose reaches high levels in the bloodstream instead of entering the muscle and other cells where it belongs. Along with insulin resistance, faulty interactions among the pancreas, liver, and larger endocrine system may also be a part of the problem.

Insulin resistance: how and why
How does the body resist using the insulin it produces? There are many possible factors, not all of them well understood, and not all of them present in all cases of type 2 diabetes.

> **66**
> In the past, neither patients nor their doctors paid much attention to [type 2] disease. Today, though, we treat type 2 diabetes more aggressively.
> —David M. Nathan, M.D., Massachusetts General Hospital
> **99**

One factor may be an imperfect match between a person's insulin and his or her cells' *insulin receptors*. This means that it is harder for cells, no matter how hungry they are for glucose, to utilize the insulin to gain access to sugar circulating in the bloodstream. Or there may not be a sufficient number of receptors, so that available insulin goes unused and glucose remains in the blood. Over time, this consistent resistance from cells may in turn cause the sluggish pancreas mentioned above: The pancreas may try for years to solve the problem by *over*producing insulin, but may eventually burn out and produce far less.

In some people, the pancreas may release insulin too slowly during digestion. If insulin is not released quickly enough after eating for blood-sugar levels to return to normal within about three hours, then these levels remain too high for too long. Or the underlying hormonal system that prompts the pancreas to make more insulin may not be getting its message through.

The liver plays an important role in controlling blood-sugar levels, but it takes its cues from the pancreas. Sometimes a problem occurs in this system, leading to or exacerbating type 2 diabetes. Normally, the liver stores excess glucose for future use; the pancreas signals the liver to store glucose, which helps keep glucose levels normal, particularly after eating, when the liver picks up extra blood sugar. In type 2 diabetes, the pancreas may mistakenly allow the liver to release stored glucose even when the amount of sugar in the blood is already high. This lack of proper control leads to abnormally elevated blood sugar.

Watch Out!
As many as one-third to one-half of all people who have type 2 diabetes don't know that they do. Symptoms may be subtle or unnoticeable at first, which is why this condition is sometimes called "the silent killer."

Unofficially...
Before the modern understanding of diabetes and insulin, physicians found that the only treatment that kept patients alive for a year or two longer than expected was a starvation diet. By cutting calories to 500 per day and virtually eliminating sugars and starches, doctors found that sugar in urine decreased and weight stayed normal longer.

The role of obesity in type 2 diabetes

A final significant difference between types 1 and 2 is that body size and fitness may have a hand in causing type 2 disease. The American Diabetes Association states that "The most important environmental trigger of type 2 diabetes appears to be obesity." We have medical definitions of obesity: weighing more than 20 percent over your desirable weight or (a more recent measure) having a Body Mass Index (BMI) of 25 or above (see Appendix D for more information on the BMI). But most of us don't need charts, graphs, or formulas to tell us we're carrying too much body fat; the mirror gives us that information. What we do need to know is that close to 80 percent of all people with type 2 diabetes are overweight. As obesity becomes more common in American children, we may see an increase of type 2 diabetes in children.

Excess body weight seems to promote insulin resistance; again, the reasons for this are not crystal clear, other than recognizing that larger bodies may simply require larger amounts of insulin. On the other hand, it appears that increased *lean* body mass, or muscle, can enhance insulin receptivity (see Chapter 9).

Note that obesity alone does not cause diabetes. There are many overweight Americans, but only about 20 to 25 percent of them develop diabetes. In people who are already predisposed to insulin resistance or low insulin production, however, an increase in body mass may be the straw that breaks the camel's back.

The fundamental difference between the two types of diabetes

Type 1 results when a damaged pancreas shuts down insulin production entirely. In contrast, type 2 diabetes is the result of several possible problems that are more subtle and that may interact, such as insufficient insulin production, due either to pancreas burnout or too few beta cells; slow insulin release; faulty signaling of the liver; resistance to insulin produced; and increased demands made upon the pancreas by excess body mass.

Gestational diabetes mellitus (GDM)

About 2 to 5 percent of pregnant women develop *gestational diabetes mellitus* (GDM) during their last trimester, typically around the twenty-fourth to twenty-eighth week. In most cases, GDM is temporary and clears up after delivery; however, having GDM increases a woman's chances of later developing type 2 (but not type 1) diabetes. About 35 to 50 percent of women with GDM will develop type 2 diabetes in the following five to twenty years, especially if they are overweight.

GDM arises because the placenta normally produces large amounts of hormones that guide the fetus's physical development. In all pregnant women, these hormones interfere to some degree with insulin action, so that all pregnant women are somewhat insulin resistant. When GDM develops, it is because the woman's pancreas cannot cope with this new insulin resistance, which demands that more insulin be produced to keep blood-sugar levels normal. The pregnant woman's larger body size may also increase her insulin needs.

Frequently, women with GDM do not have dramatic symptoms, so The American Diabetes Association advises doctors to routinely screen all women over the age of 25 in the twenty-fourth to twenty-eighth week of pregnancy. Women who have previously had GDM are at greater risk and may be tested earlier.

Watch Out! Stressful events may cause the body to release extra sugar into the bloodstream, preparing the body for "fight or flight." This can cause temporarily high blood-sugar levels that resemble diabetes.

Also at increased risk for GDM are women who are obese; over age thirty; Latina, African American, or Native American; women who have a family history of diabetes; and women who have previously delivered a baby weighing over nine pounds.

Most birth defects develop during the first trimester of pregnancy. Gestational diabetes develops later in pregnancy, and therefore it is not associated with a higher incidence of birth defects. Nor does GDM greatly increase the child's risk for developing diabetes. But GDM can increase the risk for miscarriage. It can also cause the baby to grow too large, for reasons described in Chapter 12 in the section on pregnancy. This can lead to a complicated delivery and other risks to the newborn infant. For these reasons, it is very important to monitor and treat GDM.

In 80 percent of cases, GDM can be treated simply by having the woman reduce the amount of carbohydrates in her diet or by breaking down carbohydrate servings into smaller, more frequent portions. This should reduce her need for insulin, so that her stressed pancreas can handle the job. If lowered carbohydrate intake prompts her body to burn fat for energy, however, she may produce too many ketones and will need to increase her intake of carbohydrates again. In that case, she may need to begin using injected insulin to maintain healthy blood-sugar levels.

Again, GDM is not a life-threatening complication of pregnancy, but it must be treated. Please see the section in Chapter 12 for more details on gestational diabetes.

Other forms of diabetes

Like gestational diabetes, some cases of diabetes do not fall neatly into the type 1 or 2 category due to their uncommon causes. For instance, diseases that affect the pancreas can cause diabetes. Pancreatitis, pancreatic cancer, cystic fibrosis, and hemochromatosis are all diseases that can severely impair the pancreas and decrease insulin production. Surgical removal of the pancreas for any reason will do the same.

Certain medically prescribed steroids, such as prednisone or the *glucocorticoid* drugs, which are used to treat some types of arthritis, asthma, lupus, and other autoimmune diseases, can trigger type 2 diabetes by raising blood-sugar levels beyond the pancreas's capacity to supply insulin. Some diuretics prescribed for hypertension can also induce diabetes.

Finally, some genetic disorders that affect the body's hormonal or metabolic systems, like Turner's syndrome, Prader-Willi syndrome, or the presence of genetically abnormal insulin molecules, are associated with higher incidences of diabetes as well.

Risk factors, causes, and myths about diabetes

If you have diabetes, you may wonder why. Were you born with it? Is it because of what you eat or how much you weigh? What does age have to do with it, if anything?

First, let's dispel some myths.

Probably the most prevalent myth about how diabetes develops is the notion that you can get it from eating too much sugar. For the record: This isn't true. Too much sugar may well cause tooth decay and potbellies, but it can't give you diabetes. Ingesting lots of sugar is not the same thing as having dangerously high blood-sugar levels. The average, healthy pancreas produces enough insulin

Unofficially...
An Egyptian medical document written around 1500 BC describes a malady of "passing too much urine." Without understanding the physiological reasons for this, observers then knew that sufferers of this condition had very sweet urine. In fact, one way they tested for this illness was to see if ants from anthills were attracted to urine poured nearby.

to metabolize large amounts of sugar; extra calories from sugar that are not needed right away for energy will be stored, primarily in fat cells but also as glycogen in the liver.

Another myth is that you can catch diabetes from someone who has it. This is patently untrue. Diabetes is not contagious. Nor can you get diabetes from a blood transfusion, another myth. Finally, you cannot develop diabetes from obesity alone, as many persist in believing; other risk factors must be present.

When it comes to understanding what makes a person at risk for developing diabetes, it's far simpler to cross out the wrong answers than to clearly state the right ones. Diabetes is a complex disease with complex causes. Even when we know that an autoimmune response has destroyed beta cells and induced diabetes, as in type 1 cases, we cannot as yet say why one person develops this autoimmune response in the first place, while another person, perhaps even a relative of the first, does not.

Here's the best of what we do know about risk factors associated with diabetes.

Risk factors for type 1 diabetes

Keep in mind that type 1 diabetes begins as an autoimmune attack on beta cells in the pancreas. What factors might predispose an individual to have this problem?

Family history and genetics

You are more likely to develop type 1 diabetes if it runs in your family—if your mother, father, sibling, or a grandparent has it. If one parent has type 1, your risk of having it too is about 5 to 10 percent. If both parents have it, your risk is about 20 percent. But as many as 85 percent of people with type 1

Watch Out!
The American Diabetes Association urges people with diabetes to be actively involved in personalizing their treatment plans. Your plan needs to be suitable for your goals and lifestyle. You'll have to speak up if you feel you've been handed a plan you can't live with. If it's one you can't follow, it won't help you.

diabetes have no known family history, and certainly no single "diabetes gene" has yet been identified. Rather, it appears that several genes may increase one's susceptibility to diabetes.

One set of genes that helps to control the immune system's knowledge of what is "self" and what is "foreign invader" is important in type 1 diabetes because it is the immune system that mistakenly kills healthy beta cells, as if they were "foreigners". Some people may inherit types of these immune system genes (called *human leukocyte antigen* genes, or *HLAs*), which may make them more vulnerable to diabetes. Ninety-five percent of people with type 1 diabetes have a particular type of HLA called the *DR3 form*, or a type called the *DR4 form*, or both.

What must be kept in mind, however, is that 45 percent of people who do *not* have diabetes also have the DR3 or DR4 HLAs. Clearly, there is no inevitable correlation between having these gene variants and getting type 1 diabetes. What's more, researchers have identified other gene sets that may increase susceptibility, further complicating matters. But the risk is higher for people with this particular genetic characteristic who also have a family history of type 1 diabetes. Where a family history exists, genetic screening for HLA variants may help predict whether a given individual is likely to develop diabetes.

Ethnicity

Type 1 diabetes occurs more frequently in Caucasians, especially those of Northern European descent. Scandinavia has the highest rates of type 1 diabetes in the world. The reasons for this are not entirely known, but type 1 is also more common in

Unofficially...
The first clue to the causes of diabetes emerged in 1889, when two German physiologists, who were studying fat metabolism, removed a dog's pancreas. The dog quickly developed type 1 symptoms. Prior to this, many doctors thought diabetes was a kidney disease.

colder climates (both in the United States and worldwide) and it develops more frequently in winter than in summer. It is rarer in most Asian, African, and Native American populations (in contrast to type 2 diabetes).

Age

Type 1 diabetes is more common in people who are under age thirty, although it can occur in adults up to age forty and older. The risk is highest between the ages of eleven and fourteen, and the rate drops off after puberty. The risk of developing type 1 diabetes at age fifty or older is about 1 percent, but it can occur in older and even elderly people.

Weight

Type 1 diabetes is not associated with or caused by being overweight. In fact, one symptom of type 1 diabetes may be marked weight loss, brought about by the body's burning of fat for energy because lack of insulin makes sugar unavailable to cells.

Viral triggers and other possible causes

Some theories hold that the autoimmune response that destroys beta cells may be prompted by exposure to certain pathogens. There is some evidence that viruses trigger autoimmune diseases like type 1 diabetes. Many people who develop type 1 have recently had a viral infection, and increases in the incidence of type 1 have been recorded following virus epidemics. This may explain in part the greater frequency of type 1 occurrence in colder climates; viral infections are more common in winter.

The viruses thought to be associated with type 1 diabetes are the Coxsackie family and those that cause mumps and German measles. Their role in causing diabetes is unclear. The immune system may

> ❝
> In populations living near starvation, or living in cycles of feast or famine, which would probably include many of our ancestors, diabetics might be better off than nondiabetics. They have a different sort of metabolism, one that becomes a disadvantage only when food is present in abundance all of the time. [Perhaps diabetes] becomes a disease *only in relation to lifestyle and environment.*
> —Dr. Andrew Weil, author of *Spontaneous Healing* and *Natural Health, Natural Medicine*
> ❞

confuse GAD (glutamic acid decarboxylase, a protein produced by beta cells) with these viruses, prompting it to attack beta cells. Or these virus types may somehow cause a change in the molecular structure of some pancreatic cells, making them appear foreign to the immune system. Other external factors that scientists believe may induce type 1 diabetes are:

- **Cow's milk.** In very young infants, under the age of three months, the whole proteins in cow's milk are not absorbed by the digestive tract. Outside the gut, these proteins may stimulate the immune system to make antibodies against them. One study has found that children with type 1 diabetes have higher levels of antibodies to a specific protein in cow's milk. If such children develop infectious illnesses, these antimilk antibodies may be triggered mistakenly to destroy beta cells.

- **Oxygen free radicals.** Health-conscious baby boomers may be familiar with this term, which refers to destructive molecules that occur throughout the body as a by-product of many biochemical processes. Oxygen free radicals are able to destroy or alter healthy cells and DNA, and they may play a role in genetic mutations, cancer, autoimmune disorders, and aging. The body creates defensive enzymes that can defuse free radicals. Some researchers believe that nutritional supplements providing antioxidant benefits, such as beta-carotene, vitamin C, and vitamin E, may boost this defense. But stresses to the body, like smoking, a high-fat diet, and environmental toxins, may seriously lower our resistance to free radicals.

Watch Out!
Because type 2 diabetes is more common in middle-aged people, adults experiencing symptoms may dismiss them as signs that "I'm just getting old." Don't do this! Be aware of type 2 symptoms and take them seriously.

The insulin-producing cells in the pancreas normally have only small amounts of defensive enzymes. If environmental or other stressors further reduce these enzymes in the pancreas, then damage done by oxygen free radicals may be a cause of type 1 diabetes.

- **Certain drugs and chemicals.** These include *pyriminial*, or Vacor, a type of rat poison; *pentamidine*, used to treat pneumonia; and L-*asparaginase* and *streptozotocin*, both used to treat cancer.

Risk factors for type 2 diabetes

You will recall that in type 2 diabetes the pancreas does produce insulin, but the body cannot make use of the insulin produced, a condition known as *insulin resistance*. The following are factors thought to predispose people to develop insulin resistance and type 2 diabetes.

Family history and genetics

The American Diabetes Association states that "The link to genetics seems even stronger in type 2 diabetes than in type 1." Studies of identical twins show that if one twin has type 1 diabetes, there is a 25 to 50 percent chance that the other will develop it as well. If one twin has type 2 diabetes, however, the chances that the other will have it go up to 60 to 75 percent! If one of your parents has type 2, you have a 25 to 30 percent chance of developing it. If both your parents have type 2, your risk could be as high as 50 to 75 percent.

As with type 1 diabetes, researchers have not pinpointed a single gene for type 2 diabetes. Some research, however, points to a genetic error that may play a role: Some people produce too much of a

66
A year ago, I was at risk for serious health problems from diabetes and I didn't even know it. But thanks to early detection, I have taken steps to control my type 2 diabetes, which will hopefully help to prevent or delay the onset of devastating complications. I urge those who recognize their risk for diabetes to see their doctor for a simple blood test.
—Jerry Mathers, former star of TV's *Leave It To Beaver,* addressing the press at an American Diabetes Association conference.
99

protein called *PC-1*, which can desensitize insulin receptors and cause insulin resistance. Many people with type 2 diabetes have far more of this protein than do people without diabetes. Also, the genetic roots of obesity are becoming better understood. It may be that "obesity genes" will be shown to be linked to type 2 diabetes. Mice that are genetically engineered to become obese are prone to type 2 diabetes.

Ethnicity

There is a definite link between ethnicity and type 2 diabetes. This tends to bolster evidence that this condition is inheritable. African Americans, Asian Americans, Latinos, and Native Americans have higher rates of type 2 than do Caucasians: about 60 percent higher in African Americans and about 110 to 120 percent higher among Latinos. Native Americans have the highest incidence of type 2 diabetes in the world. In some Native American groups, such as the Pimas, rates among adults are as high as 50 percent. It may be that, as Native American peoples become assimilated into modern American culture, the transition from their traditional foods to a far richer diet has overstressed their metabolism. At the same time, Latino groups that share genes with Native American groups, such as Mexican Americans, have higher rates of type 2 than do Latino peoples who do not share these genes, such as Cuban Americans.

Age

Now we have another reason to avoid growing up: Our chances of developing type 2 diabetes undeniably increase with age. Half of all new cases of type 2 occur in people over age fifty. The rest are most prevalent among those who are forty or over, although type 2 can occur in younger adults. Nearly 11 percent of Americans over age sixty have type 2 diabetes.

As cells age, they are more likely to become insulin resistant. By age fifty or so, larger numbers of people experience elevated blood-sugar levels. And typically, older people have less lean muscle mass and relatively more fat cells. This changing ratio seems to affect blood-sugar metabolism.

Gender

Type 2 diabetes may be slightly more common in women than men. This may be because only women develop gestational diabetes, which leads to type 2 diabetes in about 40 percent of women with GDM.

Weight

This is another very powerful factor: About 80 percent of people who have type 2 diabetes are overweight (although not all overweight people have diabetes). If you have a family history of type 2 diabetes, being overweight can definitely increase your chances of developing the condition. And you needn't be grossly obese, as journalist Deborah Chase discovered. A health writer, Chase chose her foods carefully and was only about fifteen pounds overweight. But both her parents, both paternal grandparents, and two paternal aunts had had type 2 diabetes, and Chase developed it in her mid-forties. (Deborah Chase tells her story in "The Disease That Goes Undiagnosed," *Ladies' Home Journal*, November, 1997.)

Excess weight seems to interfere with cells' receptivity to insulin. The fat body is not as insulin-efficient as the lean body. Part of the problem may simply be that bigger bodies require larger amounts of insulin—more insulin than some pancreases can produce. But too much fat can promote insulin resistance, even in people with the normal number of beta cells and whose pancreases are producing average amounts of insulin. Conversely, increasing muscle or lean body mass helps the body to use insulin effectively. (See Chapter 9 for more on exercise.)

Patterns of body fat distribution may also indicate higher type 2 risk, where other risk factors are present. If you carry extra fat centrally, that is, above the hips, you are more susceptible to type 2 diabetes. This may partly explain its higher incidence among African Americans, in whom obesity and especially central-body obesity is more common than among Caucasians.

Older age, higher levels of body fat, sedentary lifestyles that cause loss of muscle—with this triumvirate of type 2 risk factors, it's no wonder that this disorder has become increasingly common in the past fifty years. Baby boomers: Beware of type 2!

Can diabetes be prevented?

Thinking about risk factors leads naturally to the question of prevention. Can diabetes be prevented?

Preventing type 1 diabetes

For type 1 diabetes, this is a difficult question because we are only beginning to understand the roots and processes of autoimmune disorders. Medical science is a long way from being able to prevent such diseases as rheumatoid arthritis, lupus, multiple sclerosis, thyroiditis, and Lou Gehrig's disease (or ALS), to name but a few autoimmune conditions. In the case of diabetes, however, advances in genetic screening and in early detection of beta cell damage may come together with new

Watch Out!
Many people assume that problems with sexual functioning, like impotence, are complications of type 1 diabetes only. However, they are also associated with type 2 diabetes, as is neuropathy, or nerve damage, in the feet.

drug treatments. These drugs will suppress the overzealous immune system and stop type 1 diabetes in its earliest stages. (See Chapter 17 for more on type 1 prevention research.)

Preventing type 2 diabetes

Unofficially...
In February of 1997, the Sansum Medical Research Foundation in Santa Barbara, California, announced the Santa Barbara Diabetes Project, a collaboration of researchers determined to find a cure for type 1 diabetes by the year 2000. See Chapter 17 for details.

Prevention of type 2 diabetes is a different matter. Consider how many of the risk factors apply to you. If you are an older adult, non-Caucasian, overweight (even moderately), have had gestational diabetes, have a family history of type 2 diabetes, or any of the above, then obviously *now* is the time to start losing weight and getting some exercise (under a doctor's direction; see Chapters 8 and 9).

It is also very important to have your blood-sugar levels checked regularly, which means you should be scrupulous about having a complete physical exam every year. Many people with type 2 disease have had slowly rising blood-sugar levels for some time prior to receiving their diagnosis. (See the discussion of impaired glucose tolerance in Chapter 3.) If your doctor finds that your blood sugar is somewhat high, take heed: Full-blown type 2 diabetes could be just around the corner for you. Turn around and head in the other direction! Take steps to help your body be a more efficient user of insulin, and healthier overall. This won't prevent a process that may already have started, but it could very well keep your problem from getting worse.

The pancreas transplant: a cure for diabetes?

At present, the only medical treatment we have that can be considered a cure for diabetes is the pancreas transplant. In this procedure, part or all of a donor pancreas is surgically implanted in the abdomen of the recipient. When successful, this operation may indeed cure diabetes. Glucose levels become normal and the patient no longer requires insulin injections.

Unfortunately, the limits of our current medical technology, along with the scant supply of donor organs, makes the pancreas transplant an inappropriate treatment for the majority of diabetics. Most of us are familiar with the usual risks of transplant procedures: The body's immune system may reject the new organ, and the immunosuppressive drugs prescribed to prevent this gravely weaken the recipient's resistance to infections and cancer.

Transplant surgery is also very expensive, costing in the tens of thousands of dollars. The surgery itself also takes a big toll on the body. Close to 15 percent of pancreas transplant recipients die within five years.

The combined kidney-pancreas transplant

Doctors are more likely to recommend a pancreas transplant if a kidney transplant is planned (providing a donor pancreas is available). The kidney transplant also requires a delicate operation and immunosuppressive treatment. The doctor may suggest that since the patient must undergo this surgery anyway, it may make sense to perform a combined kidney-pancreas transplant.

Just the facts

- In type 1 diabetics, the pancreas produces no insulin, and insulin injections are necessary.
- In type 2 diabetics, the pancreas produces insulin, but the body may be insulin resistant, or the pancreas may not make as much insulin as is needed.

- Uncontrolled high blood sugar is the cause of serious health complications in both type 1 and type 2 diabetes.

- About 90 to 95 percent of all diabetics have type 2 diabetes.

- Being middle-aged, overweight, Latino, African American, or Native American and having a family history of type 2 diabetes are all risk factors associated with type 2 diabetes.

- While type 1 diabetes produces sudden symptoms that are hard to ignore, type 2 diabetes develops gradually, often with mild or no obvious symptoms.

GET THE SCOOP ON...
When to suspect diabetes ▪ The symptoms of
diabetes ▪ How high blood-sugar levels cause
symptoms ▪ When diabetes is "silent" ▪ Blood
tests for diabetes" ▪ Coping with a diagnosis
and starting treatment

Could I Have . . .?
Diagnosing Diabetes

Chapter 3

W hen you first picked up this book, did you open immediately to this chapter? Do you have a hunch or a concern that you or someone you care about might have diabetes? Perhaps it's dawned on you that you're never without a soft drink, some juice, or a big glass of water in your hand—yet the thirst persists. All that liquid keeps you running to the bathroom, and it's really beginning to wear on you. Your mom's dad had diabetes. Then there's the weight loss. It seems that no matter how much you eat, nothing "sticks" and you're always famished. And it can't be normal for a young person to feel so tired all the time.

Or maybe you've gained quite a bit of weight in the last few years. Hey, you're in your forties. Is that why you've been feeling so rundown lately? Just part of getting old? Maybe that explains the occasional blurry vision, but you were up last night worrying about it because it seems to be happening more often. Besides, your feet were aching. That's a new

Timesaver
Do you know
exactly what
services are or
aren't covered by
your health-care
plan? It will save
you lots of time
if you know this
information
before you need
medical care.

one. Is it the extra weight? Maybe you're just bloated, retaining water. You've been drinking water by the gallon, it seems. At first you blamed it on El Nino—record heat—but it's February . . . .

Maybe you've been feeling just fine. But you read somewhere about the risk factors associated with type 2 diabetes, and quite a few apply to you—age, ethnicity, weight, family history. Hmmm. Is it possible to have diabetes and not know it?

Diabetes: different types, similar symptoms

The first thing you need to know about diabetes symptoms is that you must see your doctor as soon as possible if you think you may have the disease. Symptoms of type 1 diabetes can rapidly escalate to emergency proportions, while the signs of type 2 diabetes tend to be more subtle, developing over longer periods of time. Both types are treatable but serious illnesses requiring prompt medical attention. Remember that routine blood tests done as part of your regular checkup can alert your doctor to abnormalities. This is one more reason to get regular physical exams.

The second thing to know is that type 1 and type 2 diabetes share most of the same symptoms, even though they are different disease processes. The reason for this is that the defining feature of all diabetes is abnormally high blood-sugar levels, and it is this that causes diabetic symptoms.

Symptoms of type 1 diabetes

As explained in Chapter 2, type 1 diabetes is a condition in which the pancreas stops producing insulin, leaving the person with type 1 diabetes with no internal source of insulin and no natural means for getting blood sugar out of the bloodstream and into body cells. Scientists believe that it is caused by an autoimmune reaction, perhaps triggered by a virus, that causes the body's immune system to mistakenly attack cells in the pancreas that create insulin. Type 1 diabetes is typically, but not always, a disorder of childhood and young adulthood (adults under thirty).

The primary symptoms of type 1 diabetes are

- Increased hunger
- Weight loss
- Excessive thirst
- Frequent urination, often including urinating at night
- Fatigue
- Blurred vision
- Increased infections and decreased resistance to infections (for example, sores that become infected and don't heal; recurrent eye, bladder, or vaginal infections; and recurrent infections, such as yeast or boils, in skinfolds, such as the inner thigh and groin, or under the breasts.)

Before taking a look at how high blood sugar causes these symptoms, it's worthwhile to consider one way in which type 1 symptoms tend to differ from those of type 2, and that is rapidity of onset, or *acuteness*.

Unlike type 2 diabetes, type 1 diabetes tends to come on suddenly and dramatically because the pancreas has completely shut down insulin production. While the disease process in the pancreas may take years to reach this point, when it does happen the body is thrown into an emergency situation. There is simply no insulin whatsoever, and blood

Bright Idea
Your mental health is important to your general health. Make a point of reserving at least fifteen minutes of each day just for you. Do something you like! Or just sit back and close your eyes.

glucose rapidly accumulates. Due to this rapid, unchecked rise, type 1 symptoms can emerge quickly, within a matter of weeks or months.

Acute diabetic ketoacidosis (DKA)

Without insulin, the body becomes starved for glucose and begins burning stored fats in an attempt to fuel cells. This leads to the buildup of ketones in the blood. Ketones are a biochemical by-product of fat burning. Under normal conditions, small amounts of ketones are always present in the blood. In high amounts ketones are toxic, however, causing blood to become dangerously acidic (because ketones are acidic). This can cause a condition called *diabetic ketoacidosis*, or DKA.

DKA can make a person very sick, and can even be fatal. Along with thirst, increased urination, and dehydration, DKA usually causes nausea and vomiting (which exacerbates dehydration and fatigue). The person with DKA will also show signs of "air hunger," rapid, labored breathing as if he or she had just been exercising. This is the body's attempt to expel the excess acid. Another symptom is a sweet, fruity odor on the breath, which is caused by the burning of ketones.

We mention DKA not because it always occurs in type 1 diabetes, but because it will eventually develop *in any untreated case of type 1 diabetes*. Before insulin treatment was developed in the 1920s, people with type 1 diabetes inevitably developed DKA, which led to coma and death. DKA can be a first symptom of type 1 diabetes simply because the person may not have been diagnosed and treated yet. Symptoms like excessive thirst or urination may have been ignored, or may have come on so suddenly that there was no time to treat the diabetes before

DKA began. Today, if DKA develops, it is usually treated in the hospital or the emergency room, and is not usually fatal.

Many people with type 1 diabetes never experience DKA because their disease was diagnosed before DKA could develop, and they have properly managed their disease since diagnosis. Generally, DKA occurs only in people with poorly controlled or undiagnosed diabetes. Since people with type 2 diabetes do produce at least some insulin, they usually do not develop DKA. However, in some African American people, DKA can be the first symptom of type 2 diabetes, although this is rare.

How high blood sugar causes the symptoms of type 1 diabetes

What does blood sugar have to do with thirst, urination, blurred vision, or fatigue?

Let's look at each of these symptoms separately:

- **Excessive thirst.** The kidneys respond to very high blood sugar by producing more urine in an attempt to flush excess sugar from the body. A call goes up for more and more water to meet the demands of greater urine production. As more urine is produced, the cells and the blood become dehydrated, further aggravating thirst.

- **Frequent urination.** This is the result of excessive urine production, described above. Note that the creation of more urine is not an effective method for controlling blood-sugar levels. The kidneys respond only after sugar levels are already about double normal levels, and increased urination cannot bring levels down to normal.

- **Increased hunger.** Remember that there is too much sugar in the blood because, without

Watch Out!
How are you coping with stress? Research shows that hormones produced in the body during times of stress can increase your cholesterol level and promote the buildup of plaque in arteries and veins. People with diabetes have a higher incidence of heart disease.

adequate insulin, sugar is not getting into the cells to fuel them. The body interprets this cellular hunger as starvation and triggers hunger signals to stimulate eating. (On the other hand, high ketone levels can cause nausea and loss of appetite.)

▪ **Weight loss.** In the face of glucose starvation, the body begins to raid its stores of fat and protein (muscle tissue). As these stores shrink, the diabetic loses weight. And when glucose is excreted in the urine, significant numbers of calories are lost.

▪ **Fatigue.** This is due to the fact that in diabetes, cells are starved for nutrients because glucose is not getting into cells. Glucose is the body's premiere energy source, especially for brain and muscle cells. When cells don't get glucose, they have little energy.

▪ **Blurred vision.** Increased urination dehydrates the body, which can cause moist membrane tissues to shrivel. This can happen to the lens of the eye, blurring the vision. Also, excess sugar in the blood can cause swelling in delicate structures such as the lens of the eye, also resulting in blurred vision. This type of vision impairment is not permanent and is to be distinguished from the serious, long-term complications of diabetes that can cause vision loss and blindness. (See Chapter 4.)

▪ **Increased infections.** This happens for two reasons. One is that sugar-saturated blood is a perfect breeding ground for bacteria and fungi. The other reason is that along with other cells in the body that are weakened by lack of glucose, the cells making up the immune system (white

Bright Idea
If you have recently been diagnosed with diabetes, put off buying new eyeglasses or contact lenses until your blood-sugar levels have been stable for at least one month. Before then, high blood sugar may affect your vision, making your lens prescription useless.

blood cells and antibodies) are weakened as well. Robbed of energy, the immune system can't keep its guard up.

The "honeymoon" phase

It's interesting to note that in some people who have just been diagnosed with type 1 diabetes and who have begun insulin treatment, the pancreas may temporarily increase insulin production. This usually begins within several months of starting treatment, and lasts anywhere from three to twelve months. During this "honeymoon phase," blood-sugar levels are less erratic, and the doctor may prescribe smaller dosages of injected insulin or fewer injections. This is necessary in order to prevent too much insulin in the body, which causes very low blood sugar.

It is not entirely clear why some 20 percent of newly diagnosed type 1 diabetics experience this period of improvement. Rarely, does a similar "honeymoon," or remission, occur in people with type 2 diabetes, most often in people of African American descent. It may be that, at the time of diagnosis, a small number of beta cells are still turning out insulin. When injection treatment begins, these few "holdouts" may get a chance to rest and renew their insulin production. For a while it's enough. But be aware that eventually insulin production dwindles again, blood-sugar levels become volatile, and more external insulin must be supplied. Like all honeymoons, this one must end.

Symptoms of type 2 diabetes

The main feature distinguishing type 1 and type 2 symptoms is that type 2 symptoms most often develop slowly, becoming evident over months or

66
A lot of people asked me, Doesn't it seem so unfair? But when I found out I had diabetes, I saw it as a wake-up call: Randy, start taking good care of yourself! Here's your chance.
—Randy, age forty-seven, with type 2 diabetes
99

years. Type 2 does not normally make a dramatic, urgent appearance in a person's life. Indeed, type 2 can be asymptomatic, that is, it can be present without causing noticeable symptoms. While the symptoms of type 1 rapidly reach a severity that sends people to their doctors, type 2 symptoms can be absent or mild and easily (and dangerously) attributed to overweight or aging. Diabetic complications may be present by the time type 2 diabetes is diagnosed. For this reason, type 2 diabetes is sometimes called a "silent killer."

Don't forget that type 2 diabetics do produce insulin, sometimes a little, sometimes a lot, depending upon the person. The problem for type 2 diabetics is insulin resistance; for various reasons their bodies do not respond to the insulin produced, so their blood glucose levels are too high. The fact that at least some insulin is made by the pancreas accounts for the typically muted symptoms and slower progression of type 2 diabetes. It also means that type 2 diabetics do not develop diabetic ketoacidosis.

All of these facts point again to the importance of regular physical checkups, even though you feel well, in order to identify any asymptomatic or mildly symptomatic problems. There are, however, definite symptoms of type 2 diabetes that are certainly noticeable and that you must not brush off. Although overt symptoms may be mild, the serious complications of uncontrolled blood sugar could already be developing and, in fact, will develop if the diabetes is not treated. Symptoms of type 2 diabetes can include

- Increased thirst
- Frequent urination, including at night

- Fatigue and drowsiness
- Blurred vision
- Weight loss
- Pain, tingling, or numbness in the legs or feet
- Skin problems, such as dry, itchy skin or acne
- Slow healing of cuts or wounds
- Increased infections, including recurrent urinary tract (bladder) or vaginal infections and fungal infections of the skin

Any of these symptoms calls for medical attention, especially (but not exclusively) if the person experiencing them is overweight, over forty, African American or Latino, has a family history of type 2 diabetes, or previously has had gestational diabetes.

As with type 1 diabetes, the symptoms listed above for type 2 diabetes are caused by abnormally high blood glucose levels. The way this happens is briefly explained above, under type 1 symptoms, except for the symptom of pain or numbness, which indicates nerve damage, or *neuropathy*, caused by uncontrolled blood-sugar levels. Neuropathy is discussed at greater length in Chapter 4.

Nerve damage caused by diabetes almost always is the result of many years, usually ten or more, of elevated blood sugar. This is why it is not an initial or acute symptom of type 1 diabetes, which does not go undetected over time the way type 2 diabetes often does. No one knows exactly how excess blood sugar damages nerves. It may be that too much blood sugar swells nerve cells or adheres to their surfaces, "gumming up the works." It may also be that nerve damage is caused by the impaired circulation that can occur in diabetes. Nerve cells, like others, require adequate amounts of oxygen

Unofficially...
Actress Dina Merrill's son has type 1 diabetes. She is a founder of the Juvenile Diabetes Foundation.

and nutrients in order to function and survive. If circulation slows or halts, the health of cells is diminished.

Table 3.1 gives the major defining characteristics of both types of diabetes.

TABLE 3.1   WHICH TYPE OF DIABETES IS IT?

Symptoms and characteristics	Do I have type 1 diabetes?	Do I have type 2 diabetes?
Age 10 at diagnosis	Probably	Probably not
Age 20 at diagnosis	Probably	Not likely, but possibly
Age 30 at diagnosis	Probably	Not likely, but possibly
Age 40 at diagnosis	Maybe	Maybe
Age 50 at diagnosis	Probably not	Probably
Age 60 at diagnosis	Probably not	Probably
Age 70 at diagnosis	Probably not	Probably
Underweight at diagnosis	Probably	Probably not
Normal weight at diagnosis	Maybe	Maybe
Frequent urination, increased hunger, and thirst before diagnosis	Yes	Maybe
Large amount of ketones in urine	Yes	Unlikely
Family history of type 1 diabetes	Yes	Maybe
Family history of type 2 diabetes	Maybe	Yes (Strong Indicator)
Previous gestational diabetes	No	Yes
Use Insulin	Yes	Maybe
Use Oral diabetes medication	Rarely useful	Yes
Controlled with diet	No	Maybe

Symptoms of gestational diabetes

Gestational diabetes mellitus (GDM) refers to high blood sugar that develops in a pregnant woman who previously did not have diabetes. Women with type 1 or type 2 diabetes who become pregnant do not have GDM; their diagnosis remains what it was prior to pregnancy.

Gestational diabetes is often asymptomatic. Symptoms that are noticeable may be similar to those of type 2 diabetes, except for those indicating nerve damage, which would not have time to develop in GDM. Frequent urination, a hallmark of diabetes, occurs early in most pregnancies and increases as the fetus grows, and this can also mask the presence of GDM.

GDM occurs because the placenta produces hormones that reduce insulin's effectiveness, thereby creating insulin resistance. In most women, the normal pancreas can compensate successfully by producing the right amounts of insulin to overcome the resistance. For some reason, however, the pancreas in 2 to 5 percent of pregnant women is not up to the task. This may explain why women who develop GDM are at greater risk for developing type 2 diabetes later. GDM itself, however, is by definition temporary and disappears when pregnancy ends.

Gestational diabetes usually occurs during the second half of pregnancy, too late to cause birth defects in the developing fetus. However, GDM increases the risk of miscarriage, as well as premature birth and complications for the newborn. For these reasons, and because there may be no obvious symptoms, doctors routinely check pregnant women for GDM, typically during weeks twenty-four to twenty-eight of the pregnancy. Since many

Bright Idea
The Internet address for the American Diabetes Association is www.diabetes.org. The Web site is full of useful information, including online copies of ADA magazines and links to other relevant sites.

pregnant women who do not have GDM have sugar in their urine, urine tests for sugar are not reliable in diagnosing GDM. Instead, a test called an oral glucose challenge is administered (see the following discussion of tests for diabetes).

Like all forms of diabetes, GDM poses serious health threats due to elevated blood-sugar levels. It can usually be treated with dietary changes, but diets that are too low in calories may be dangerous during pregnancy. If dietary changes do not control blood-sugar levels, insulin injections may be necessary. (Oral diabetes medications cannot be taken during pregnancy.)

There is more information about GDM, and diabetes and pregnancy, in Chapter 12.

One sure method: blood tests for diabetes

Diabetes can be confusing. It is one illness that takes several forms. The different types of diabetes share some symptoms, but not all. Some symptoms are impossible to ignore; others creep up on you, causing few immediate problems but signaling potentially devastating consequences.

High blood glucose is the underlying cause unifying these symptoms. If your doctor suspects you have diabetes, he or she will test your blood for high levels of sugar. Urine tests are not used to diagnose diabetes, although a high level of sugar in the urine may indicate that blood tests are in order. Alone, however, sugar in the urine is not sufficient to diagnose diabetes. Sugar can appear in the urine for other reasons, for instance, during pregnancy.

There are three possible blood tests for the diagnosis of type 1 and type 2 diabetes. If you have one test and the results are positive, it is best that you have the results confirmed by a different test. The tests are:

■ **The random plasma glucose test.** This is called *random* because it tests blood drawn at any time, whether the person being tested has just eaten or not. If you have some symptoms of diabetes, your doctor will look for a glucose level of 200 milligrams (mg) to each deciliter (dl) of blood. A level of 200 mg/dl or much higher, sometimes as high as the 400s, indicates diabetes.

■ **The fasting plasma glucose test.** This test is usually done twice to confirm a diagnosis of diabetes. The blood is drawn specifically after the patient has eaten nothing other than water for at least eight hours prior to the test. The purpose of this is to see how high the blood-sugar level is at its lowest, long after the last meal has been digested. In healthy people, the blood-sugar level following fasting will be 110 mg/dl or lower. In diabetics, the fasting blood-sugar level will be (on two testings) 126 mg/dl or higher.

Until 1977, the cutoff reading was 140 mg/dl, but the new criterion set by the American Diabetes Association is 126 mg/dl. It is hoped that this will result in earlier detection of diabetes, which improves the chances for preventing complications.

■ **The oral glucose tolerance test (OGTT).** Your doctor may want to use this diagnostic test. First, a fasting blood sample is taken and the sugar level checked. The patient then drinks a measured amount of a specially prepared, very sweet liquid. After a period of at least two hours, the blood-sugar level is checked again to determine how well the person's insulin has handled the sharp rise in glucose caused by taking the sweet drink on an empty stomach. Diabetes is diagnosed if the blood-sugar level at two hours after the drink is 200 mg/dl or greater.

The test for gestational diabetes, called the *oral glucose challenge*, is similar. The pregnant woman is given a sugar-rich preparation and her glucose levels are then checked at prescribed intervals. The amount of liquid given, however, as well as the diagnostic mg/dl criteria, are somewhat different from those for the fasting plasma glucose test. For more information on the oral glucose tolerance test for GDM, see Chapter 12.

"Borderline" diabetes and impaired glucose tolerance (IGT)

If you have type 1 diabetes, there is no chance that you will be diagnosed with "borderline" diabetes. In type 1, the lack of insulin in the body causes clear-cut symptoms; if they're vague or mild at first, this doesn't last long, and blood-sugar levels will rapidly become very high.

So-called "borderline" diabetes is more of an issue for people who fit the risk profile for type 2 diabetes—those who are over forty, overweight, who have a family history of type 2 diabetes, and especially (but not exclusively) African Americans, Native Americans and Latinos with these characteristics.

Let's say you haven't noticed any symptoms of diabetes in yourself; in general, you feel all right. You've had your blood drawn as part of your annual physical exam, so that many things can be checked, like cholesterol, liver function, iron levels, and so

Moneysaver
You may be able to reduce insurance plan costs by purchasing insurance at group rates through a professional, fraternal, alumni, or other association such as the American Association of Retired Persons.

forth. You're surprised to hear from your doctor that your fasting blood-sugar levels are higher than normal, over 110 mg/dl but not as high as the 126 mg/dl that indicates diabetes. Your doctor may then order an oral glucose tolerance test to get more information.

If the OGTT shows blood-sugar levels from 140 to 200 mg/dl at two hours, your doctor may diagnose *impaired glucose tolerance*. Impaired glucose tolerance is not diabetes, and it does not guarantee that diabetes will develop. But it *may* mean that your risk for developing type 2 diabetes is increased.

It is one thing to be formally diagnosed with impaired glucose tolerance. It is another thing to be told you have "borderline diabetes," "a touch of diabetes," or any other vague, nonmedical term that suggests a partial or small case of diabetes. There is no such thing. Ask your doctor specifically whether you have diabetes or not, what exactly your diagnosis is, and what specific treatment he or she recommends based upon his or her diagnosis. Do not accept unclear statements that may encourage you, if unintentionally, to minimize your legitimate concerns about problems with your blood-sugar levels. If you have been diagnosed with IGT, consider asking your doctor to refer you to The Diabetes Prevention Trial. See Chapter 16 for details.

When you are diagnosed with diabetes

Don't kid yourself. If you have received a diagnosis of diabetes, you're in the midst of an emotional reaction, whether you choose to acknowledge it or not. Your reaction may be obvious: You cry, shout, curse; you talk nonstop to friends; you curl up in a ball on your favorite chair; you sit and stare; you lie awake nights, worrying about your future and

Unofficially...
About 35 to 40 percent of people with impaired glucose tolerance go on to develop diabetes.

wondering how and why this has happened to you. You might even feel some relief at finally knowing why you haven't been feeling well.

Or your reaction may not be obvious at all: You go about your business calmly, as if nothing unusual has happened. "Diabetes? Me? No way. Big deal. I'll deal with it later. Everything is status quo. Because I'm not going to let all the fear, anger, and sadness get to me. I've got too much to do!"

This is called being in denial. Denial and diabetes are a dangerous mix.

Whether you're ready to acknowledge your feelings or not, at least know that they're there. And they're perfectly normal. Think about it: You've just been told that your body has stopped functioning normally, and that something you have taken for granted, blood-sugar control, is now something you must consciously manage every day. To top it off, it's possible that your situation could worsen; if you don't stay on top of all this new stuff you're supposed to do, you could develop life-threatening complications. Besides fear and anger, you feel a painful sense of loss—loss of health and the sense of normalcy. No wonder many people deny their feelings and even deny that anything is wrong.

But the feelings are there, rightfully so, and acknowledging them is probably your first step in coping with diabetes. You are entitled to these feelings, and one of the best things you can do for yourself is first to acknowledge you have them, and second, to express them in appropriate ways. Most people do this by opening up to friends and family members. You can also acknowledge your feelings to yourself, which is one way to give them a hearing. Sometimes it helps to write feelings down. A diary or journal can be a great "ear."

> **"**
> Sometimes she'd just like to forget she has this disease. And I tell her, hey, I can understand that. Who wouldn't wish now and then that they would wake up one morning, and poof, it would just be gone?
> —Claire, age thirty-four, mother of Laurie, age twelve, with type 1 diabetes
> **"**

How you may feel

Be on the lookout for anger masked by depression, or turned against the self in destructive ways. You may feel as though your body has betrayed you, so why should you take good care of it? But the fact is that your body very much needs your care if you have diabetes. Try to be aware of your feelings and allow yourself to have them, but don't use them as an excuse to ignore or delay your necessary treatment.

Moreover, having a chronic illness can challenge your sense of self-esteem. You may feel like "damaged goods." If you've always had trouble valuing or respecting yourself, having diabetes may make you feel worse. Again, try to be aware of this, rather than expressing it through poor self-care. Ironically, having to think consciously about managing your diabetes may be a golden opportunity to act on your own behalf as a person and to appreciate your value more strongly.

Don't hesitate during this period (or at any time) to seek professional counseling if you feel it could help you manage your feelings about having diabetes. Your doctor will most likely have suggestions about finding competent caregivers. Be sure to check into your insurance coverage for mental health services. (See Chapter 7 for more information on finding a mental health professional.)

The point is that dealing with strong feelings is a normal, necessary part of coping with diabetes. Don't judge yourself for reacting strongly; don't mistake having feelings for a lack of progress. They're part of the progression, part of adjusting to the new facts.

Watch Out!
If you are struggling with depression, seek help. Recent research shows that people who are depressed are more likely to develop heart disease, and are more likely to smoke, overeat, and drink excessively.

Adjusting to a new reality

Accepting feelings is one thing you can do to help yourself begin to adjust. Another is to be aware that you may feel overwhelmed by the complexity of diabetes. You should expect to feel that there is more to know about the disease and its treatment than you can possibly learn. It seems like there is a mountain of scientific and technical information; how will you ever scale it? It's very important to remind yourself that you need and deserve time to assimilate anything beyond the basics of self-care. Remember that your treatment plan has not yet become a habit, and before long, it will. As this happens, it will be easier to take in more information and refine what you know. The confusion you feel at first will resolve, and the components of treatment, which right now may seem like jigsaw puzzle pieces jumbled together in a box, will come together into one big picture.

Be especially patient with yourself if you have to learn to self-inject insulin. This can be an upsetting, even terrifying prospect for many people. You deserve the full support of the health-care professionals who will teach you this skill. You must learn it, but you are entitled to have some feelings about it. Even if your regimen does not include insulin, you will probably have to make lifestyle changes, maybe big changes, in your diet and activity level. This is difficult for anybody. Give yourself credit for accepting this, even before you begin to implement changes.

Don't fall into the trap of feeling guilty or bad if you don't achieve perfect blood-sugar control, now or even after you become more skilled at self-care. This is especially important for people with type 1 diabetes, who face greater challenges in stabilizing their blood-sugar levels.

Talk with your doctor or diabetes educator about appropriate, healthy, realistic goals for daily management. Ask for your doctor's perspective on how daily ups and downs relate to long-term treatment goals. Aim to do the best you can; you know that your health is at stake. Understand, however, that you cannot expect to replicate perfectly the minutely tuned workings of a healthy pancreas. But doing your best will be doing a great deal.

If someone close to you has been diagnosed with diabetes

If someone close to you has recently been diagnosed with diabetes, the best thing you can do is to listen to his or her feelings on the topic. The downside of this is that you may not want to hear about it. You may find yourself wishing that your loved one would just buckle down and take this more in stride. Feeling this way is understandable, but remember that if you don't have diabetes, you have little idea of what it's actually like to adjust to having it.

The upside is that listening doesn't involve any special knowledge on your part. In fact, one of the worst things you can do right now is try to offer your friend advice ("You really ought to . . . " or "If I were you . . ."). Don't feel you should try to fix or control your friend's feelings or his or her situation. You can't. What you can do is

- Give him or her your time, which, after all, is precious.
- Listen without commenting, except to say that it must be painful and difficult, and that his or her feelings are understandable.
- Ask your loved one to say more about these feelings, and listen even more.

- Now and then, try to reflect back to your friend what you're hearing about the experience: "So learning you have diabetes makes you feel like your health is out of your control?"

- Reassure your loved one that, although diabetes is serious and frightening, it is absolutely manageable and treatable.

- Never nag or remind your friend to follow doctor's orders! This is the diabetic's responsibility, not yours. And scare tactics don't work.

- Offer or be willing to attend an educational meeting or doctor's appointment with your friend.

- Educate yourself in the basics of diabetes self-management so that you have a sense of what your loved one is going through.

Don't forget to be proud of yourself for being there for this person. Remember that he or she would do the same for you and perhaps, in another context, already has.

For a closer look at diabetes and personal relationships, see Chapter 14.

First steps in developing your diabetes care plan

Diabetes is a complex disease requiring a team approach to treatment. In addition to a medical doctor who specializes in diabetes (usually an *endocrinologist*), you will also be working with a registered nurse or nurse practitioner, who is certified in diabetes education (signified as *C.D.E.*), and a registered dietitian (signified as *R.D.*), preferably one who is also certified in diabetes education. Additionally, you may see an eye doctor, a podiatrist (foot-care specialist), and an exercise specialist.

There will be more detailed information on this treatment team in Chapter 7. Our focus here is on aspects of getting started on this new phase of life: treating your diabetes.

The first step is to understand that you, not the doctor, play the starring role on your treatment team. In diabetes, the primary practitioner is the patient himself. Understanding and accepting this can be one of the biggest adjustments that the newly diagnosed person has to make. Most of us tend to expect doctors to tell us what is wrong, prescribe the appropriate treatment, and essentially take full responsibility for the outcome. Diabetes doctors do, of course, prescribe the treatment. But it is largely the patient's actions that determine the outcome.

What's more, whenever possible the patient should have a say in the overall treatment plan. In order for a daily treatment plan to be effective, it must be something the patient can live with.

If taking an active role with doctors is new to you, you might begin by discussing this very fact with your doctor:

- Ask how your doctor feels about your asking questions, stating preferences, or voicing doubts. You may be pleasantly surprised by the response you receive. Diabetes practitioners know that responsibility for the day-to-day management of diabetes belongs to the patient. A competent practitioner will support patient involvement.

- Take a written list of questions with you to appointments, write down the answers, and be mentally prepared to ask for clarification if the answers you get don't seem clear. Your top priority is your health. It's worth speaking up for it.

Unofficially...
Did you know that pet owners tend to experience less stress and depression?

Don't leave burdened with unspoken questions; they won't just disappear, and your self-care may suffer.

Having recognized this, however, keep in mind that the professionals involved in your care have a lot of information that they must impart to you, especially in the beginning. You'll need to do your share of listening. It's reasonable to expect to speak up about 40 percent of the time and to spend the rest of the time listening.

What to expect: initial treatment of type 1 diabetes
The immediate objective of your treatment will be to supply insulin to your body in order to bring your blood sugar down to as normal a level as possible while avoiding the low blood sugar caused by too much insulin. You and your team will be monitoring your response to insulin therapy. You will be taught to inject yourself with insulin. If the patient is a young child, parents are taught to administer injections.

Usually, persons newly diagnosed with type 1 diabetes are started on two to three injections a day, one before breakfast and one before supper, and perhaps a third at bedtime. As you begin insulin therapy, two to three shots are easier to manage than the four to five daily injections of more intensive treatment. Intensive treatment may be started within the next several months, after your blood-sugar levels have stabilized and you begin to get the hang of administering injections and timing your meals.

You will be taught how to take blood samples and how to monitor your glucose levels. Learning how and why to monitor your glucose is an essential part of self-care. Your diabetes educator will help you

> " Having diabetes is hard sometimes. But it's really helped me to focus on my priorities, on what I want to do with my life.
> —Sarah, age twenty-seven, with type 1 diabetes "

take a number of samples and supervise your evaluation of them to ensure that you know how to evaluate your glucose levels.

The diabetes educator, or a registered dietitian, will give you instruction on what foods to eat and how to time meals and select foods based on your blood glucose testing and insulin dosages. During this initial phase of treatment, you will be introduced to these key components of type 1 management:

- Timing of blood glucose tests (you should have a basic understanding of when to do them and why).

- Timing of meals (you should have a basic understanding of how this affects blood-sugar levels and your need for injections prior to eating).

- Choice of foods and amount of calories to be consumed (you should have a basic under-standing of the impact different foods have on blood-sugar levels).

- Timing of insulin shots (you should understand when to inject yourself and why).

- Frequency of insulin shots (you should have a basic understanding of what the options are and the pros and cons of different frequencies).

- Dosage and type of insulin used (you should have a basic understanding of how much insulin to use and when to choose shorter- or longer-acting types).

It is the balancing and interaction of these com-ponents that help to control blood sugar.

As a new type 1 patient, it can seem like an awful lot to learn. You should expect to receive at least ten hours of patient education.

You should also expect that you and your team will make changes in your regimen in the months ahead, tailoring it to changes in your insulin needs and your level of comfort with the treatment plan.

What to expect: initial treatment of type 2 diabetes

There is no one standard treatment for type 2 diabetes. People with type 2 diabetes can differ greatly in terms of how much insulin they produce; how resistant they are to insulin; and in age, weight, and lifestyle. It is very important to tailor treatment plans for type 2 diabetes as closely to the individual patient as possible.

That said, you can expect your treatment plan to focus on nutrition and exercise as the first lines of defense:

- Most people with type 2 diabetes are overweight; losing even 5 to 10 percent of body weight can enhance insulin sensitivity. So the first treatment goal may often be to lose a moderate amount of weight.

- Even for type 2 diabetics of normal weight, proper diet and regular exercise are the preferred treatment choice, so the first step will probably be a thorough assessment of your current diet and activity level. What you eat and whether you are active both have a major impact on glucose levels.

- Your team will help you to choose a type or types of exercise that are consistent with your current overall health. Since many people with type 2 diabetes have had the disease for some time prior to diagnosis, it is essential that your doctor check you for any signs of damage to your eyes, kidneys, heart, feet, and nervous system before making treatment recommendations.

Bright Idea
For extra help in understanding all you need to know about diabetes self-care, contact the local branch of the American Diabetes Association for information on diabetes education classes in your area that meet the Association's National Standards for diabetes education.

- Even gentle, moderate exercise, like walking, can be highly beneficial. You won't be asked to run marathons. What's more important in most cases is that exercise be done at least three times a week for thirty to forty minutes.

- In the realm of diet, expect the focus to be on how foods, especially carbohydrates and portion sizes, affect your glucose levels. You will not be told to eliminate starches and sugars. Instead, you'll learn to establish "carbohydrate goals." Your diabetes educator or dietitian will help you decide on ways to alter your eating, through food choice, portion size, meal frequency, and food combinations, so that your hunger is satisfied without sending your glucose levels skyrocketing. This will include information on the way fats, protein, and fiber factor in to blood-sugar control.

People with type 2 diabetes, like those with type 1 diabetes, learn to monitor blood sugar as part of their treatment. It's essential for tracking the effects of dietary and exercise changes. Your team will recommend how often to test your glucose levels, based upon the degree of your diabetes and the lifestyle changes you make. Frequency of testing can vary widely among individual patients, and will certainly change with any adjustments to your treatment plan.

Finally, your doctor may prescribe oral medications that will either enhance insulin secretion, increase the effectiveness of your insulin, or slow down the absorption of carbohydrates from the intestines, depending on the medication used. In recent years, doctors have been more inclined to prescribe medications to patients earlier in the course of their disease because evidence has mounted showing that tighter blood-sugar control definitely helps prevent long-term complications of diabetes. Nevertheless, most doctors turn to pharmacological treatment only after nutritional and exercise prescriptions have failed to keep blood sugar at near-normal levels.

OK, which of my favorite things in life do I have to give up first?

Believe it or not, the answer to that usually is "Not one."

Nutrition will be discussed at length in Chapter 8. But here's some good news: Eliminating or restricting all sugar is no longer the primary focus of the diabetic diet. Research has shown that it is the overall amount of carbohydrates of all types in the diet that is important, not the specific source or type of carbohydrate. All carbohydrates—bread, pasta, potatoes, fruit, hard candy, you name it—raise glucose levels. The goal, then, is to monitor the amount of carbohydrates you eat overall.

This does not mean that you can freely indulge in large amounts of sugar, but it does give you a little leeway. You can adjust your carbohydrate intake to include a treat as long as you keep your overall limit in mind. And that includes moderate alcohol consumption, unless other considerations prevent it.

Just the facts

- Type 1 and type 2 diabetes share many symptoms.
- Type 1 diabetes usually emerges acutely, while type 2 often develops insidiously.

Moneysaver
The American Diabetes Association publishes an annual *Buyer's Guide to Diabetes Supplies*. Check out the latest offerings and most competitive prices.

- Type 2 diabetes may be asymptomatic, or "silent," for many years, while complications of diabetes may develop.
- For all types of diabetes, blood tests are the only accurate tests.
- There is no such thing as "a touch of diabetes."
- Sugar restriction is no longer the cornerstone of nutrition therapy for diabetes.

GET THE SCOOP ON...
What are the complications of diabetes ▪ The
role of blood-sugar control ▪ Diabetes and
heart disease ▪ Diabetes and your eyes ▪
How diabetes affects the legs and feet ▪
Coping with complications

Getting Serious: Potential Complications of Diabetes

Chapter 4

The symptoms of diabetes make clear the huge impact of elevated blood-sugar levels on the entire body. Left untreated or poorly controlled, chronic high blood sugar can do serious harm to the circulatory system, the nervous system, the kidneys, and the eyes. Conversely, when blood sugar is well controlled over time, the risk for serious complications is significantly reduced. This is true for both type 1 and type 2 diabetes.

The Diabetes Control and Complications Trial (DCCT)

In 1993, the American Diabetes Association announced the results of a nationwide study, the Diabetes Control and Complications Trial (DCCT), that followed 1,441 people with type 1 diabetes for more than six years. The purpose of the study was to measure the effects of "tight" or "intensive" insulin treatment on the development of diabetes complications, in comparison to less rigorous treatment. (Intensive treatment involves frequent daily glucose checks and multiple insulin injections. It is discussed in Chapter 5.)

The goal of intensive treatment is to keep blood-sugar as close as possible to that of a nondiabetic person. Does intensive treatment, with tighter control of blood-sugar levels, lower the risk for serious complications? The DCCT results proved that the answer is a resounding yes. This study showed that keeping blood-sugar levels as close to normal as possible reduces the overall risk for serious diabetes complications by as much as 50 percent. The incidence of eye disease was reduced by 76 percent, nerve damage by 60 percent, and kidney damage by up to 56 percent.

The DCCT did not include people with type 2 diabetes, but there is every reason to believe that the results apply to this group as well. This is supported by the results of The United Kingdom Prospective Diabetes Study, or UKPDS, reported in September of 1998. The UKPDS followed more than 5,000 newly diagnosed people with type 2 diabetes for an average length of ten years. The UKPDS found that intensive blood sugar control results in decreased incidences of eye, kidney, and nerve complications, heart attack, and sudden death. The study also found controlling blood pressure has an even greater impact on reducing risks for these complications.

The message is loud and clear that the long-term complications of diabetes, types 1 and 2 alike, can be delayed or prevented by careful control of blood-sugar levels. This is good news in light the seriousness of diabetes complications.

What are the complications of diabetes?

You may not be a smoker. You may get regular exercise. You may even be a premenopausal woman. Nevertheless, if you have diabetes, your risk for developing vascular disease (atherosclerosis, or hardening of the arteries) is two to three times that of a nondiabetic person. Among diabetics (including premenopausal women, heart disease occurs more frequently, more severely, and earlier in life than among nondiabetics. Atherosclerosis accounts for 80 percent of deaths in people with diabetes. The risks are even higher, of course, in diabetics who smoke, are obese, or have high blood pressure or high cholesterol.

Vascular disease can affect circulation in the brain, causing strokes. People with diabetes are five times more likely to have a stroke than nondiabetics. Stroke accounts for 6 percent of deaths in people with diabetes under age forty-five. Peripheral vascular disease, which hampers circulation in the limbs, can cause chronic ulcers on the legs and feet, ulcers that become infected and do not heal. Over half of amputations performed in the United States that are not due to accidents and trauma occur in people with diabetes.

Diabetes can also damage the eyes and the kidneys. It is a leading cause of blindness in adults in the United States, and it increases the risk of glaucoma and cataracts. Diabetes is also a major cause of end-stage kidney disease; about 40 percent of people starting dialysis in America have diabetes.

Finally, having diabetes can predispose you to serious bacterial and fungal infections that may be difficult to treat and can develop anywhere in the

"
I finally, finally quit smoking, because I knew that, with diabetes, my risk for heart disease is higher than average. But the great thing is, my husband quit, too! He said he doesn't want his second-hand smoke ruining my health.
—Angela, age forty-six, with type 2 diabetes
"

body. Some of these infections, such as pseu-
domonas bacterial infections and certain fungal
infections, are rare in the general population. In
people with diabetes, however, high blood sugar
encourages the growth of fungal organisms and bacteria.

It may seem that the deck is stacked against you
if you have diabetes. Remember your ace in the
hole: good, consistent self-care, including frequent
blood-sugar monitoring. Serious complications are
not inevitable, and if they develop they often can be
managed. You do have a measure of control.
Prevention and management of complications is discussed later on in this chapter. Some of the chronic
complications of diabetes are summarized on the
following page.

Macrovascular complications: the heart, brain, and circulatory system

Macrovascular complications are the effects of diabetes
on veins, arteries, and blood flow throughout the
body. Diabetes seems to hasten and worsen atherosclerosis, the hardening of the arteries caused by the
accumulation of fat-based plaque on the inner walls
of blood vessels. No doubt you are familiar with
many of the factors that can lead to atherosclerosis:
a high-fat diet, high levels of cholesterol and triglycerides in the blood, lack of exercise, high blood
pressure, and smoking cigarettes. Having diabetes is
also a risk factor for cardiovascular disease.

It is not entirely clear how diabetes accelerates
cardiovascular disease. High blood sugar may
interfere with the movement of blood fats, or *lipids,*
into cells, or excessive blood sugar may make
lipids sticky, causing them to adhere more readily to
vessel walls. Diabetes may cause blood platelets,

Unofficially...
Although not yet
available, neuro-
protective drugs
that are specifi-
cally designed to
protect nerves
from inflamma-
tory damage are
being tested for
treatment of dia-
betic neuropathy.
An anti-seizure
medication,
Neurontin, has
also been used
to treat painful
neuropathy.

Chronic Complications of Diabetes

Vascular Diseases (Affecting Veins and Arteries)
Macrovascular
- Heart disease; atherosclerosis
- Stroke; transient ischemic attacks
- Circulatory disorders in legs, feet

Microvascular
- Eye disease: retinopathy
- Kidney disease: nephropathy
- Nerve disease; neuropathy

Neuropathy (Nerve Damage)
- Peripheral neuropathy
  - Nerve damage in legs, feet
  - Nerve damage in arms, hands
  - Foot ulcer due to nerve damage
  - Charcot's foot
- Mononeuropathy
- Nerve damage to one specific nerve or nerve group
- Muscle atrophy due to nerve damage
- Autonomic neuropathy
  - Gastroparesis: Nerve damage affecting the stomach
  - Diabetic diarrhea: Nerve damage affecting the intestines
  - Diabetic constipation: Nerve damage affecting the intestines
  - Neurogenic bladder: Nerve damage affecting the bladder
  - Impotence, sexual dysfunction
  - Impaired reflexes of the heart and circulatory system
  - Decreased symptoms and awareness of hypoglycemia

Mixed Vascular and Nerve Damage Complications
- Ulcers of the leg and foot

responsible for normal blood clotting, to overproduce a clotting factor and impede blood flow. In any case, the result is clogged, less elastic arteries that are less able to dilate as needed to increase blood flow.

When the coronary arteries that supply blood to the heart muscle become partly blocked, the reduced blood supply to the muscle of the heart wall makes it harder for the heart to pump. This can cause chest pain (*angina pectoris*), especially upon exertion. If coronary arteries are completely blocked, areas of heart tissue die. This is a heart attack, or *myocardial infarction*.

Similarly, in cerebrovascular disease, obstructed arteries can cause areas of the brain to weaken or die. Where blood supply is diminished, neurological functioning is temporarily disturbed, usually evidenced by such symptoms as numbness in an arm or an inability to speak clearly. These events are short-lived and are called *transient ischemic attacks*, or *TIAs*. A stroke occurs when an artery to the brain is completely blocked and the brain cells served by that artery die.

Watch Out!
High-heeled shoes cause excessive pressure on the metatarsals, the small bones at the base of the toes. People with diabetes are particularly vulnerable to foot ulcers in this area.

Finally, hardening of the arteries can cause blockages in the long arteries supplying the legs and feet. This is *peripheral vascular disease*. Partial arterial blockage can lead to leg or buttock pain, called *claudication*. If there is a complete blockage in a leg artery, blood tends to bypass it by going through other arteries. Extreme obstructions of circulation, however, could cause gangrene. In diabetics, the greater risk is that impaired circulation in the leg and foot will combine with nerve damage (discussed below), causing insensitivity to wounds, slow healing, death of skin around wounds, and advanced infection which can spread into the bone.

Microvascular complications: the eyes and kidneys

The term *microvascular* refers to the tiniest, most delicate blood vessels in the body. These are essential to providing blood flow to equally delicate organs and structures, for instance, the retina of the eye and the inner filters of the kidney.

Eye damage

Generally, damage to the eyes takes a minimum of five years to develop once diabetes begins. It can progress with few or no obvious symptoms, however, so it is extremely important for all people with diabetes to receive regular eye examinations by ophthalmologists who are trained to spot diabetic eye disease. (An ophthalmologist is a medical doctor who specializes in diagnosing and treating eye disease.)

Fifteen years following diagnosis, more than 90 percent of people with type 1 diabetes will show some degree of damage to the retina, as will over 55 to 80 percent of people with type 2 diabetes. Fortunately, if there is vision impairment, laser surgery techniques can in many cases prevent further loss of vision.

People with diabetes are at greater risk for developing cataracts (clouding of the eye's lens) and glaucoma (excessive pressure within the eyeball). The most common and potentially serious complication of diabetes affecting the eyes, however, is *diabetic retinopathy.*

The retina is the membrane at the inner back of the eye upon which images are projected. Like all parts of the body, the retina depends on a blood supply for healthy functioning. Retinopathy develops when there is damage to the tiny blood vessels supplying the retina. There are two major forms of retinopathy.

Nonproliferative retinopathy (sometimes called *background retinopathy*)

This condition is the earlier stage of retinopathy and is extremely common in diabetics who have had the disease for five years or more. It usually does not

Unofficially...
In 1991, Italian and Belgian researchers reported promising results in using Vitamin E to slow the accumulation of *advanced glycosylation endproducts*, or *AGEs*, the molecular combinations of glucose and protein thought to cause many long-term complications of diabetes.

affect the vision, unless it causes macular edema, discussed below.

In nonproliferative retinopathy, blood vessels in the retina weaken and balloon out or collapse. Blood, other fluids, and fats can leak into the eye through these microaneurysms, in some cases causing blurred vision (but not blindness). Secretions may collect in the retina and form microscopic clumps called *hard exudates*, visible only through an instrument called an *opthalmoscope*.

Nonproliferative retinopathy seriously affects the vision only when it causes leakage into the macula, a nerve-rich spot in the center of the retina that is responsible for focused central vision. Leaks into the macula cause it to swell, creating macular edema, which is treatable with laser techniques. A test called a fluoroscein angiogram, performed by an ophthalmologist, can detect early leakage.

Proliferative retinopathy

Background retinopathy can progress to a more serious stage known as *proliferative retinopathy*. In this condition, new blood vessels are created (proliferate) in an attempt to keep the retina richly supplied with blood. These new vessels are fragile and their growth exerts pressure on the tissue-thin retina. The increase of fragile vessels greatly increases the risk of hemorrhages into the normally clear vitreous fluid of the eyeball, which can completely obstruct sight. Blood may be surgically drained from the eyeball, restoring vision, but in proliferative retinopathy, hemorrhages are highly likely to recur. Repeated bleeding, scarring, and blood vessel growth can ultimately lead to a detached retina. Surgical interventions may repair the damage in some cases.

> "
> At first I thought, I'm giving up all my personal freedom just to take care of my blood sugar! But gradually it dawned on me the freedom I'd give up if I lost a foot, or my eyesight.
> —Tony, age forty-two, with type 1 diabetes
> "

Many people with type 2 diabetes have high
blood pressure. They should be aware that high
blood pressure can exacerbate retinopathy.

The box below contains important eye care tips.

Eye Care Tips

Follow these important eye care tips to reduce
your risk for eye problems:

- Have a complete eye exam every year,
  done by an ophthalmologist (a medical
  doctor) trained to diagnose and treat eye
  disease). Remember, eye damage often
  has no symptoms in its earliest stages.
- See an ophthalmologist at once if you
  have any of these symptoms:
  - Blurred or double vision
  - Narrowed field of vision
  - Seeing dark spots
  - Feeling of pressure or pain in the eyes
  - Difficulty seeing in dim light
- Have your blood pressure checked often
- Do not smoke

Kidney damage

Your kidneys perform the vital, round-the-clock
function of filtering toxins out of the bloodstream
and into the urine for removal from the body. The
kidneys also control the ratio of water, salt, and
potassium in body fluids, prompting the body to
excrete excess salt or water as needed to keep just
the right balance. This gives the kidneys a central
role in controlling blood pressure as well. Finally,
the kidneys help to maintain normal levels of acid-
ity, phosphorus, and calcium in the body, and they

play a role in keeping your red-blood-cell count normal. They are small, but very important, organs.

The tiny filtering structures within the kidneys are called *nephrons;* kidney disease is called *nephropathy.* Diabetic nephropathy is caused by damage to the extremely delicate blood vessels or capillaries supplying the nephrons. Eventually the nephrons themselves become thickened and clogged. It is not known exactly how this occurs. High blood pressure, frequent urinary tract infections, and chronic overuse of nonsteroidal analgesics (like ibuprofen and acetamenophen) can all contribute to nephropathy.

Kidney damage can progress for many years with no overt symptoms of illness. The kidneys have so much filtering capacity that at least 80 percent of kidney tissue must be damaged before serious problems begin. Before that time, however, certain symptoms can be detected in your urine.

Damaged kidneys "leak" protein into the urine, both dietary protein and that which results from the use and repair of muscle tissue. An excessive amount of protein in the urine is called *proteinuria* if it persists over time and is found on repeated testing. (Protein in the urine can be a temporary, normal effect of stress, other illnesses, or exercise.)

People with diabetes should be checked annually for proteinuria from the time they are diagnosed. The most sensitive test for proteinuria measures *microalbuminuria,* tiny particles of the protein *albumin* in the urine. This test detects kidney damage in its earliest stages. Another very accurate test, which measures how well the kidneys are handling protein, is the *blood creatinine* level.

Nephropathy that goes undetected and unchecked ends in kidney failure, or end-stage renal

Unofficially...
Certified diabetes educator J. Shawn Faulk points out that one of the most dangerous complications of diabetes is "diabetes fatalism," a negative, apathetic attitude toward self-care.

disease. The kidneys are no longer able to filter toxins and waste products, which begin building up in the blood. Along with extreme proteinuria, symptoms of kidney failure may include high blood pressure, pronounced swelling of the feet or legs, anemia, exhaustion, nausea, vomiting, and increased or reduced urine production. The level of potassium in the blood may become high, requiring that potassium-rich foods be restricted.

As kidney damage progresses, the blood can become too acidic. The person must eventually begin dialysis treatment, which is a method for replacing the filtering function of the kidneys. Dialysis is a lifesaving treatment that must be performed several times weekly for life. There are two types of dialysis: *hemodialysis* and *peritoneal dialysis.* The first uses specialized equipment through which the patient's blood can circulate for filtration. The second involves the draining of fluids allowed to accumulate within the abdominal (peritoneal) cavity.

Complications of the nervous system: neuropathy

Nerve damage is a very common, rather mysterious complication of diabetes. Like other complications, nerve damage usually takes years to develop; it is rarely seen within the first five years of diagnosis. People with type 2 disease who have gone undiagnosed while the disease progressed may have signs of nerve damage, or *neuropathy,* at the time of diagnosis.

No one knows exactly how diabetes harms nerves. High levels of glucose may disrupt the chemical balance within nerve cells, impairing their ability to transmit electrical signals. Glucose

Bright Idea
Some people find that pain and muscle cramping caused by neuropathy of the legs or feet can be eased by a little walking, especially before bed. Or try the "tiptoe" exercise: Hold on to the back of a chair and slowly raise and lower yourself on your toes. Leg cramps that occur at night are sometimes relieved by quinine pills.

molecules may stick to the cells of the membranes that sheath the nerve fibers. These sheathing membranes, called the *myelin,* insulate nerve fibers and allow the conduction of electrical signals. If the myelin is hampered, nerve function is impaired. Or microvascular disease may restrict blood flow to nerve cells, depriving them of oxygen and impairing their function.

Depending upon the nerves affected, the symptoms of diabetic neuropathy can be temporary; they can change from mild to severe, and back again. They can persist. Symptoms vary with the type and location of the damage and its severity. Neuropathy is diagnosed based on the patient's description of his or her symptoms. The doctor may also check for nerve damage using an *electromyogram* test, which measures the strength of nerve impulses by electrically stimulating nerves, or by checking the decreases in sensitivity to touch, using specialized microfibers to stimulate nerve endings.

Polyneuropathy is nerve damage that can occur in many parts of the body, or that affects entire systems of the body. This tends to develop slowly over time, sometimes going unnoticed until the neuropathy worsens. Polyneuropathy is the most common diabetic neuropathy. *Mononeuropathy* is damage restricted to one particular area and nerve, or to a group of single nerves. The nerve is impaired suddenly, perhaps due to pressure or blocked circulation, causing marked, often painful symptoms. It is not as common in diabetes as polyneuropathy.

The following are the three categories of diabetic neuropathy.

Peripheral symmetrical polyneuropathy (generally called *peripheral neuropathy*)

This is the most common of diabetic neuropathies, called "peripheral" because symptoms first appear at the extremities of the body, principally the toes and feet. In more severe cases fingers and hands may be affected. Peripheral neuropathy is caused by gradual damage to the longest nerves, which seem to be the first affected by diabetes. Peripheral neuropathy is symmetrical in that it appears simultaneously on both sides of the body, although it is possible that symptoms on one side may not feel identical to those on the other.

Peripheral neuropathy rarely impairs motor functioning or movement. Instead, symptoms are usually sensory in nature, for example:

- **Numbness, tingling, or pain in the toes.** Symptoms may be very subtle at first, even imperceptible to the person affected; it may take a doctor's examination to discover a problem.

- **Skin hypersensitivity.** For example, the light pressure of bed sheets or socks may cause a painful or burning sensation.

- **Leg cramps, especially at night.** The uncomfortable sensations may come and go.

- **Strange, odd, or difficult-to-describe sensations,** called *parothesias* by doctors.

More advanced neuropathy can be very painful, but as the nerve damage progresses, pain diminishes and numbness sets in. This can range from contact numbness—impaired sensitivity to light or moderate touch—to profound numbness, or feet that feel dead, usually accompanied by coldness of the feet. In severe cases, peripheral neuropathy can spread to areas of the abdomen, causing sensory impairment there, as well.

It's worth emphasizing that many people who have peripheral neuropathy may not be aware of it. If there is no pain and only mild or superficial numbness, the nerve damage may go unnoticed, progressing all the while. It is very important for all diabetics and their health-care practitioners to check the feet regularly for signs of neuropathy.

Charcot's foot

One possible consequence of peripheral neuropathy and numbness of the feet is *Charcot's foot,* a condition in which bones in the foot become deformed. Numbness, diminished reflexes, and poor muscle tone in the foot cause people to misstep repeatedly or position the foot badly while walking and standing. This structural stress can be subtle, but over time it bends and damages bones, often causing them to protrude under the skin on the sole of the foot. This can lead to pressure spots on the skin, sores, and foot ulcers.

Autonomic neuropathy

Long nerves also regulate the body's autonomic functions, such as breathing, the heart beat, pupil dilation, perspiration, and stomach and intestinal function. These nerves, too, may be affected over time by diabetes. Like peripheral neuropathy, autonomic neuropathy is polyneuropathy in that it affects many nerves and functions. Autonomic neuropathy can affect virtually any of the organs under autonomic control.

Cardiovascular autonomic neuropathy

This can cause irregularities of the pulse rate and can mute or block the warning pains signaling heart attack. It can also interfere with the heart's performance during exercise.

Normally, when you change from a lying or sitting position to standing, your blood pressure rapidly adjusts to the change in position. With autonomic neuropathy, however, arterial reflexes may become weaker or delayed. Blood "pools" in the legs, causing faintness or dizziness upon standing (*orthostatic hypotension*).

Gastrointestinal autonomic neuropathy

The normal movements of the stomach and bowel may become impaired. *Gastroparesis* may develop, in which the stomach becomes sluggish or less active in response to the presence of food. The muscular contractions that move food into the intestines are weak or erratic. Food remains too long in the stomach and nausea or poor appetite can result. Most bothersome and risky is that gastroparesis makes blood-sugar control more difficult by slowing down digestion. This makes it harder to predict rises in glucose and corresponding insulin needs.

When neuropathy affects the intestines, constipation may occur (*low bowel motility*), alternating with diarrhea (*high bowel motility*).

Urinary tract autonomic neuropathy

Damage to nerves controlling the bladder may cause a slackening of that organ, resulting in slow or dribbling urination, incomplete emptying of the bladder, and increased risk for urinary tract infection. Recurrent infections can harm the kidneys. The sensation of bladder fullness may be impaired, and "overflow" incontinence may occur. In severe neuropathy, the bladder may become incapable of emptying properly, which, besides being a serious

Unofficially...
According to some studies, hypnosis as a means of treating chronic pain provides total relief in 15 to 20 percent of subjects. To locate a medical doctor who is a qualified hypnotherapist, call the American Society of Clinical Hypnosis, in Des Plaines, Illinois, at (708) 297-3317.

problem in itself, can cause kidney damage due to the buildup of pressure.

Sexual dysfunction

Symptoms are erectile impotence in men and, possibly, vaginal dryness, pain during intercourse or diminished sexual response in women. Women with diabetes are also more likely to have vaginal fungal infections, which can be painful. Keep in mind that many factors other than autonomic neuropathy can affect sexual functioning, for instance hormonal imbalances, vascular disease, many medications, and psychological problems.

Sweating

Autonomic neuropathy may impede or accelerate sweating in different parts of the body. Activities that normally do not cause sweating may trigger it, such as eating ("gustatory sweating").

Hypoglycemia unawareness

This is an especially serious symptom of diabetic neuropathy. The nerve damage has muffled the inner alarm system (the response to adrenaline) that is triggered when blood-sugar levels become dangerously low, which can happen if too little food has been eaten, too much insulin is present, or exercise has been too vigorous or done on an empty stomach.

Severe low blood sugar, or *hypoglycemia*, can lead to loss of consciousness, convulsions, and death; it is discussed in Chapter 5. Low blood sugar is an emergency, and there should be many warning signs when it occurs, including acute, uncomfortable symptoms such as shakiness, heavy sweating, clamminess, anxiety, or jitteryness. Autonomic neuropathy may dull a person's experience of or awareness of these signs, putting that person in danger.

Mononeuropathy (focal neuropathy)

Mononeuropathy is less common in diabetics than polyneuropathy. While polyneuropathy affects the body diffusely, is symmetrical, and develops gradually, often with mild symptoms (in early stages), mononeuropathies affect a single nerve or a set of single nerves (the latter case is referred to as *mononeuropathy multiplex*). Only the body area supplied by the specific nerve or nerve set is affected (hence the term *focal neuropathy*), and symptoms are not necessarily symmetric.

Mononeuropathy develops suddenly and is usually obvious. Depending upon the nerve affected, there may be sensory disturbances (numbness or pain), muscle weakness, or both. Unlike polyneuropathy, mononeuropathy is self-limiting, that is, it clears up instead of steadily progressing, usually after blood-sugar levels are brought under better control. Most cases last anywhere from several weeks to a year or so.

Mononeuropathy can affect potentially any nerve and many parts of the body. Examples of mononeuropathy commonly seen in diabetes include

- **Bell's palsy.** A cranial (head) nerve controlling facial muscles is temporarily affected, causing drooping in one area of the face.

- **Eye muscle palsy.** A nerve supplying an eye muscle is affected, suddenly causing a crossed eye and double vision.

- **Carpal tunnel syndrome.** The median nerve of the forearm, running through the wrist, is squeezed, causing weakness and pain in the hand, wrist, and forearm. Carpal tunnel syndrome is a nerve compression syndrome that is more common in people with diabetes.

- **Femoral neuropathy (diabetic amyotrophy).** A set of nerves in the pelvis that serves the upper legs is compressed, causing weakness of the hips and upper legs.

Foot ulcers and other complications

Sadly, diabetes is famous for causing ulcers of the foot and leg. It should be clear that the combination of vascular and neurological complications described so far places people with diabetes at great risk for developing sores that will not heal. Peripheral numbness blunts pain, so that injuries are not felt, while poor circulation prevents healing and abets infection. (Remember that the blood carries essential nutrients, oxygen, and immune-system cells to infection sites.) It is no surprise, then, that infections of the lower extremities are one of the most frequent causes of hospitalization for people with diabetes.

Proper foot care and suitable footwear, however, can help prevent serious damage to the feet. The figures below illustrate helpful foot care tips.

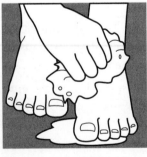

Wash your feet daily with luke-warm water and soap.

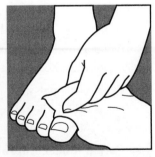

Dry your feet well, also between the toes. Treat fungal infections between the toes as soon as they develop.

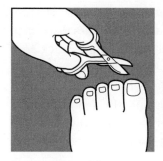

Cut your nails straight across.
Ingrown nails, calluses, and
corns should be treated by a
podiatrist.

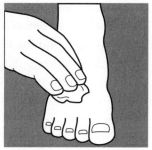

Keep the skin supple with a
moisturizing lotion, but do not
apply it between the toes.

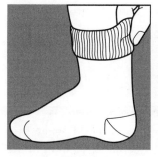

Change daily into clean, soft
socks or stockings, which are
neither too big nor too small.
Wear cotton or wool socks
that "breathe" and wick away
moisture.

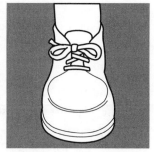

Keep your feet warm and dry.
Wear leather or canvas shoes.
Always wear shoes and sandals
that fit. Avoid sandals with
straps between the toes.

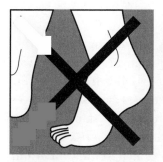

Never walk barefoot—either in-
or outdoors.

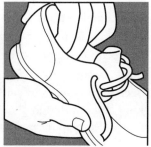

Examine your shoes every day
for cracks, pebbles, nails, and
other irregularities, which may
irritate the skin.

Bright Idea
Take off your shoes and socks at every doctor's appointment. This will remind you and the doctor to do a foot check.

Besides neuropathy and vascular disease, foot deformities can contribute to the formation of ulcers. People with diabetes have a higher incidence of foot deformities due to Charcot's foot (described above in the discussion of peripheral neuropathy) and due to inflammation and shortening or contractures of muscles and tendons. This can also occur in the hands and fingers. (See "Limited joint mobility," below.)

While usually not painful, contractures change the shape of the foot and can cause imbalances of pressure, leading to areas of inflammation, rawness, pressure sores, and ulceration. Neuropathy and poor circulation in the foot may also cause overly dry skin, which is more vulnerable to cracking and infection.

Gums and teeth

Vigilance against gum disease, or *gingivitis*, is crucial for people with diabetes. Excess blood sugar provides a feast for bacteria, decreases your immune response, and increases your risk for infection anywhere in the body. Don't forget that this includes your mouth and gums. People with diabetes are also vulnerable to yeast infections of the mouth, called *thrush*.

Skin complications

Dry skin is not typically a symptom of diabetes except in cases of extreme dehydration due to very high blood sugar. Decreased circulation and decreased sweating can cause dry skin, however. Keep in mind that fissures in the skin may easily become infected. This is especially a risk if you suffer from athlete's foot, "jock itch," or any other fungal infection of the skin. Be sure to moisturize dry

skin, guard against sunburn and other burns, and
protect your lips from chapping. Skin conditions
that may arise as a result of repeated insulin injections include

- **Bruising.** Small, harmless bruises may occur at
  injection sites. You may be able to prevent them
  by applying pressure to the site immediately following injection. Or try pulling the skin taut at
  the site before injecting. These techniques discourage blood from spreading under the skin.

- **Insulin hypertrophy.** A small patch of excess fat
  may accumulate at frequently used injection
  sites. This is because insulin stimulates fat tissue
  growth. Rotating injection sites may help prevent this harmless side effect.

- **Lipoatrophy.** Fat tissue at frequently used injection sites may recede, or atrophy. There may be
  an indentation around the site, or some fibrous
  tissue. If an area is noticeably atrophied, insulin
  absorption from that site may be impeded.
  Another site should be used. Lipoatrophy is
  more common when animal-derived insulin is
  used. Using human analogue insulin at the
  affected site may help.

Skin conditions associated with diabetes that are not related to insulin injection

Here are some other skin conditions associated with
diabetes:

- **Necrobiosis lipodica diabeticorum (NLD).** This
  condition can occur early on in the course of
  diabetes, usually type 1, so it is not considered a
  long-term complication. NLD is a patch of vio-
  let- or purple-colored skin occurring on the
  shin, ankles, or feet. It typically ranges from

Bright Idea
To keep dry skin
moist, try these
lotions: Eucerin,
Alpha-Keri,
Carmol 2.0, or
DiabetiDerm. Ask
your pharmacist.

dime-sized to three or four inches across. It is painless and usually becomes less florid in color over time.

- **Acanthosis nigricans.** This is a darkening of the skin pigment around the neck, shoulders, underarms, under the breasts, and in the groin. The skin becomes "velvety" in appearance, and small skin "tags" may appear. It appears most commonly in people of African descent who have type 2 diabetes. It may be associated with a high level of insulin resistance (a cause of type 2 diabetes) and with polycystic ovaries syndrome.

Limited joint mobility

Watch Out!
Too many seams or detailing in the upper portion of a shoe (or in socks) can cause dangerous pressure points on your feet that may lead to foot ulcers.

Chronic high blood sugar may cause changes in muscle and tendon tissues, which become saturated with sugar over time (known as *glycation*). When these tissues are affected, or where there is nerve damage, muscle atrophy and tendon contractions may occur, along with thinning of bones and changes in skin around joints (so-called "waxy skin"). These processes usually affect the hands and feet. Deformities of the toes and feet may predispose the foot to pressure sores and ulcers. The tendons of the hand may thicken, contract, or become inflamed, causing pain and restricting the motion of the wrist and fingers. "Trigger fingers," or fingers "frozen" in a bent position, may result.

Limited joint mobility reflects chronic high blood sugar, and therefore may be a warning of the presence of other long-term complications such as vascular, kidney, or eye disease. Your doctor will examine your hands and feet for signs of stiffness or contracture.

Preventing and managing complications

No one with diabetes can take the threat of complications lightly. Gone are the days, however, when having diabetes was considered a grim and certain path to blindness or amputation. Today we know far more about preventing complications, treating them, and halting or slowing their progress.

The single most powerful factor in preventing long-term complications is excellent control of blood-sugar levels. High blood sugar defines the disease of diabetes and is at the heart of all its symptoms and complications. Any doubts or controversy on this matter were put to rest by the results of the Diabetes Control and Complications Trial (see the beginning of this chapter). Close behind blood-sugar control are the following significant prevention measures:

- **Controlling high blood pressure.** High blood pressure, or *hypertension*, strains the micro- and macrovascular systems, including the heart, blood vessels and tiny capillaries, and kidneys. In diabetes, hypertension may exacerbate retinopathy and nerve damage. The results of The United Kingdom Prospective Diabetes Study, described earlier in this chapter, demonstrate the importance of controlling high blood pressure.

- **Following your meal plan.** Eating with diabetes in mind is a healthy way for anyone to eat. There is no specific diabetic diet, but in general it is a low fat, low cholesterol diet high in fiber— in short, it is heart and kidney friendly, good for managing glucose levels, and keeps weight down. Keep in mind that excessive dietary protein puts a strain on your kidneys.

Bright Idea
High blood pressure increases your risk for developing complications. In 1997, a landmark study called "Dietary Approaches to Stop Hypertension" found that a diet high in vegetables and fruits, and low in total fat, can substantially lower blood pressure.

- **Quitting smoking.** This is essential. Not only does smoking seriously damage your lungs, it narrows the blood vessels throughout your body. As a diabetic, you must avoid anything that compromises your circulation. Smoking promotes cardiovascular disease, which can cause heart attack and stroke.

- **Regular exercise.** Regular aerobic exercise keeps your heart strong and your circulation toned, and it lowers glucose levels as well (more energy expended equals more glucose burned). There is also evidence that healthy muscle cells enhance insulin absorption or decrease insulin resistance. Remember that exercise must be balanced with eating and medication or insulin use in order to prevent low blood sugar.

- **Glycosylated hemoglobin test (also called the hemoglobin A1c test).** This test lets you know how well you're controlling your blood-sugar levels on average over time. Have the test two to four times per year, depending on whether you use insulin and your overall blood-sugar management. (See Chapter 5 for more details.)

- **Foot checks.** Check your feet every day for signs of fungal infection, skin cracks, redness, heat, coldness, swelling, numbness, or pressure sores. Never attempt to cut calluses or to correct ingrown toenails yourself; see a podiatrist or other foot specialist.

- **Regular medical exams.** These are crucial to prevention. See your doctor at least once every three months; have your bare feet examined at each visit and have a glycosylated hemoglobin test. Have your eyes examined at least once a year, more often if you are pregnant or if your last eye exam was abnormal. See your dentist every six months, and have a microalbumin test every six months to monitor kidney health. Have your cholesterol and triglycerides checked once a year.

A schedule, below, summarizes how often you should have specific medical examinations.

Diabetes Care Schedule

Every 3 months:
- Regular visit to your doctor
- Glycosylated hemoglobin test
- Bare feet examined by doctor

Every 6 months:
- Dental exam (all people with diabetes)
- Kidneys: Microalbumin test

Every year:
- Cholesterol/triglycerides (more often if your levels are abnormal or to check the effects of treatment for high levels)
- Eyes: Dilated pupil examination an ophthalmologist (more often if pregnant or if last exam abnormal)

Treating long-term complications

There is much you can do to lead a long and healthy life with diabetes. If complications develop—and, unfortunately, they may, despite good self-care—you and your health-care team have some options for treating them or for discouraging them from getting worse. Let's look at treatment possibilities for each major complication.

Treating cardiovascular complications

Standard dietary and exercise prescriptions are very beneficial, such as decreasing dietary fats and

Bright Idea
Use a moisturizing lotion on your feet every day (except between the toes) to prevent cracks in the skin.

getting regular aerobic exercise. These should be tailored to each individual. Losing excess weight is very beneficial in treating vascular disease and for lowering the risk for progression of the disease.

Controlling high blood pressure is very important in diabetes and in managing cardiovascular disease. Some medications prescribed for hypertension, however, should not be used by people who have diabetes, or should be taken in lower doses than those for nondiabetics. This is because some blood pressure medications can raise levels of glucose or blood fats, or can decrease sensitivity to low blood sugar.

At proper doses, thiazides, ACE inhibitors, alpha and beta blockers, and calcium channel blockers can be used to treat hypertension in diabetics. There is good evidence that ACE (*angiotensin-converting enzyme*) inhibitors may protect against kidney damage (see Chapter 16).

Medications to lower blood fats (cholesterol and triglycerides) can be used in managing cardiovascular disease. Generally, doctors will recommend the statin class of drugs. Recent studies have shown that these drugs can reduce the plaque that blocks vessels that supply blood to the wall of the heart. Nicotinic acid-based drugs may interfere with blood-sugar control.

Your doctor may prescribe low-dose aspirin treatment (81 to 325 milligrams daily), which can protect against heart attack by reducing blood platelet action (clotting). Regular exercise also helps to control cholesterol.

If necessary, surgery such as angioplasty or atherectomy may be performed to open blocked arteries or to provide alternative blood flow routes around severely blocked vessels (bypass surgery). In

recent years, laser techniques have made angioplasty a far less invasive surgery than it once was.
Experimental laser techniques and the use of small
fiberoptic scopes are now under research and may
also revolutionize bypass surgery.

Treating retinopathy

In the case of nonproliferative retinopathy, the recommended treatment is tighter blood-sugar control
to curb progression, as well as stopping cigarette
smoking and controlling high blood pressure. If the
nonproliferative symptoms become more severe,
laser surgery (*photocoagulation*) may be used to stem
the tiny hemorrhages occurring in the retina or to
correct macular edema. Laser treatment is also used
in some cases for treating full-fledged proliferative
retinopathy. It stops the bleeding from the retina as
well as the production of new blood vessels. Laser
treatment has been shown to reduce the risk of
severe visual impairment by about 60 percent.

If the retina is very damaged or detached,
surgery called *vitrectomy* may be indicated over photocoagulation. The retina is repaired, scar tissue
removed, and the clouded vitreous fluid in the eyeball is replaced with clear saline solution.

Treating nephropathy

As with cardiovascular complications, treating diabetic kidney damage may include controlling high
blood pressure, which can be treated by drugs (thiazides, alpha and beta blockers, calcium channel
blockers, and ACE inhibitors). There is evidence
that ACE inhibitors not only lower blood pressure
but may also act directly on the kidneys, protecting
them from damage. (See Chapter 16.) Indeed, the
current standard of care is to prescribe ACE

My diabetes edu-
cator really got
through to me
about the impor-
tance of glucose
control. One
thing I do every
so often is
review with him
my blood test
technique, to
make sure I'm
getting a good
sense of my
sugar levels.
—Peggy, age
thirty, with type
2 diabetes

inhibitor drugs as soon as microalbuminuria is detected.

Too much concentrated protein in the diet can seriously burden the kidneys. You may consider reducing or modifying your protein intake; consult your doctor or dietitian. You may also want to reduce salt intake, reduce your potassium intake, and increase your calcium intake. Calcium pills, as well as pills containing active Vitamin D, may be necessary if kidney disease progresses. (Healthy kidneys produce active Vitamin D.) Injections of a hormone called erythropoeitin may also be necessary. Normally, the kidneys produce this hormone, which causes the production of red blood cells.

If the kidneys begin to fail, there are only two treatment options: dialysis or a kidney transplant.

Treating neuropathy

As yet, we have no technique for reversing nerve damage. But if caught in time, diabetic neuropathy can be stopped or slowed by tightening blood-sugar control. The unpleasant symptoms of nerve damage can also be alleviated.

Unexpected treatments for neurological pain

The pain that often accompanies peripheral neuropathy may be relieved by taking the following:

- A tricyclic antidepressant such as *amitryptyline* (Elavil), *nortriptyline* (Pamelor), *desipramine* (Norpramin), or trazadone (Desyrel).

- The anti-epileptic drugs *phenytoin* (Dilantin), *carbamazapine* (Tegretol), and *gabapentin* (Neurontin).

- Drugs that control heart arrhythmia, such as *mexilontine* (Mexitil).

Less surprising treatments for neurological pain

Here are some more conventional treatments which may be used to treat the pain that often accompanies peripheral neuropathy.

- Aspirin and other standard analgesics may be used. (Painkillers that can be toxic to the kidneys must be avoided or taken in safe dosages.)

- A topically applied cream containing capsaicin, the chemical in peppers that makes them taste hot, can be used to relieve painful areas. It works by causing the nerves to deplete themselves of a chemical called *substance P,* which is necessary for the perception of pain. Capsaicin creams (such as Zostrix and ArthiCare) seem to be most effective on pain that is restricted to relatively small areas. They usually take three to four weeks to become effective and must be applied three to four times a day. Never use capsaicin creams on broken skin, and wash your hands after applying them. Avoid getting them into your eyes.

Other treatments for neurological pain

Finally, a few more treatments that can be explored:

- Electrical stimulation of painful nerve endings may be effective, such as TENS units (transcutaneous electrical nerve stimulation) or ESCS (electrical spinal cord stimulation). TENS appears to relieve pain by increasing blood flow to the affected nerves, while ESCS stimulates nerves in the spinal cord that inhibit pain signals. These treatments may be especially effective if combined with drug therapy.

- Acupuncture has been used to good effect by people suffering neuropathic pain. See Chapter 10 for more information on acupuncture.

Bright Idea
Relaxation training and guided imagery are two treatments for pain that some people find very effective. Talk to your doctor about finding a qualified practitioner, or contact the Academy for Guided Imagery, P.O. Box 2070, Mill Valley, California 94942, (415) 389-9324

Other troubling symptoms and their treatments

Diabetes may cause other symptoms such as impotence, stomach and intestinal complications, constipation, diarrhea, bladder problems, dizziness, and hypoglycemia unawareness. Here are some suggested treatments for each.

- **Impotence.** This may be treated with vasodilators injected into the penis or delivered by penile suppositories, inflatable implants, and the oral medication *sildenafil* (Viagra). Soon, an impotence medication that can be applied to the surface of the penis may be available. Your doctor should be sure that other medications, for example hypertension medications, are not causing or aggravating impotence. Sildenafil should not be used by men who have heart disease, especially men taking nitroglycerin products. See Chapter 12 for more information on impotence treatments.

- **Stomach and intestinal complications.** Gastroparesis can be managed by changes in eating habits, notably eating small, frequent meals or increasing soft and liquid foods. High fiber diets can aggravate gastroparesis, so sources and types of dietary fiber should be carefully selected or avoided. Medication such as *cisipride* or *metaclopramide* can treat gastroparesis. Insulin pumps (see Chapter 5) can be used to help slow the release of insulin when digestion is delayed.

- **Diabetic constipation.** This is treated with standard laxatives or stool softeners.

- **Diabetic diarrhea.** This can be treated with Lomotil. Occasionally, antibiotic treatment is in order, or treatment with *cholestyramine*, a drug that lowers cholesterol.

- **Bladder problems.** These can be treated with training in special bladder control exercises or through timed urination schedules. If necessary, self-catheterization can be used to empty the bladder. Drugs that decrease bladder spasm, or surgery to the bladder sphincter, can treat more advanced bladder neuropathy. There are also drugs to treat overly strong urges to urinate.

- **Dizziness or faintness upon standing (orthostatic hypotension).** This condition can be relieved by adjusting fluid and salt intake. Medicines that improve blood vessel constriction (*vasoconstrictors*) are helpful. These prevent pooling of blood in the legs. Doctors may also prescribe drugs that help the body to retain salt and water, keeping blood pressure adequately high.

- **Hypoglycemia unawareness.** This may improve if blood-sugar levels are purposely allowed to remain somewhat elevated for two weeks (under a doctor's supervision), then brought to normal levels again, a treatment that seems to resensitize the patient to the signs of low blood sugar. Some people who use insulin pumps discover that they become more sensitive to low blood sugar levels.

New treatments for diabetic neuropathy

Drugs called *advanced glycosylation endproduct (AGE) inhibitors* may stop or slow the bonding of glucose molecules to nerve axon cells. Similarly, *aldose-reductase inhibitors (ARIs)*, which block an enzyme that causes the accumulation of sugar by-products,

Watch Out!
On a day-to-day basis, we probably don't notice elevated blood-sugar levels. But if they persist over time, our hearts, kidneys, eyes, and nerves will notice.

may protect nerves if used early in the course of neuropathy. A drug called *memantine* may protect nerve cells from harmful inflammation; it awaits clinical trials. Scientists have isolated a nerve growth factor that is now being tested as a treatment for diabetic neuropathy.

Treating foot ulcers

The best "treatment" for foot ulcers is to prevent them. If you develop a stubborn foot ulcer, however, there are a number of treatment options. The most common treatments are

- Antibiotic therapy.
- Rest and elevation of the foot.
- *Debridement,* the removal of dead tissue from around the wound, promoting growth of healthy tissue.
- *Casting:* foot casts protect the ulcerated area and provide uniform pressure, which is beneficial to healing.
- *Vascular surgery* (if very poor circulation is slowing down healing) or, if foot deformities are causing pressure sores and ulceration, orthopedic surgery may be considered.
- *Skin grafting:* new techniques that use laboratory-cultured skin hold promise for treatment of chronic foot ulcers.
- *Topical gel treatment: becaplermin* (Regranex) has been developed with platelet-derived growth factor (PDGF), which stimulates new tissue growth in wounds that don't heal (providing there is adequate circulation to the area).
- *Hyperbaric pressure chambers,* like the ones used to treat sick scuba divers, have been used to treat

foot ulcers. The object is to promote healing by increasing oxygen flow to the wound. It is unclear how effective this treatment is.

Throughout this chapter the importance of good, consistent blood-sugar control has been stressed, whether the diagnosis is type 1 or type 2 diabetes. Proper blood-sugar management is your strongest weapon in the war on long-term complications. It is also important to remember, however, that early detection of problems is essential to slowing or even halting the progression of diabetes complications. Do your best, within reason, to keep your blood-sugar levels as normal as possible, and check in with your team on a regular basis to evaluate signs of problems.

Seven warning signs you must not ignore

The American Diabetes Association recommends that you see your doctor as soon as possible if you notice

- Blurred vision, spotty vision, or "floaters"
- Extreme fatigue that can't be explained
- Pain in the leg during movement
- Numbness or tingling in the hands or feet
- Chest pain during exertion
- Sores that don't heal
- Headaches that won't go away (which could signal high blood pressure)

Just the facts

- People with type 2 diabetes are at risk for long-term complications just as people with type 1 diabetes are.

Bright Idea
Many communities have clinics devoted entirely to treating diabetic or chronic wounds. Check with your doctor or local American Diabetes Association for one in your area.

- Keeping blood-sugar levels as close to normal as possible, as consistently as possible, is the best defense against the development and progression of complications.

- Diet, exercise, blood-pressure control, and not smoking are powerful preventive factors.

- Daily foot care is essential to the health of all diabetics.

- Complications are not inevitable and in most cases they can be prevented or treated.

The Balancing Act: Treating Diabetes

GET THE SCOOP ON...
Thinking like a pancreas ▪ Monitoring your
blood sugar ▪ Diabetic emergencies ▪
Identifying hypoglycemia ▪ The basics of insulin
therapy ▪ "Tight" glucose control

PART II

Managing Your Blood Glucose Levels: Type 1 Diabetes

Chapter 5

So how do you turn your brain into a happy, healthy pancreas? That's what the task of treating diabetes can feel like: You've got to train yourself to think like a pancreas, to be aware of and react to all the factors that can affect your blood-sugar levels, and to do what's necessary to keep those levels consistently within healthy ranges. It means trying to balance the amount of glucose in your blood with the amount of insulin available to deal with that glucose, whether you inject insulin or take medications to enhance the action of the insulin you produce.

Your long-term goal is to prevent or slow the development of complications like kidney disease, eye disease, heart disease, nerve damage, and foot ulcers. Your day-to-day goal is to keep blood sugar near a level that is your golden mean, and to avoid reaching levels that are too low or too high. Both hypoglycemia (low blood sugar) and hyperglycemia (high blood sugar) can cause serious acute complications.

High blood sugar is the defining symptom of diabetes, and testing for levels is a part of life for every person with diabetes. How frequently one tests one's glucose levels depends upon the diagnosis and the treatment plan agreed upon. In this chapter we'll take a look at different treatment regimens commonly used in treating type 1 and type 2 diabetes.

Acceptable blood-sugar levels

Watch Out!
Double-check your health-care insurance. What medical equipment is covered? What treatments, if any, are designated as experimental, and therefore not covered?

Just what are normal or acceptable blood-sugar levels? Levels in the person without diabetes will be within the range of 70 to 140 mg/dl throughout the day, showing peaks after meals, and averaging out to about 85 mg/dl (eighty-five milligrams of glucose in one deciliter of blood). In the person with well-controlled diabetes, levels can easily exceed 150 mg/dl following meals, and the average level may be around 130 mg/dl. Ideally, the fasting blood-sugar level in well-controlled diabetes is 120 mg/dl. In less well-controlled diabetes, blood-sugar levels may swing dramatically and abruptly from very low, 60 mg/dl, into the 200s or higher.

Most people with diabetes, especially type 1 diabetes, cannot expect to achieve perfectly normal, nondiabetic blood-sugar levels. Don't ask this of yourself; it's not realistic, and being "perfect" is not essential to managing your diabetes responsibly. Any reduction in high glucose levels is good! At the same time, the more consistently you keep your levels within the ranges you and your health-care team have decided upon, the better your chances of avoiding complications.

You're in charge

Diabetes is largely a self-managed disease. For this reason, it is very important that treatment goals be tailored to each person's diagnosis, lifestyle, age, overall health status, living situation, and personal motivation. Other factors include your history or pattern of low or high episodes and your degree of hypoglycemia awareness.

In your role as pancreas, you will balance

- When you eat and how many carbohydrates you eat, with

- Whether you have exercised or plan to exercise, along with

- When you had your last injection or pill, and

- When you will need to have another. You'll also consider

- When you will be eating again,

- Where you will be eating again, and

- How large a meal you will eat.

If you have the flu or problems with digestion, you'll have to be sure that blood-sugar levels don't fall too low, even if it's difficult to eat—and you'll stick to your normal insulin regimen. You'll be mindful of anything that may cause your glucose level to rise or fall, including where you are in your menstrual cycle, if you are a woman. You will keep your blood sugar stable by adjusting your diet, activity level, medications, or insulin injections accordingly.

Your greatest tool

In meeting this challenge, your strongest ally will be your own motivation to stay as healthy as possible.

66

I have a tendency to be kind of compulsive and want to do everything perfectly. At first I applied that to my diabetes care. Now, though, I'm not going for perfect sugar control; I'm going for better sugar control. I'm doing really well, and I'm a lot happier.
—Sarah, age twenty-seven, with type 1 diabetes

99

Next to this, your greatest tool is regular monitoring of blood glucose levels.

Your blood glucose levels tell the story: whether you are "high" or "low"; whether what you just ate had a big or small impact on your levels; the impact of exercise; whether you are taking enough insulin or medication; whether you're using the right type of insulin; and whether you are taking it frequently enough to maintain good control.

Diabetic emergencies, or acute complications

No matter what type of diabetes you have or what your treatment plan is, a primary goal of your treatment is to prevent the dangerous, potentially lethal medical emergencies that can develop when blood-sugar levels drop too low or shoot too high. It's essential to understand these conditions, and it's a good idea to keep them in mind while learning about blood-sugar control.

Hypoglycemia

Unofficially...
In the days before self-monitoring of blood was common, people with diabetes often didn't know if they were heading into a hypoglycemic episode until their blood sugar was so low that symptoms appeared. Today, frequent self-monitoring reduces the risk for hypoglycemia.

Hypoglycemia (sometimes called an *insulin reaction*) is low blood sugar. Your brain requires a constant supply of glucose in order to function properly. If blood sugar drops near or below 60 mg/dl, this is an emergency situation for the brain, and immediate action is necessary to raise the amount of blood glucose.

Low blood sugar is the most common acute complication of diabetes. A person with type 1 diabetes may experience as many as one or two mild hypoglycemic episodes per week. Mild hypoglycemia is defined as blood-sugar levels of 50 to 60 mg/dl. Moderate hypoglycemia refers to levels between 50 and 20 mg/dl, and severe hypoglycemia is 20 mg/dl or below. Keep in mind, however, that it is the type and severity of symptoms, not necessarily the blood-sugar level, that define the severity of hypoglycemia. Some people, especially young children or the elderly, may have severe hypoglycemia even when blood-sugar levels are not drastically low. Hypoglycemia must be treated by symptoms, not by numbers!

Hypoglycemia rarely progresses to the point of being fatal, but it is very unpleasant and can impair thinking, judgement, and motor functioning, putting you in a hazardous state.

Symptoms of hypoglycemia

As soon as the body senses that blood-sugar levels are dangerously low, it attempts to correct the situation by prompting the liver to break down the glycogen it has stored and release it as glucose. (The presence of this glucose in the blood is called the Somogyi effect.) In this emergency situation, the body uses adrenaline (or epinephrine) to signal the liver.

Adrenaline is one of our "fight or flight" hormones. The rush of adrenaline explains the typical initial symptoms of hypoglycemia:

- Rapid heartbeat
- Shakiness (for example, trembling hands)
- Sudden perspiration that may be profuse
- Feeling cold or clammy
- Hunger
- Anxiety, having a sense that something is wrong

If blood sugar continues to drop, the brain is further affected and symptoms of moderate hypoglycemia develop:

- Dizziness
- Mental confusion (fogginess, lightheadedness)

- Difficulty concentrating

- Headache

- Slurred speech

- Drowsiness or more extreme fatigue

- Clumsiness

- Emotional symptoms. Many people experience symptoms like irritability, sudden anger, or tearfulness, leading those close to them to feel that they are not acting like themselves. A person with hypoglycemia may seem distant, or become argumentative, even belligerent. He or she may insist that nothing is wrong and argue against or even physically resist taking treatment for the condition.

Bright Idea
Keep a "hypo-glycemia action plan" clearly posted in your home, so that roommates, family members, and guests can quickly refer to it. Personalize the instructions; for example, state what your emergency sugar source is and exactly where in the house to find it.

When hypoglycemia is life threatening

Severe hypoglycemia, in which the brain is starved for glucose, causes pronounced mental disorientation, and the person affected is not able to treat his condition. It must be treated immediately; if severe hypoglycemia goes untreated, it can lead to coma and death. But keep in mind that even moderate hypoglycemia can be life threatening, because mild disorientation or slowed reaction time can cause accidents, especially during driving or recreational activities.

Hypoglycemia can easily occur during sleep, when food intake has stopped and if the bedtime insulin or medication dose is too high. Low blood sugar can cause nightmares or profuse night sweats.

Causes of hypoglycemia

Common causes of hypoglycemia are

- Taking too much insulin.

- Eating too little food (due to illness or an eating disorder).

- Waiting too long to eat.

- Eating too few carbohydrates (the main source of glucose) or vomiting food.

- Getting too much exercise or unplanned exercise.

- "Tight" or intensive insulin therapy. (We discuss the different insulin regimens later in the chapter.)

- Drinking alcohol; alcohol interferes with the liver's normal response to low blood sugar, which is to break down glycogen and release it as glucose.

- Increased energy demands upon the body that use up more glucose (for example, pregnancy or recovering from major illness or surgery).

- Chronic liver or kidney disease.

- Newly diagnosed diabetics who have just started treatment may feel "low" when their blood-sugar levels first drop from very high to near-normal, but not low, levels.

All of these factors have a hypoglycemic (glucose-lowering) effect, which is why balancing of diet, exercise, insulin, and other factors is so important.

Hypoglycemia and insulin reactions

We should emphasize that the single most common cause of hypoglycemia is taking too much insulin. This is why hypoglycemia is often referred to as an *insulin reaction*. Think of it as insulin doing its job too well when there is not a lot of glucose in the blood. Different types of pharmaceutical insulin differ in how quickly they begin to work and how long it takes their action to peak. Using fast-acting insulin can increase the risk for hypoglycemia because its effectiveness may peak before digestion is complete and before larger amounts of glucose have been released into the blood. Slower-acting insulin can cause hypoglycemia if too large a dose is taken at night or food intake is inadequate during the peak in the insulin's action.

Other causes of hypoglycemia

Other causes of hypoglycemia are alcohol consumption and digestion problems, such as gastroparesis (discussed in Chapter 4). Alcohol suppresses the release of stored glucose from the liver. What's more, being in an altered state due to alcohol, marijuana, or other drug use can make you unaware of early hypoglycemia. Gastroparesis, or delayed emptying of the stomach, slows digestion, which in turn slows or halts the entry of glucose into the bloodstream.

Hormonal shifts can also affect blood-sugar levels; women may notice that their levels are more erratic during certain phases of their menstrual cycle. Progesterone tends to impede the action of insulin; progesterone levels rise in the second half of the menstrual cycle, after ovulation has occurred, then drop quickly when menstruation begins. Low blood sugar can occur if insulin doses are not adjusted to these cyclic changes.

Some people who have had type 1 diabetes for many years may have depleted stores of glucagon, the hormone that triggers the release of stored glucose when the blood-sugar level drops. These people have an increased risk for developing hypoglycemia.

Hypoglycemia and type 2 diabetes

People with type 2 diabetes who take insulin or certain oral medications for blood-sugar control are vulnerable to hypoglycemia (see Chapter 6).

Identifying mild, moderate, and severe hypoglycemia

You should know the signs of hypoglycemia, and how these change if it worsens. Again, hypoglycemia should be diagnosed and treated by its symptoms; the blood-sugar levels given are not absolute.

- **Mild hypoglycemia.** Blood sugar is 50 to 60 mg/dl. Symptoms are shakiness, nervousness, rapid heart beat, lightheadedness, and dizziness.

- **Moderate hypoglycemia.** Blood sugar is less than 50 mg/dl. Symptoms are lack of coordination, blurred vision, nausea, headache, profuse sweating, drowsiness, stubbornness, and confusion.

- **Severe hypoglycemia.** Blood sugar is 20 mg/dl or less. Symptoms are unconsciousness, possibly seizures.

Keep in mind that individuals may react differently to different blood-sugar levels. For instance, in a person with impaired circulation to the brain, a blood-sugar level of 60 to 70 mg/dl may cause symptoms of hypoglycemia, because the diminished blood supply means that less glucose reaches the brain.

Below is a summary of symptoms and treatment for mild, moderate, and severe hypoglycemia.

Treating hypoglycemia

You should treat hypoglycemia as soon as you notice symptoms. While symptoms are still mild, it's good to do a quick blood test if possible. Sometimes stress can have effects that feel similar to "going low." Testing your blood each time you suspect hypoglycemia will help you to identify genuine symptoms. If it is not possible to do a test, however,

Watch Out!
Are you a coffee drinker? Keep in mind that "coffee nerves" can feel like the symptoms of mild hypoglycemia. Don't confuse the two.

Recognizing and treating mild, moderate, and severe hypoglycemia:

Mild hypoglycemia
- shaking
- sweating
- hunger
- blood sugar 50 to 60 mg/dl

Self-treat with 10 to 15 grams carbohydrate:
- 4 to 6 oz. real fruit juice or non-diet soda
- 5 hard candies (except Precose users)
- 1 tablespoon honey
- ¼ cup raisins
- 2 to 4 glucose tablets

Follow in 15 minutes with protein and carbohydrate, such as 8 oz. milk with crackers or bread. Continue testing every half hour.

Moderate hypoglycemia
- headache
- fast heartbeat
- mood change
- blood sugar < 50 mg/dl

Assistance may be required. Take or give 20 to 30 grams carbohydrate:
- 8 glucose tablets
- 8 oz. real fruit juice or non-diet soda
- 2 small boxes of raisins

Follow in 15 minutes with protein and carbohydrate, such as 8 oz. milk with crackers or bread. Continue testing every half hour.

Severe hypoglycemia
- unresponsiveness
- unconsciousness
- convulsions
- blood sugar ≤ 30 mg/dl

Emergency measures are generally required, including injection of glucagon and calling 911. Severe hypoglycemia can result in seizures and coma if untreated.

Hypoglycemia must be recognized and treated. Learn to recognize the signs of hypoglycemia, and teach them to friends and relatives. Always keep a carbohydrate snack on hand to treat mild to moderate hypoglycemia.

Note that some people with diabetes do not feel or show symptoms of mild or moderate hypoglycemia. When in doubt, test your blood sugar.

do not hesitate to take steps to raise your blood-sugar levels.

As soon as you notice symptoms, you must get a good 10 to 15 grams of rapidly digestible carbohydrate into your body. This is the equivalent of:

- 4 to 6 ounces of fruit juice or non-diet soda
- 8 Lifesaver candies, 6 jelly beans, or 10 gumdrops
- 4 packets of granulated sugar or a tablespoon of honey
- ¼ cup dried fruit, such as 2 tablespoons of raisins
- 6 saltines
- 2 or 3 commercially prepared glucose tablets

If you have active insulin in your body at the time you first notice hypoglycemia (for example, from a recent shot of short-acting insulin or a morning shot of long-acting insulin), add a glass of milk to your carbohydrate dose. The glucose generated more slowly from the milk protein will ensure that your blood sugar stays at a normal level once it has risen, even though your insulin is peaking or active.

Sugary foods containing fat, like ice cream, rich pastries, or buttery frosting, are not good choices because fat slows the introduction of sugar into the bloodstream. Treating mild hypoglycemia calls for concentrated sugars that can be rapidly absorbed. Always carry an appropriate carbohydrate dose!

Hypoglycemia occurring at night can be treated with carbohydrate intake, followed by a snack containing carbohydrate and protein, like milk and crackers, to ensure steady blood-sugar levels into the morning.

Once the carbohydrate has been supplied, rest for fifteen or twenty minutes and check your blood-sugar level again. It should not be under 90 mg/dl. Notice the way you're feeling; have the uncomfortable symptoms subsided? You may need to eat your next meal right now, or have a second snack, one including some protein. Continue to rest until symptoms improve.

Moderate hypoglycemia is treated in the same way, but it may require additional portions of the carbohydrate given and it may take longer for the person affected to recover. If you are alone, let someone know what's happened and ask that person to check in with you later.

An important message for users of *acarbose* (precose) and *miglitol* (glyset)

If you take either of the oral diabetes medications *acarbose* (Precose) or *miglitol* (Glyset), some of the carbohydrates we list above for treating hypoglycemia will not work for you. These medications prevent certain sugars from being rapidly absorbed; that's how they help you keep your blood sugar down. But if you become hypoglycemic, you need your blood-sugar level to go up quickly, so you need to eat carbohydrates that can be rapidly absorbed even though you are taking acarbose or miglitol. For you, the correct carbohydrates for treating hypoglycemia are

- 3 to 4 glucose tablets
- 1 tube of glucose gel
- 1 tablespoon of honey
- ½ cup of real orange juice (not orange drink)
- ⅓ cup of real grape juice (not grape drink)
- 2 tablespoons of raisins

Loss of consciousness

The person suffering from severe hypoglycemia is unable to treat him- or herself and requires emergency assistance. This person will exhibit impaired consciousness, lack of consciousness, and inability to swallow. The first thing to do is to provide emergency care, then call for emergency medical assistance. Under these circumstances, it is dangerous to attempt to give carbohydrates orally, especially liquid, as the person may choke, vomit, or drown.

The best response is to give the person an injection of glucagon, the hormone that stimulates the liver to release glucose. The diabetic person should always have glucagon on hand, and people closest to that person should learn how to prepare and administer glucagon injections. (Emergency kits containing prepared syringes are available.) Keep the affected person's head elevated slightly while giving the injection, and turn it to the side in case the person vomits upon regaining consciousness.

See Appendix D for step-by-step instructions on how to prepare and administer an emergency glucagon injection.

If it is not possible to provide an injection of glucagon, carefully try to rub some honey, cake icing from a tube, or a commercial glucose preparation such as InstaGlucose inside the cheek or under the tongue of the affected person.

The severely hypoglycemic person will need medically supervised care to bring glucose levels back up and stabilize insulin levels. This may require intravenous delivery of insulin and even hospitalization.

Frequent episodes of hypoglycemia, or episodes that recur at certain times of the day, must be discussed with your physician. It may be necessary to change the timing, type, or amount of insulin or oral medication.

Hypoglycemia unawareness

In some people, the signals of hypoglycemia are dull or imperceptible. This can be due to nerve damage (neuropathy) affecting the autonomic nervous system caused by long-term diabetes, discussed in Chapter 4. A lack of definite symptoms, however, may not be caused by diabetic neuropathy. Some people simply may not have pronounced symptoms, especially if they have had repeated hypoglycemic episodes. Repeated "lows" can dull the alarm system in some people, even those who have not been diabetic for long. And repeated episodes of low blood sugar can deplete the pancreas of the hormone, glucagon, which signals the liver to respond to drops in blood sugar.

You must be aware of the possibility of slipping into lows with little or no warning. Frequent blood-sugar monitoring can help you to identify hypoglycemia unawareness. If you find that your level can drop below 60 to 55 mg/dl without triggering symptoms of hypoglycemia, you must discuss this with your health-care team as soon as possible. Your team may prescribe temporary changes in your daily blood-sugar goals, perhaps allowing them to remain a bit elevated, to try to re-sensitize the body to drops in glucose.

A final caveat

We've devoted a lot of space to the topic of hypoglycemia because it is such a common complication of diabetes, and also because even mild hypoglycemia poses risks to safety, if only the risk that it will rapidly progress if not promptly treated. This

Bright Idea
Blood glucose awareness training, or BGAT, is a recently developed technique that teaches people how to improve their awareness of hypoglycemia symptoms. Ask your doctor or diabetes educator about BGAT.

brings us to one final caveat: Do not make the mistake of over-treating hypoglycemia! Eating too much sugar all at once may cause glucose levels to soar.

Remember that during hypoglycemia, your liver breaks down glycogen and releases it as glucose into the blood stream—causing a rise in blood sugar, called the Somogyi effect. This, in combination with eating too much sugar, can cause rebound *hyper*-glycemia (high blood sugar). You may then give yourself too much insulin or take other steps to bring down your very high level, and presto, you're back at risk for hypoglycemia. It's understandable that the discomfort or anxiety of hypoglycemia may prompt you to gorge on sugars, but the best treatment for low blood sugar is to stick to the plan recommended by your health-care providers.

Keep checking your glucose level after eating your treatment carbohydrates. This is the best way to know whether your glucose is stabilizing as it should.

The dawn phenomenon

You may find that your blood sugar is high in the mornings. This can happen due to the *dawn phenomenon*, which is the daily early-morning release of the hormone *cortisol* and growth hormones. These hormones happen to have an adverse effect on insulin action, allowing blood-sugar levels to rise. Speak to your health-care team if you notice persistent high morning levels. You may need to eat less carbohydrate in the evening or at breakfast, or adjust your bedtime or pre-breakfast insulin dose. The dawn phenomenon may be more pronounced in people on an intensive insulin regimen or who use an insulin pump, but it is also easier to treat, by adjusting the insulin dose.

Diabetic ketoacidosis (DKA)

This complication is most likely to occur in people with type 1 diabetes. People with type 2 diabetes, even those on insulin, don't develop DKA because they produce at least some insulin of their own that offers protection against diabetic ketoacidosis.

DKA is a life threatening, emergency condition caused by sustained high blood-sugar levels of (typically) 250 mg/dl or more.

DKA is almost always caused by lack of insulin (as in undiagnosed type 1 diabetics) or by insufficient insulin treatment. Before the advent of pharmaceutical insulin in the 1920s, all people with type 1 diabetes eventually developed DKA, went into a coma, and died.

Insufficient insulin can result from

- Missed injections or failure of an insulin pump to deliver insulin.

- Use of expired insulin.

- An increase in the body's insulin requirements due to illness or infection.

Serious illnesses like pneumonia or heart attack can have these effects; when the body is under extreme physical stress, insulin activity may be overwhelmed by stress hormones like adrenaline. In any case, blood sugar accumulates to extremely high levels.

Why "ketoacidosis"?

With little or no insulin available to help absorb all this glucose into body cells, cells become starved for energy. In desperation, the body turns to its back-up energy source, stored fat. The burning of fat causes the production of ketones, acidic compounds that begin accumulating in the blood, making it dangerously acidic. This is ketoacidosis. The body attempts to correct this situation, as well as get rid of the excess blood sugar, by producing lots of urine. Dehydration, fatigue, and extreme thirst result.

Symptoms of DKA

Fatigue, excessive thirst, and excessive urination are the first signs of DKA, along with a blood-sugar reading of 250 mg/dl or higher. Other symptoms are nausea and vomiting. A more specific symptom is shortness of breath or panting, called *air hunger*. Another classic symptom is a sweet or fruity odor to the breath, reminiscent of Juicy Fruit gum, caused by the excess ketones.

Ketones and DKA

At the first sign of high blood sugar (240 mg/dl and above), you should do a urine test for elevated ketones. Urine samples are tested with chemically treated paper called *reagent strips*. (Make sure your strips have not expired.) Occasionally, some ketones are present in urine for other reasons, especially in the morning before breakfast, or if carbohydrate intake has been limited. But high levels of urinary ketones, when present with other signs of hyperglycemia or DKA, can signal the need for immediate medical treatment.

Treating DKA

DKA is entirely reversible if caught in time and if treated under medical supervision. Standard treatment consists of providing adequate insulin, replenishing fluids and electrolytes (especially potassium), and intravenous feeding if necessary. Treatment may or may not require hospitalization, depending upon the severity of the case (but DKA *always* requires prompt professional care)

Hyperglycemic hyperosmolar nonketotic syndrome (HHNS)

This condition is most commonly seen in older people with type 2 diabetes. It refers to grossly elevated blood-sugar levels of at least 600 mg/dl, but typically as high as 1,000 to 2,000 mg/dl. In people with little or no insulin production (type 1 diabetics), ketoacidosis will usually develop before glucose levels become this high. In type 2 diabetics, who typically produce at least some insulin, fat-burning and ketone accumulation are not as likely to spiral out of control, but blood sugars can still climb remarkably high.

When this happens, the body steps up urine production in an attempt to eliminate sugar, and severe dehydration develops. Less fluid combines with the huge amount of sugar in the blood to make the blood abnormally thick, a condition known as *serum hyperosmolality*. At this stage of dehydration, the person affected is vulnerable to mental confusion, loss of consciousness, and coma.

Some other medical conditions can predispose a person to, HHNS, for instance, kidney disease, heart attack, extensive burns, or acute infections. Some drugs and medical treatments can do the same, such as *hydrocortisone, prednisone,* beta blockers such as *propanolol* (Inderol), diuretics, *phenytoin* (Dilantin), beta blockers, and peritoneal dialysis. All these factors can markedly interfere with the body's fluid levels, the amount of glycogen released by the liver, and the action of insulin.

Treatment for HHNS must be done under medical supervision. It includes identifying and correcting any precipitating factors, thoroughly rehydrating the patient (via intravenous administration of liquids and potassium), and providing adequate insulin so that blood-sugar levels come back down.

You can prevent HHNS by regularly monitoring your glucose levels, letting your doctor know if your levels are very high or rising, drinking plenty of water, and being familiar with the potential side effects of any medication or treatment you use.

Treatment for type 1 diabetes: blood-sugar monitoring and insulin use

You now have a good sense of how and why the most common *serious* complications of diabetes occur. This should set the stage for recognizing the importance of regular self-monitoring of blood glucose and of balancing the other factors that affect glucose levels. As we've said, this balancing act is what diabetes treatment is all about.

Self-monitoring of blood glucose (SMBG)

The bottom line is that you will not be able to manage diabetes successfully without self-monitoring of blood glucose, or *SMBG*. SMBG is the window into the status of your diabetes management. Knowing your glucose level at a given time allows you to make vital adjustments in your meals, insulin use, and activity level. It is these adjustments, in concert with one another, that keep glucose stable (or that at least improve stability) and prevent the onset of both short-term and long-term complications. Remember that problems can begin brewing without any obvious signs. In particular, SMBG is your most reliable method for detecting hypoglycemia.

SMBG is especially important if you are taking three or more insulin injections daily, if you use an insulin pump, or if your blood sugar tends to be volatile. Regular monitoring is also one of the best ways to evaluate the effectiveness of your treatment

Bright Idea
Frequent blood-sugar testing can cause sore finger-tips. The Bayer Corporation has developed a lancing device that makes it easy for you to draw blood samples from other parts of your body, such as the outer thigh or edge of the palm. It's called the *Microlet Vaculance*. Ask you doctor or pharmacist, or call (800) 445-5901 for more information.

plan. By consistently knowing what your levels are, you know what changes are needed and what changes are helping. You have a real basis on which to establish or modify personal treatment goals. Blood-sugar readings can translate into specific action.

How often should you test? Your doctor will make this recommendation. Standard recommendations are discussed later in this chapter.

How blood glucose monitoring is performed

At one time, blood sugar was measured by urine tests. Urine tests are poor indicators of actual blood-sugar fluctuations, because glucose appears in the urine only after it has already reached harmfully high levels, at least 180 mg/dl. Moreover, urine tests can show only what was happening in the body several hours ago, not what is happening right now. It won't catch an imminent emergency.

During the 1970s, self-administered tests using blood were developed. The early technology involved chemically treated paper strips and color charts. Blood was dropped onto the strip, causing a chemical reaction. The resulting color was checked against the chart to "read" the glucose level. Problems arose when the strip colors did not exactly match chart colors, forcing the tester to estimate his or her glucose level. And visually impaired or color-blind people could not easily use this method.

The glucose meter

Today, SMBG is performed with a palm-sized, computerized blood glucose meter. Using a specially designed, spring-loaded lancet device, a small drop of blood is taken from a finger. Usually, the drop is applied to a paper strip and the strip is inserted into the meter for reading. Some of the newer meters need only tiny amounts of blood on the strips. With most glucose meters, the strip is inserted first, and the drop of blood is placed on an exposed section of the strip. The blood is then absorbed through the strip into the meter. The meter reads the level of glucose in the blood, and then the level is digitally displayed. (For people with visual impairment, large-type meters and meters that speak the reading are available.)

Blood glucose meters are generally very trustworthy when used properly and maintained according to manufacturer directions. Most are designed to be accurate within 10 percent of the level that the most accurate laboratory test would find. Meter readings for extremely low (below 50 mg/dl) or extremely high (above 400 mg/dl) glucose levels are much less accurate. The paper strips can vary by batch, affecting results. You may want only to use strips supplied by the meter manufacturer and follow the instructions for coding the meter for each new batch of strips.

Many meters automatically store test results, as many as 300 readings. They may also compute averages over specified time periods. It is a good idea, however, to keep a written log, or a computer file, of your SMBG readings. It's easier to track patterns by eyeballing your log. Your glucose meter manufacturer may even sell computer software that enables you to download stored information from your glucose meter to your computer, giving you many options for logging and tracking glucose levels over time on the computer.

These glucose data management programs range in price from $60 to $215. Three companies that produce them are: Medlife, Inc.,

Moneysaver
Although list prices for glucose meters range from about $50 to $100, you should actually pay much less for your meter. Meter manufacturers routinely offer discounts, rebates, and trade-in deals because they make most of their money selling blood test strips. Always compare prices (for both meters and strips) at mail-order or other pharmacies before purchasing a meter.

(888) 656-5656, Boehringer Mannheim Corp., (800) 858-8072, and MetaMedix Inc., (800) 455-4105). You may also be able to download a free data management program from the *Children with Diabetes* Web site, www.childrenwithdiabetes.org. If you own a PalmPilot and want to use it to keep track of glucose readings, call (817) 461-3480, or visit www.tweak.org to order the $20 GlucoPilot.

Consumer Reports glucose meter ratings

The esteemed consumer advocacy publication *Consumer Reports* most recently rated glucose meters in October of 1996. As of this writing, Consumers Union (which publishes *Consumer Reports*) hasn't scheduled its next review of glucose meters.

For your convenience, we provide here the 1996 *Consumer Report* ranking of glucose meters, listed in order of highest overall score. Many factors influence your choice of glucose meter, such as cost, ease of operation, size of memory, and availability of computer software accessories. Keep in mind that a high overall score from *Consumer Reports* does not necessarily mean a particular glucose meter is the best one for you.

1. Glucometer Elite
2. Lifescan One Touch Profile
3. Accu-Chek Advantage
4. Lifescan One Touch Basic
5. Accu-Chek Easy
6. MediSense Precision QID
7. Glucometer Encore
8. Accu-Chek III

For a copy of the entire 1996 *Consumer Reports* article, or to find out if a new review is planned, call (914) 378-2740.

The American Diabetes Association magazine, *Diabetes Forecast*, publishes a Buyer's Guide each fall. Although the Buyer's Guide does not rate meters, it is an excellent source of consumer information on glucose meters.

Another excellent source for current information on meters is the *Blood Glucose Meters* page on the Web site www.childrenwithdiabetes.org. We also want to mention several of the newest glucose meters on the market:

- The Accu-Chek Complete from Roche Diagnostics. This meter uses a new test strip called the Comfort Curve, which requires much smaller drops than traditional strips. The Accu-Chek Complete also is available with an excellent computer software accessory program.

- The Accu-Chek Voicemate, which "speaks" the glucose reading for those who have visual impairment.

- The Fast Take meter from Lifescan, which also features new, smaller test strips that use much smaller blood drops.

Other blood-sugar tests

SMBG measures the daily, even hourly, ups and downs of blood sugar. It is equally important to test the quality of glucose management over larger periods of time. Two tests that are done at your doctor's office or a medical laboratory accomplish this:

Bright Idea
Look for creams designed especially to soothe sore fingers. One brand to try is Can-Am Care's Formula for Fingers.

■ **The glycosylated hemoglobin test (also known as the hemoglobin A1c or the glycated hemoglobin test).** Glucose molecules normally stick to the hemoglobin in red blood cells. If high levels of glucose persist over time, hemoglobin becomes saturated with glucose, that is, the hemoglobin becomes glycosylated. A test for glycosylated hemoglobin, performed every three months, will give you a bird's-eye view of your average glucose level of the preceding six to ten weeks. This is especially important to know if you've been performing fewer SMBG tests.

The test result is given as a percentage on a scale of four to thirteen. Each percentage corresponds to an average daily glucose level. For instance, a 10 percent glycosylated hemoglobin result corresponds to an average daily glucose level of 250 mg/dl. Scores of 8 percent to 9 percent are usually cause for concern. For people with diabetes, scores of 7 percent and below are considered excellent. These scores usually correspond with well-controlled diabetes, measured in part by consistent fasting glucose levels of 120 mg/dl. In non-diabetics, the usual reading is about 5 percent.

Regular blood glucose monitoring gives important information that's used to make needed changes in medicine, food, and exercise. But regular glucose testing may not give you and your doctor an accurate picture of your overall diabetes control. A different test is used for that: the glycosylated hemoglobin test, or Hemoglobin A (often written as HbA).

The figures on the next page illustrate the test's findings.

Timesaver
A home fructosamine test called "Glucoprotein" was approved by the U.S. Food and Drug Administration in 1997. Your diabetes management team can talk with you about whether this is an appropriate adjunct to your SMBG.

■ **The fructosamine test, which is similar to
the glycosylated hemoglobin test** (No, it has
nothing to do with fruit sugar!) It, too, checks
the degree of glycosylation, but not in hemoglobin; it targets other blood proteins, primarily
albumin. The other difference is that the
fructosamine test measures overall changes in
glucose level over a period of two to three
weeks, as opposed to several months. This
means that the effects of changes in your treatment plan can be quickly assessed. Another
time when quick assessments may be important
is during pregnancy.

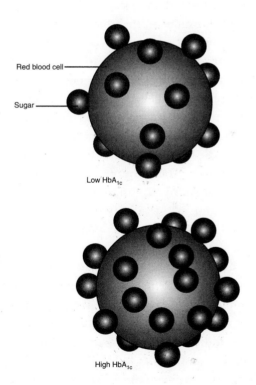

Red blood cell

Sugar

Low HbA$_{1c}$

High HbA$_{1c}$

← Note!
Sugar (small
balls) sticks to
the red blood
cells in the blood
(large balls). The
accumulation of
sugar damages
body tissues. The
more sugar there
is in the blood,
the more damage
occurs. The
amount of sugar
stuck to the red
blood cells can
be found with
the glycosylated
hemoglobin test,
which shows the
average blood
sugar level over
the last 3
months.

Insulin use: the basics

The goal of insulin use is to mimic the action of the pancreas, which normally puts out a *continuous baseline* amount of insulin, fortified by *bursts of additional insulin* at any time during the day that glucose levels rise.

Ideally, then, your insulin treatment must serve two purposes: to provide a steady, continuous baseline (or *basal*) amount of insulin throughout the day, and also to provide bursts (or *boluses*) of insulin whenever blood sugar rises, namely, following meals.

Medical science has developed rapid-acting, short-acting, intermediate-acting, and long-acting pharmaceutical insulins so that diabetics can generally predict the peaks and plateaus of insulin activity, corresponding to the basal rate and boluses secreted by the normal pancreas. They can also decide how frequently they want to inject insulin.

More frequent shots equal tighter glucose control and greater similarity to normal pancreatic functioning. The healthy pancreas is a master of quick adjustments. You cannot adjust quickly to changes in insulin needs using only long-acting insulin and one shot a day. On that plan, you're locked into living around one peak in insulin activity.

This is not to say that any particular regimen is the best one for you. Only you and your physician can determine that. Our point here is to explain the underlying rationale of insulin treatment programs.

Before continuing, it's important to note that while insulin is classified as faster- or slower-acting, determining the action times of insulin is not an exact science. Actual rates of absorption can differ not only among individuals, but often within the

Watch Out!
Glucose meter readings can drift into inaccuracy. To test for this, you must use a control solution in your meter once a month. It contains a standardized amount of glucose, and will tell you if your meter is giving readings that are too high or low. Call the manufacturer's 800 number if this is a problem.

same person on a given day, by roughly 20 to 40 percent. This is another reason why consistent SMBG is so important; unfortunately, people with diabetes can't take insulin patterns for granted.

Types of insulin

Pharmaceutical insulin comes from three sources:

- It may be extracted from the harvested pancreases of cattle;

- It may be extracted from the harvested pancreases of pigs; or

- It may be synthetic human insulin, created by recombinant DNA techniques in which genetic material that produces human insulin is inserted into rapidly multiplying bacteria.

Insulin from animal sources is becoming less widely used, and soon may no longer be available. Although highly purified, animal insulin is more likely to cause allergic reactions or antibodies to insulin, especially if beef preparations are used. Animal insulin is also more expensive. Nowadays, synthetic human insulin is more commonly used and, thanks to genetic engineering, it is available in abundance. In general, synthetic human insulin (or just "human insulin") is usually more quickly absorbed than animal insulin. This may or may not be desirable, depending on your body's unique responses to insulin and your treatment plan.

Insulin preparations also differ as to

- The rate of onset, or time elapsed before they are effective, that is, able to lower glucose levels;

- The amount of time before peak effectiveness is reached;

- The duration of maximum effectiveness; and

- The total duration of effectiveness.

Moneysaver
There are many order-by-telephone companies that deal exclusively with diabetes supplies, including insulin. They offer competitive prices and the convenience of mail-order delivery to your home. Check American Diabetes Association magazines, like *Forecast*, or the ADA's Web site, www.diabetes.org.

Based on these characteristics, all insulin, regardless of its source, is made to be rapid-acting, shortacting, intermediate-acting, or long-acting. Each person has a somewhat different response to insulin; only SMBG can tell you how a particular insulin acts in your body.

Insulin type	Onset (hours) effective	Peak (hours) duration	Usual maximum (hours)	Usual duration (hours)
Short acting				
Human Lispro	Within 15 minutes	1 to 1 ½	4 to 5	4 to 5
Human Regular	0.5 to 1.0	2 to 3	3 to 6	5 to 7
Intermediate acting				
Human NPH	2 to 4	4 to 10	10 to 16	14 to 18
Human Lente	3 to 4	4 to 12	12 to 18	16 to 20
Long acting				
Human Ultralente	6 to 10	14 to 24	18 to 20	20 to 36

Short-acting insulin

There are two types of short-acting insulin, *Regular* and *lispro* (Humalog), a newer, faster-acting insulin. (Lispro is sometimes classified separately as rapid-acting insulin.)

- **Lispro insulin.** This new synthetic human insulin is very short-acting. It is effective by about fifteen to thirty minutes, peaks in one to two hours, and may be effective for three to four hours.

   Lispro insulin becomes effective almost as quickly as natural insulin does. This means it improves the accuracy of timing insulin with eating. It also allows for rapid adjustment to eating a larger than usual amount of carbohydrates, allowing greater flexibility and glucose control. Because it peaks quickly, it may reduce the risk of hypoglycemia (although it may increase that risk in a diabetic whose stomach empties slowly, or who has eaten too few carbohydrates).

■ **Regular insulin.** Regular insulin is effective by thirty minutes to one hour, peaks in two to four hours, and is effective for six to eight hours. Regular insulin is available in human and pork preparation form.

Intermediate-acting insulin

There are two types of intermediate-acting insulin: *NPH* and *Lente*. Both are cloudy preparations because substances have been added to slow down the insulin's action (a fish protein substance, *protamine*, is added to NPH, while zinc is added to Lente).

■ **NPH** is effective by one to four hours, peaks in four to ten hours, is effective for ten to sixteen hours, and may be effective for fourteen to eighteen hours. The graph on page 143 shows the action of NPH and Lente insulin (one figure is used because the action of these two insulins is very similar; Lente's peak is flatter, less pronounced, than NPH's).

■ **Lente** (Novolin L, Humulin L) is effective by two to four hours, peaks in four to ten hours, is effective for twelve to sixteen hours, and may be effective for sixteen to twenty hours. Novolin L may peak later and last slightly longer than Humulin L. Your physician can suggest the best one for you.

Note! ➔
Lispro insulin is
an insulin ana-
log. It has a very
rapid onset of
action—about
15 minutes. It
peaks in 1 hour
and lasts about 3
hours in the
body. Lispro
insulin should be
taken right
before a meal.

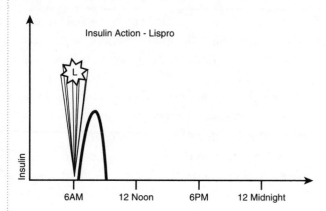

Note! ➔
Regular insulin is
referred to as a
short-acting
(clear) insulin
because it lasts
only about 5 to
6 hours. It starts
working about
45 minutes to an
hour after injec-
tion and peaks
in about 2 hours.
Regular insulin is
usually taken 30
to 45 minutes
before a meal.

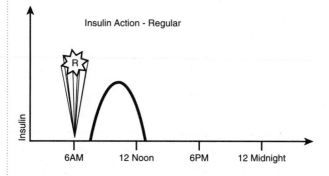

Long-acting insulin (also called *ultralente* insulin)

Ultralente insulin is effective in four to six hours, reaches peak effectiveness in fourteen to twenty-four hours, and is usually effective for twenty-four to thirty-six hours. The action time of Ultralente is slow and sustained, so no sharp peak in activity occurs, that is, its action pattern is flatter.

Like NPH and Lente insulin, Ultralente is cloudy because of an additive (zinc) that slows down its action time. The graph on page 144 shows the action of Ultralente insulin.

Mixing insulins

It is very common to mix Regular or lispro (short-acting or rapid-acting) with NPH or Lente

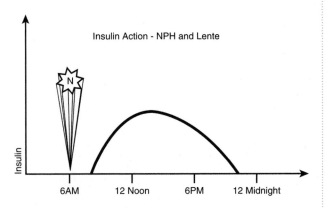

Insulin Action - NPH and Lente

← Note!
NPH and Lente
are intermediate-
acting insulins.
They generally
start working
about 1 to 3
hours after injec-
tion, peak at
about 8 hours,
and last about
20 hours. Both
NPH and Lente
insulins are
cloudy, not clear,
due to additives
(protamine and
zinc, respec-
tively) that slow
down the
insulin's action.
Lente's onset of
action is almost
identical to
NPH's, but
slightly slower
and with a less
pronounced peak.

(intermediate-acting) insulin in order to combine an immediate bolus effect with an extended baseline effect. This is a common pre-breakfast injection. The Regular or lispro insulin covers breakfast, while the NPH or Lente provides coverage through lunch. Typically, the mix is 70 percent intermediate-acting and 30 percent short-acting; 50/50 mixes are also used. Both mixes are available in premixed preparations, or you may be trained to mix insulins yourself. Longer-acting insulin is usually not mixed with Regular because it can alter the absorption of Regular insulin, with unpredictable results. If these two insulins are used at the same time, they are usually injected separately. Never mix insulins without the recommendation and knowledge of your doctor. You may develop your own "designer" mix of insulins, with your doctor's help.

See Appendix D for step-by-step instructions for mixing insulins. The most important instruction is that the clear and faster-acting insulin must always go into the syringe before the slower-acting, cloudy insulin.

All of the insulin types are manufactured by several companies under various trade names. Your

Note! →
Ultralente insulin is the longest-lasting insulin available. It starts working about 2 to 4 hours after injection, peaks at about 16 hours and lasts about 32 to 36 hours. Ultralente insulin contains more zinc than Lente insulin, which slows down its action time and makes it appear cloudy, not clear.

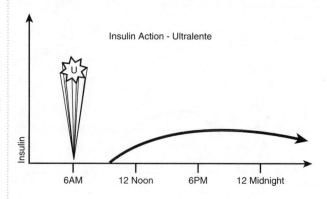

doctor can recommend the best brands for you. Table 5.1 summarizes the brands of insulin sold in the United States.

Insulin strength

In the United States, most insulin is packaged in 100 units per milliliter of fluid, or U-100 strength. A U-500 strength is available for people with severe insulin resistance who have very high glucose levels.

Syringes are made to accommodate U-100 and U-500 insulin. Using the wrong syringe could mean mismeasuring your dose, so be sure to use the right syringe. Insulin strengths in Europe and elsewhere may be different, typically U-40. You'll need to keep this in mind while traveling abroad. See the discussion of travel in Chapter 8.

Handling insulin

Unopened insulin bottles should be kept in the refrigerator. Do not expose insulin to temperatures below 36°F or above 86°F. An opened bottle can be kept at moderate room temperatures, away from direct sunlight, for as long as a month. If you find it takes you longer than that to use a bottle, keep it refrigerated. A few types of mixed insulin have a much shorter life span because of the action of one

TABLE 5.1 INSULINS SOLD IN THE UNITED STATES

Product	Manufacturer	Strength
Rapid-acting (onset < 15 min; usual duration 3 to 5 hours)		
Human analog		
Humalog (insulin lispro)†	Lilly	U-100
Short-acting (usual onset 0.5 to 2.0 hours; usual duration 4 to 6 hours)		
Human		
Humulin R (regular)*†	Lilly	U-100
Novolin R (regular)*†	Novo Nordisk	U-100
Velosulin human (regular, buffered)	Novo Nordisk	U-100
Pork		
Iletin II R (regular)	Lilly	U-100, U-500
Purified pork R (regular)	Novo Nordisk	U-100
Intermediate-acting (usual onset 3 to 6 hours; usual duration 12 to 20 hours)		
Human		
Humulin L (lente)	Lilly	U-100
Humulin N (NPH)*†	Lilly	U-100
Novolin L (lente)	Novo Nordisk	U-100
Novolin N (NPH)*†	Novo Nordisk	U-100
Pork		
Iletin II L (lente)	Lilly	U-100
Iletin II N (NPH)	Lilly	U-100
Purified pork L (lente)	Novo Nordisk	U-100
Purified pork N (NPH)	Novo Nordisk	U-100
Long-acting (usual onset 4 to 6 hours; usual duration 18 to 24 hours)		
Human		
Humulin U (ultralente)	Lilly	U-100
Premixed combinations		
Human		
Humulin 50/50 (50% NPH, 50% regular)	Lilly	U-100
Humulin 70/30 (70% NPH, 30% regular)*†	Lilly	U-100
Novolin 70/30 (70% NPH, 30% regular)*†	Novo Nordisk	U-100

* Indicates availability in cartridges for pens, in addition to vials.
† Indicates availability in "prefilled" disposable pens, in addition to cartridges and vials.

insulin upon the other. Be sure you know the life span of the insulin you use and follow the manufacturer's instructions for handling.

Unopened insulin can be stored in the refrigerator until its expiration date. Opened bottles can be stored in the refrigerator for three months and should then be discarded. Opened bottles can be kept at room temperature for one month; then discard any unused insulin. Don't handle insulin roughly; this may encourage clumping.

Insulin appearance

Don't use insulin that looks strange. Regular and lispro insulin are clear. NPH, Lente, and Ultralente are cloudy, but they should be uniformly cloudy when gently shaken or swirled. There should be no clumps or chunks of material, no change of color, and no crystals.

Insulin that looks strange may be faulty, but it's possible you have been storing or handling it improperly. Your pharmacist should be able to clarify this for you.

- Look at your insulin carefully before you use it. Don't use insulin that doesn't look right.

- Regular insulin should be clear and have no color. Do not use Regular or lispro insulin if it looks cloudy, thickened, even slightly colored, or if it has any solid particles in it.

- All other insulins should have an even, cloudy appearance after gentle shaking—they look a lot like skim milk.

Do not use NPH, Lente, 70/30, 50/50, or Ultralente insulins if

- Insulin stays at the bottom of the bottle after gentle shaking.

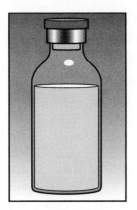

Correct appearance of insulins. All insulins (except Regular) should look uniformly cloudy after gentle shaking.

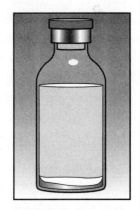

Insulin at the bottom of the bottle. Do not use if insulin stays at the bottom of the bottle after gentle shaking.

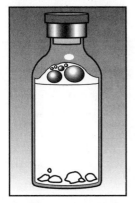

Clumps of insulin. Do not use if there are clumps of insulin in the liquid or on the bottom after gentle shaking.

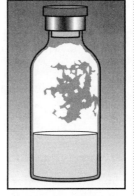

Bottle appears frosted. Do not use if particles of insulin on the bottom or sides of the bottle give the bottle a frosted appearance.

- There are clumps of insulin in the liquid or on the bottom after gentle shaking.

- Solid particles of insulin stick to the bottom or sides of the bottle after gentle shaking. This makes the bottle look "frosted" on the inside.

If your insulin doesn't look right, don't use it. Take it back to your pharmacy.

Injecting insulin: basic principles

Insulin must be injected into fat tissue that is *subcutaneous*, or just below the skin. Muscle tissue should be avoided. Good body sites for subcutaneous injections are the abdomen (except close to the navel), the buttocks, the upper/outer thighs, and the upper underarms.

See Appendix D for step-by-step instructions for preparing and administering an insulin injection.

As stated previously, insulin is most quickly and evenly absorbed from the abdomen. In general, it's best to choose one body area consistently, then rotate sites within that area. Keep injection sites several inches apart, and avoid moles or scars, which can interfere with absorption.

Following the abdomen, absorption is fastest from the upper arms, then the thighs, and finally the buttocks. You may want to take advantage of the different absorption rates at different times, for instance, injecting in the buttock before bedtime, for slower overnight absorption.

Note that absorption will be more rapid if muscles near an injection site are vigorously exercised, for example, the thigh or buttock muscles. Body warmth can also affect absorption, by dilating veins and increasing circulation—after a hot shower, for instance. You'll need to keep these influences in

Watch Out!
To avoid injury to household members and trash handlers, you *must* properly dispose of syringes, needles, and lancets (called *sharps*). Please see "Instructions for Safe Sharps Disposal" in Appendix D.

Front

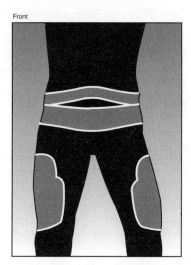

Back

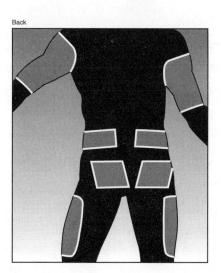

← Note!
These figures show the most appropriate areas for insulin shots. Remember to rotate sites within each area, as described on the following page, to prevent overuse of one site. No one site should be used too often. If you are pregnant, you may wish to avoid some of the abdominal sites. Ask your doctor.

Rotating Sites

Here are some tips for healthy injection site rotation:

- Use all the sites in one area before changing to another. For example, use all the sites in both arms before moving to your thighs. This will help keep your blood sugar more even from day to day.
- If you take more than one shot each day, use a different area for each shot. For example, you might give your morning shot in your abdomen and your evening shot in your thigh.
- Starting in a corner of an area, move down or across the injection sites in order. This will make it easier to remember where you gave your last shot.
- When you've used all the sites in an area, move to another.

Insulin enters the blood:

- Fastest from the abdomen (stomach).
- A little slower from the upper arms.
- Even more slowly from the thighs. (Exercise can speed up insulin entry from the thighs.)
- Most slowly from the buttocks.

At times, you may want to choose an injection site based on how quickly or slowly insulin is absorbed from it. For example, when you'll be eating very soon after a shot, you could use a site on your abdomen, so that the insulin will be more quickly available.

mind as you balance your insulin needs with eating and exercise.

Aids to injection

Fortunately, the technology of self-injection has greatly improved over time. Today, needles are microfine and lubricated, allowing for virtually painless injections. Devices are now available that make injections easier or eliminate the need for syringes:

- **Automatic injectors** insert the needle painlessly without your having to see it. Some are designed to inject the insulin for you as well, so that you do not operate the syringe plunger.

- **Infusers** are special small catheters that are inserted into an injection site and remain for several days, reducing the number of times the skin must be pierced. Insulin is delivered through the catheter into the injection opening. Care must be taken that infections do not develop.

- **Jet injectors** are a needle-free delivery device. A high-pressure "shot" of insulin passes through the skin. They are easy to use, but they may cause bruising and they must be disassembled for frequent, thorough cleansing. Jet injectors are also expensive.

- **Insulin pens** replace multiple syringes holding different doses. The pen holds a needle and a cartridge containing 150 units of your pre-scribed insulin. When you need an injection, you set the pen for the correct insulin dose. The pen makes a clicking sound as you set the dose, which may help visually impaired people to set the right amount. The pen also eliminates the need to draw insulin from a jar into a syringe.

- **On the horizon?** Injections may soon become a thing of the past. The first large scale clinical trials of a powdered, inhaled form of insulin began in the fall of 1998. Preliminary results proved highly successful. Insulin pills may also become available. Ask your doctor or the American Diabetes Association about the status of these innovations.

A few words about the insulin pump (or CSII, Continuous Subcutaneous Insulin Infusion)

The insulin pump is a computerized device, about the size of a beeper, that can be attached to your

Timesaver
Ask your pharma-cist about pen-sized cases for carrying pre-filled syringes. These will enable you to avoid carrying insulin vials or measur-ing out doses away from home.

belt, a nearby pocket, a garter, or other clothing. It is filled with a one- or two-day supply of short-acting insulin—Regular (Velosulin Buffered Human) or human lispro. The pump is programmed to provide a steady basal supply of insulin around the clock, delivered through a flexible plastic tube attached to a needle inserted under the skin of the abdomen.

When you know that you will need more insulin in your bloodstream—say, within twenty minutes of eating dinner—you activate the pump to release a bolus in the amount you deem appropriate (based on your blood-sugar level, meal size, and so forth). Some pumps allow you to control the timing of the bolus delivery.

The insulin pump combines basal flow of tiny amounts of short-acting insulin with boluses of short-acting insulin, supplied just as the body needs them. And the basal dose can be programmed to vary at different times throughout the day. For these reasons, the pump more or less closely mimics normal insulin secretion.

Insulin pumps include failsafe features such as alarms for low battery, clogged tube, empty reservoir, and "runaway" (overdose) insulin delivery. The pump can be easily detached from the insertion tube for activities like showering, swimming, or lovemaking (you can also purchase a waterproof pump cover for swimming or bathing). Usually, it can safely remain detached for an hour or two, although that depends upon how active you are while it's off, whether or not you eat, and anything else that affects blood-sugar levels.

The insulin pump is a wonderful device, but it is not for everyone. To begin with, CSII is a form of intensive insulin treatment, which has certain

Unofficially...
Most people who use an insulin pump find that their total daily dose of insulin is 50 to 75 percent less than their prior total dose on an injection regimen. The pump is able to deliver smaller amounts of insulin than is possible using syringes.

advantages and disadvantages, as discussed below. Intensive insulin treatment means better glucose control and potentially reduced risks for complications, but it also demands frequent glucose monitoring.

What's more, insulin pumps are expensive. Pumps and their equipment currently cost about $5,000, although your health insurance may cover part or all of this cost. (Remember that your insurance company will need a letter from your physician attesting to your medical need for the pump.) Maintenance can cost up to $300 per month.

It takes time and commitment to learn how to use and care for the pump. You'll need special instruction in how to use it. You may use a training pump filled with saline solution for several days while you continue to take insulin injections, allowing you to become familiar with pump operation. Once you begin to use insulin with the pump, you will need intensive follow-up appointments to make sure that the insulin delivery rates are correctly adjusted.

You must also become skilled at counting the carbohydrates in meals in order to give yourself the correct dose of insulin. Infections can occur at the insertion site, and the tubing kinks can interfere with insulin delivery and trigger the clogged-tube alarm. If insulin flow-rate is very low, it may not get through the tubing into your body. This could cause a rapid rise in blood sugar, as there will be no stored subcutaneous insulin in your body.

We've just told you some of the problems that can come with using the insulin pump. The fact is, however, that insulin pumps are beginning to grow in popularity, and we predict a steady rise in the

> 66
> The insulin shots were dictating my life. I had to take them at certain times of the day, I had to eat my meals at certain times of the day. Now, I can eat three hours later if I want to. I have more freedom with the pump.
> —Nicole Johnson, Miss America 1999, with type 1 diabetes
> 99

number of people who use insulin pumps. The advantages of using the insulin pump are

- Needle-free insulin delivery.

- If used properly, the pump can help you achieve excellent glucose control and near-normal glucose levels, which will decrease your risk for developing chronic complications.

- Many people can use less insulin with the pump, because it can dispense smaller (but still effective) amounts than syringes can. Also, as glucose levels become near-normal, the body's sensitivity to insulin is increased, so that smaller amounts of insulin may be effective (although you may need slightly more insulin in the early morning hours, due to the dawn phenomenon).

- Because the pump uses only short-acting or rapid-acting insulin, insulin use is timed to meals, not vice versa, so meal and exercise schedules are very flexible as well.

- Many people who use the pump have improved awareness of symptoms of hypoglycemia.

- Because the pump can help you to achieve excellent glucose control, it may be a good choice for women who are pregnant or planning to become pregnant.

If you think the insulin pump might be right for you, talk it over with your doctor and consider it carefully before making a decision.

Injection and glucose monitoring schedules

How often you perform SMBG is closely associated with how often you inject insulin. Most people increase the frequency of injections (or begin insulin pump therapy) because they want to achieve

Bright Idea
Today, the leading manufacturer of insulin pumps is MiniMed, Inc. of Sylmar, California. For information about MiniMed insulin pumps, call (800) 933-3322, or visit the company's Web site at www.minimed.com. Another manufacturer is Disetronics Medical Systems at(800) 688-4578, www.disetronics.com.

better, tighter glucose control. Frequent monitoring is an essential tool in achieving this goal.

Without SMBG, one can't fine-tune the factors affecting blood sugar. SMBG should be performed about thirty to forty-five minutes prior to eating, because you may need to adjust the timing of your injection based on your level. If your levels are somewhat high, around 180 mg/dl or higher, you need to inject immediately so that the insulin can begin to bring down blood sugar before you eat. If you are somewhat low, say 40 to 70 mg/dl, you should wait before you inject, so that your blood sugar does not continue to drop before you eat. If levels are normal, 70 to 120, you give your pre-meal insulin its standard time to become effective (thirty minutes for Regular and fifteen minutes or less for human lispro). If your blood sugar is very low, you may need to treat this before taking insulin. Most people who are trying to achieve "tight" blood-sugar control also test their blood-sugar level one to two hours after eating.

Many people choose to self-inject three or more times a day not only to achieve better blood-sugar control, but because it gives them greater freedom to make changes in when they eat, how much they eat, and when they exercise. Combining intermediate or long-acting insulin with "booster" shots of short- or rapid-acting insulin allows you to tailor the amount of insulin to fit your choices and timeframe. The longer-acting insulin provides background coverage, and you use shorter-acting insulin on a per-meal basis, as needed. This gives you control over insulin peaks.

Timesaver
If you are ordering diabetes supplies over the phone for the first time, have your insurance information at hand, and place your order at least several weeks before you will need supplies. The company will need to verify your insurance coverage before it can fill your order, and this may take some time.

Standard insulin and SMBG regimens

An insulin injection plan and glucose monitoring form the foundation of your daily treatment. Here are some standard recommended schedules:

- **One shot daily.** Such a plan is almost never recommended for people with type 1 diabetes because it does not provide enough insulin, nor enough bursts of insulin, to control glucose levels. It may be used in cases where the patient is very resistant to insulin therapy. It may be prescribed temporarily during the "honeymoon phase" (see Chapter 3). Some people with type 2 diabetes may take one insulin shot daily in conjunction with oral medication to improve blood-sugar control.

- **Two shots daily.** This schedule can be done in two ways, the *split* and the *split/mixed* schedules:

  The split schedule consists of two shots daily of intermediate-acting insulin, providing two peaks of insulin activity. The first injection is taken about thirty to forty-five minutes before breakfast and usually contains a larger portion of the total daily insulin dose (often 70 percent). The second shot is taken about thirty to forty-five minutes before dinner. On this schedule, SMBG is performed at least twice a day, before each shot, and perhaps before lunch or bedtime, to adjust snacking or meals if necessary.

  The *split/mixed schedule* consists of two shots daily in which short or rapid-acting and intermediate-acting insulin are mixed together(typically Regular or lispro and NPH). Thirty to forty-five minutes before breakfast, a shot containing both intermediate- and short or

Unofficially...
The National Aeronautic and Space Administration has teamed up with the Juvenile Diabetes Foundation to find noninvasive ways to take blood samples from astronauts in space. One goal is to develop needleless insulin. Insulin crystals grown in 1994 in the Space Shuttle are providing new insights that may show the way.

rapid-acting insulin, usually in a two-to-one or 70%/30% NPH/Regular or lispro ratio, is administered. The Regular or lispro insulin is quickly available for breakfast, and the intermediate insulin peaks after lunchtime. Similarly, the second mixed shot, taken before dinner, covers dinner and the nighttime period. (See Appendix D for important pointers on mixing insulin.)

The split/mixed approach provides better, more natural insulin coverage than the split approach, and it can be adjusted to personal needs by changing the insulin ratios, for example, increasing Regular insulin if you anticipate a larger meal, or if your blood sugar is high before a meal.

The split-mixed plan usually requires SMBG forty-five minutes before each meal—three tests per day, and another if exercise is performed or the meal plan changes.

A disadvantage of twice-daily regimens is that insulin from the second shot may peak during the night, causing nocturnal hypoglycemia and related problems. If this occurs, your physician can recommend adjustments.

■ **Three shots daily.** (Note: injection plans consisting of three or more shots a day are sometimes referred to as *Multiple Daily Injection regimens,* or *MDI.*) Ideally, this regimen gives you increased control over blood glucose levels, because you are providing short- or rapid-acting insulin on an as-needed basis, combined with baseline coverage from longer-acting insulin. Typically, this plan would consist of a mixed Regular or lispro/NPH morning injection, a

Regular or lispro shot before eating dinner, and an injection of NPH or Lente before bed. An alternative is to take one mixed Regular or lispro and Ultralente shot before breakfast, and one Regular or lispro shot before lunch and before supper. The Ultralente coverage should last through the day and night.

SMBG should be performed before each meal and at bedtime, with additional tests if there are changes in activity level or meals.

Watch Out!
Not all doctors have experience in working with patients on intensive insulin regimens. Make sure that your doctor has the necessary experience and is comfortable with starting you on intensive treatment.

Intensive or "tight" insulin treatment

Like other regimens, intensive insulin treatment provides basal insulin in the form of one or two injections of long- or intermediate-acting insulin, usually before breakfast, before bed, or at both times. What is different in intensive insulin regimens is that you inject short- or rapid-acting insulin three times daily, before each meal, bringing the total daily number of injections up to four or five. Such a regimen allows you to choose when to eat: Since an injection accompanies each meal, you can time your meals according to your preferences (providing your blood-sugar level is not too low, in which case you'll need to eat something right away). You won't be tied to eating only when your morning or noon injection of intermediate-acting insulin is peaking.

The insulin pump, or CSII, is also a form of intensive treatment.

The goal of intensive treatment is to mimic more closely the normal pancreas (by supplying an insulin bolus for each meal), and, ideally, to achieve near-normal blood-sugar levels throughout the day. Another goal is to increase flexibility as to meal times.

It is essential to perform SMBG frequently on intensive regimens. Your total daily dose of insulin may be higher, so you must be vigilant against hypoglycemia. (The insulin pump usually requires less insulin.) As your glucose levels are brought to stable, near-normal levels, smaller changes in glucose levels become more significant, so it's easier to go "too high" or "too low." The margin for error is narrower. People on intensive treatment do SMBG at the usual times, as well as an hour or so after each meal, especially if they have just begun this regimen. And, of course, any changes in food intake or activity call for monitoring as well, in order to keep control fine-tuned.

The Diabetes Control and Complications Trial demonstrated that tight glucose control significantly lowers the risk of developing the serious complications of diabetes. But intensive treatment is not everybody's cup of tea. You must be motivated and willing to learn how to adjust your insulin dose in response to SMBG results. You must also learn to calculate the effects of the carbohydrate contents of your meals on your glucose levels. This goes beyond simply limiting carbohydrate intake; it means tracking your body's response to different types and portions of carbohydrates. Finally, be aware that healthier blood-sugar control can sometimes cause you to gain weight, as your body makes more efficient use of calories you ingest. On the other hand, some people lose weight if their insulin dose is lowered.

If you are frustrated by ongoing swings in your levels despite your best efforts, if you have any signs of complications, if you want more flexibility in your schedule, or if you are pregnant or want to become pregnant, then intensive therapy may be the right approach for you. Never attempt to institute such a program without your doctor's help. You must be medically evaluated and properly educated before embarking upon intensive diabetes management.

Balancing food and exercise with your insulin treatment

Ideally, understanding the role and use of insulin allows you to eat so that you do not exceed the limits of your regimen's insulin effectiveness. You need to factor in exercise as well, because it can affect your glucose levels for as long as twenty-four hours afterwards.

Food and insulin

The basic principle is that there must be enough active insulin in your blood when glucose is released into the bloodstream following digestion of food. Conversely, there must not be too much insulin, or hypoglycemia may result.

The presence of active insulin is affected by

- **The timing of your last insulin shot.** When did it or how soon will it become effective?

- **Your glucose level at the time of injection.** Was it high? Low? Fine?

- **How much food you ate at a given time.** Did you eat more than you planned? Less than you planned? Will the meal result in more glucose than your active insulin can handle?

- **How rich in carbohydrates the food was.** Again, will it result in too much glucose?

Your meal plan will be designed to accommodate your tastes as much as possible within the pattern of insulin activity provided by your injection plan.

There is no one-step, surefire method for balancing food intake with insulin use. The best course is to stick to your meal plan as consistently as possible while performing SMBG. Over time, SMBG results will help you to see the relationship between specific foods and your blood-sugar levels. You'll then be freer to make healthy changes and avoid unhealthy mistakes.

Exercise and insulin

As with eating, there is no one right way to balance exercise with insulin use. Exercise lowers blood sugar, but to different degrees in different people. It will probably take some time to determine exactly how exercise affects your blood-sugar control. At first, you may want to commit to a fixed exercise schedule with fixed levels of intensity—for example, three twenty-minute walking sessions per week, following the same route each time, for six weeks. That way you can monitor yourself before and after exercise to get a general sense of how much it lowers your glucose levels, and how long after exercise you see this effect. (Again, effects can last for as long as twenty-four hours afterwards.) Only then can you adjust pre- or post-exercise insulin and meals accordingly, for example, lowering your bedtime dose of insulin if you exercise in the late afternoon, or eating a bigger bedtime snack so that you don't experience nocturnal hypoglycemia.

See Chapters 8 and 9 for detailed information on nutrition and exercise.

"Sick days": managing diabetes when you are ill

Illness stresses your body, and stress hormones inhibit the effectiveness of insulin. If you are ill, your glucose levels may rise significantly. It's very important to stick to your usual insulin injection schedule even if you are experiencing nausea,

66

Not long after I started intensive therapy, I got a fierce case of the flu. I was pretty confused about how to handle it, because nothing stayed down. Later, I sat down with my diabetes educator, and we wrote up a sick-day plan. I'm all set for next time.
—Patricia, age thirty-two, with type 1 diabetes

99

Bright Idea
Ask your doctor to prescribe an antinausea medication that is available as a rectal suppository instead of a pill or liquid. This is useful if you can't keep anything down when you are ill.

vomiting, or lack of appetite. It's also very important to monitor your glucose levels closely, probably about every four hours, and to check your urine for ketones if your blood-sugar level is higher than 240 mg/dl.

Be in touch with your health-care team if you are ill. If you have been vomiting or have diarrhea, they may recommend that you begin checking your urine for ketones, a sign of DKA. They can also suggest ways to stay nourished and hydrated while you're ill, so that you can maintain blood-sugar balance as you continue with your insulin treatment. You should have an agreement with your doctor as to what changes in glucose levels, if any, call for changes in your insulin dose. You may want to keep some antinausea medication on hand; your doctor can prescribe some. Do not take any over-the-counter medications that have not been approved by your doctor.

A sick-day plan can help keep your blood sugar (glucose) under control when you have fever, vomiting, nausea, diarrhea, coughing or head congestion.

Below are some important guidelines for coping with sick days.

Sick Days for People with Diabetes

A plan for medicine
Always check with your health care team before you change your medicine in any way. It is usually recommended not to stop taking your diabetes pills or insulin when ill, but if you are taking Precose (acarbose), Glyset (miglitol), or Prandin (Repaglinide) and are too sick to eat, do not take Precose, Glyset, or Prandin. Ask your doctor for a prescription for anti-nausea medication before you get sick.

A plan for monitoring
It is recommended that you test and record your blood sugar every 2 to 4 hours. If your blood sugar is over 240 mg/dl, check your urine for ketones.

A plan for food

If you can't eat your usual meal plan, have 1 serving of food containing 15 grams of carbohydrate every hour while awake. This will help keep your blood sugar from going too low.

Each of these foods and liquids contains 15 grams of carbohydrate:

1 cup chicken soup

½ cup apple juice

1 cup cream soup, made with water

½ cup ginger ale (not diet)

½ cup grape juice

½ cup vanilla ice cream

½ cup orange juice

½ cup Coka-Cola (not diet)

½ cup regular Jell-O

½ cup cranberry juice

½ cup cooked cereal

1 cup Gatorade

A plan for liquids

Drinking liquids is very important, especially if you are losing fluids due to fever, vomiting, or diarrhea. Let your blood sugar be your guide to choosing liquids. If your blood sugar is over 240 mg/dl, drink calorie-free liquids, such as water, broth or bouillon, sugar-free/caffeine-free soda or decaffeinated tea that won't raise your blood sugar. If your blood sugar is low, drink calorie liquids, such as regular soda, milk or fruit juices.

Call your health team if

■ You've been sick for two days and aren't getting better.

■ You've been throwing up or have had diarrhea for more than six hours.

■ Your blood sugar stays over 240 mg/dl.

■ You have ketones in your urine.

■ You have chest pain, trouble breathing, breath that smells fruity, or dry, cracked lips.

■ You aren't sure what to do.

Just the facts

- Successful diabetes management means balancing insulin injections with glucose readings, meal times, food choices, and physical activity.

- Self-monitoring of blood glucose (SMBG) is an essential tool in managing blood-sugar levels.

- Glucose lows and highs, if uncontrolled, lead to diabetic emergencies (such as hypoglycemia and DKA) that can be life threatening.

- It's possible to become hypoglycemic with no awareness of having symptoms.

- Most insulin treatment regimens seek to provide a baseline supply of insulin throughout the day, combined with additional insulin with meals.

- You have choices about how intensive your treatment will be and how closely you will comply with your treatment program.

GET THE SCOOP ON...
Weight loss and glucose control ▪ Whether
insulin in pill form exists ▪
Diabetes pills and when they are prescribed ▪
Insulin injections and type 2 diabetes ▪ When
to monitor your blood sugar

Managing Your Blood Glucose Levels: Type 2 Diabetes

ype 1 and type 2 diabetes differ in some important ways, but the ultimate goals of treatment are the same for both: to achieve good control of blood-sugar levels and to prevent the development of long-term complications. And type 2 diabetes, like type 1, is mostly a self-managed disease. You're in charge of treating your high blood sugar.

How are healthy, stable glucose levels achieved in type 2 diabetes? As with type 1 diabetes, nutrition and exercise are an important feature of treatment, and so is self-monitoring of blood glucose, or SMBG. A person with type 2 diabetes may even inject insulin; about 30 percent of type 2 diabetics do. There are, however, significant differences in how the two forms of diabetes are treated. This chapter will focus on the unique aspects of successful management of type 2 diabetes.

Chapter 6

165

Unofficially...
If you're a woman with type 2 diabetes, you're more vulnerable to developing vaginal yeast infections. Did you know that eating yogurt can help prevent yeast infections? A study printed in the November/December 1996 issue of the *Archives of Family Medicine* reports this finding. Yogurt provides calcium, too!

Medical treatment of type 2 diabetes

For the first ten to fifteen years or so of their illness, the majority of people with type 2 diabetes produce often normal amounts of natural insulin, or more. The problem is that their bodies do not use that insulin effectively; most people with type 2 diabetes are insulin resistant. Because of insulin resistance, the pancreases of many type 2 diabetics produce excess insulin for years (to compensate for the resistance) before developing obvious symptoms of diabetes. Sometimes diabetes occurs because insulin production finally starts decreasing and blood-sugar levels rise. (See Chapter 2 for more information on this characteristic of type 2 disease.) Treatment, then, focuses on treating insulin resistance as well as adjusting other factors affecting blood sugar.

Remember also that type 2 diabetes is most common in middle-aged, overweight people, and that people with type 2 diabetes with these characteristics are at increased risk for high blood pressure, high cholesterol, and cardiovascular disease. These factors also affect the way treatment is carried out.

The treatment methods most commonly recommended for managing type 2 diabetes are

- Diet modification for weight loss.

- Exercise for weight loss, cardiovascular conditioning, and to improve insulin sensitivity.

- Use of one or several oral medications that increase insulin output or that enhance insulin's effects (by decreasing or delaying the absorption of glucose from the gut; by decreasing the liver's breakdown of glycogen to glucose; or by decreasing insulin resistance).

- Use of SMBG.

- Use of insulin injections.

One factor influencing your treatment approach is the severity of your fasting glucose levels. Is your diabetes mild to moderate? This is defined as fasting glucose levels of 126 to 140 mg/dl. Making some changes in diet and exercise may be all that is necessary to improve your levels. More severe diabetes is indicated by fasting levels of 141 mg/dl to 180 and above. Medication may be prescribed along with diet and exercise.

These are not hard and fast rules. Your doctor will make the decision as to what course to try first.

Diet, exercise, and weight loss

About 80 to 90 percent of people with type 2 diabetes are overweight. Since larger body mass increases insulin resistance, and also increases the risk for heart disease, the first approach to managing type 2 diabetes is usually to begin a weight loss program. Don't despair—a loss of as few as eight pounds can significantly improve glucose levels. Again, weight loss brought about by changes in diet and exercise may be the only treatment you need to bring your blood-sugar levels down into a healthy range. Exercise can increase insulin's effectiveness even if there is no reduction in body size.

In the 10 to 20 percent of people with type 2 diabetes who are not obese, controlling the amount of carbohydrate in the diet may be sufficient, as may distributing carbohydrate intake more evenly throughout the day. Simple and refined carbohydrates have the greatest impact on glucose levels since they are quickly converted to glucose. Setting and adhering to daily carbohydrate goals is part of every person with diabetes treatment plan.

There is no single diet prescription for type 2 diabetes; each plan must be tailored to the

Watch Out!
Insulin resistance can increase if blood sugars stay high for too long. This is called glucotoxicity.

individual in question. (We discuss the principles of healthy eating for people with diabetes in Chapter 8, and we review the use of exercise in Chapter 9.)

"Diabetes pills": treatment by oral medication

The use of oral medications to control blood-sugar levels distinguishes treatment for type 2 diabetes from treatment for type 1. Let's be clear on one point before continuing: Oral diabetes medications are not oral insulin or insulin in pill form. Oral medications are a separate category of drugs and they do not replace insulin or insulin injections. Furthermore, there is as yet no form of insulin that can be taken orally. Stomach acids destroy insulin, so it cannot be swallowed. (Soon, however, oral insulin and insulin that is inhaled may be available.)

Insulin injections, and insulin injections only, supply that hormone to people whose pancreases produce insignificant amounts of insulin or none at all. Oral diabetes medications have different functions, as we shall see below.

Table 6.1, below, summarizes the oral diabetes medications.

TABLE 6.1   ORAL DIABETES MEDICATIONS

Generic name	Brand name	Usually taken	Action usually lasts
Tolbutamide	Orinase	2 or 3 times/day	6 to 12 hours
Chlorpro-pamide	Diabinese	Once a day	Up to 60 hours
Tolazamide	Tolinase	1 or 2 times/day	12 to 24 hours
Acetohexamide	Dymelor	1 or 2 times/day	12 to 24 hours
Glipizide	Glucotrol	1 or 2 times/day	12 to 24 hours

	Glucotrol XL	Varies	Up to 24 hours
Glyburide	Diabeta	1 or 2 times/day	16 to 24 hours
	Micronase	1 or 2 times/day	12 to 24 hours
	Glynase PresTab	Varies	
Glimepiride	Amaryl	Once a day	Up to 24 hours
Repaglinide	Prandin	3 times/day, before each meal	3 hours
Metformin	Glucophage	2 or 3 times/day	4 to 8 hours
Troglitazone	Rezulin	Once a day, with meal	Up to 24 hours
Acarbose	Precose	3 times/day, with meals	4 hours
Miglitol	Glyset	3 times/day, with meals	4 hours

When will your doctor consider oral medication? Again, there are no hard and fast rules. In general, though, these drugs are prescribed if

- Lifestyle changes (diet and exercise) have not brought blood sugar under control.

- You have had diabetes for less than ten years.

- Your fasting glucose levels remain high (126 mg/dl or above before breakfast, 160 mg/dl or above before bed).

- Your glycosylated hemoglobin is over 8 percent. (The glycosylated hemoglobin test is described below and in Chapter 5.)

Most oral medications are metabolized by the liver and excreted by the kidneys. If you have kidney or liver disease, your doctor may not recommend these medications for you. They must not be taken by pregnant or nursing women.

Two classes of oral diabetes medications

Oral medications that treat high blood sugar in people with type 2 diabetes come in two classes or groups. The first is the older drugs, the mainstays of type 2 treatment, called *sulfonylureas*. Sulfonylureas were discovered during World War II, when a French army doctor noticed that some soldiers given the then-new sulfa antibiotics showed symptoms of very low blood sugar. The second group of drugs, which has been developed and has come to prominence within the last five years, has no single name but consists of four medications: *repaglinide, acarbose, metformin,* and *troglitizone.*

The sulfonylureas

These drugs act by binding to beta cells in the pancreas and stimulating them to secrete more insulin. Sulfonylureas have no effect in persons with very few or no active beta cells, which can be the case in advanced type 2 diabetes. Sulfonylureas generally cannot be used by people with advanced kidney disease. The oldest of these drugs—the first-generation sulfonylureas—are *tolbutamide* (Orinase), *chlorpropamide* (Diabinese), *acetohexamide* (Dymelor) and *tolazamide* (Tolinase). Newer, second-generation sulfonylureas are *glizipide* (Glucotrol), extended-release glizipide (Glucotrol XL), *glyburide* (DiaBeta, Micronase, Glynase), and *glimeperide* (Amaryl).

All sulfonylureas are very effective in lowering glucose levels, especially when first given to patients. The older sulfonylureas are quite vulnerable to drug interactions and typically need to be taken frequently, or in high doses. The newer sulfonylureas are not likely to interact with other drugs and can be taken in lower doses. Extended-release glizipide, for example, is taken only once a day.

Since sulfonylureas are a type of sulfa drug, they may cause an allergic reaction in sulfa-sensitive people. Make sure your doctor knows if you have a sulfa allergy. Symptoms of an allergic reaction include hives, extensive or whole-body rash, wheezing, or difficulty breathing (an emergency situation).

Normally, however, sulfonylureas do not cause side effects. Some people may experience nausea, vomiting, a mild rash, or itching when first taking these medications, as well as flushing if alcohol is consumed.

Certain prescription medications, such as some sulfa antibiotics, can increase the effect of sulfonylureas. If you are taking a sulfonylurea medication and one of these medications, you may be at increased risk for hypoglycemia. Table 6.2 lists these medications.

TABLE 6.2 PRESCRIPTION DRUGS THAT INCREASE THE EFFECTS OF SULFONYLUREA MEDICATIONS

Combining any of these drugs with sulfonylureas may increase your risk for hypoglycemia:

Generic Name	Trade Name(s)
Sulfacytine	Renoquid
Sulfadiazine	Microsulfon
Sulfamethoxazole	Azo Gantanol, Bactrim Gantanol, Septra, Uroback
Sulfamethizole	Thiosulfil, Proklar, Urobiotic
Sulfisoxazole	Azo Gantrisin, Eryzole Gantrisin, Pediazole, SK-Soxazole
Chloramphenicol	Chloromycetin
Bishydroxycoumarin	Dicumarol
Phenylbutazone	Butazolidin
Oxyphenbutazone	Tandearil
Clofibrate	Atromid-S

Hypoglycemia (low blood sugar)

The main risk involved in taking sulfonylureas and other oral medication is the increased chance for hypoglycemia, due to the medications' effectiveness in lowering blood-sugar levels. (Refer to Chapter 5 for detailed information on the symptoms of and treatment for hypoglycemia.)

Newer oral medications

With the exception of one medication, called *repaglinide,* these new drugs work not by stimulating the pancreas to produce more insulin, but by helping the body to use insulin effectively. Unlike the sulfonylureas, these medications are not as likely to cause hypoglycemia. They can safely be used only by people whose pancreases still secrete some insulin, including newly diagnosed diabetics with mild to moderate diabetes.

The newer oral drugs are

▪ **Repaglinide (Prandin).** Repaglinide was approved by the Food and Drug Administration in
April 1998, and is the newest of the new oral
medications for type 2 diabetes. Repaglinide is
not a sulfonylurea, but it works similarly to the
sulfonylureas in that it stimulates the beta cells
in the pancreas to release insulin. Unlike other
oral diabetes medications, repaglinide works
very quickly, so it can be taken with meals or up
to thirty minutes before. It can be used by people who have some deterioration of their kidney
function.

Side effects of repaglinide are usually mild
and are similar to those of the sulfonylureas:
Nausea, minor weight gain, mild rash or itching,
and flushing if alcohol is consumed. Repaglinide can cause hypoglycemia, although this is

less common than with sulfonylurea use. It must be taken with meals. If you miss a meal you should not take a dose of repaglinide.

■ **Acarbose (Precose).** This medication works in the intestine, where it slows the absorption of dietary carbohydrates. This makes the post-meal rise in blood sugar slower and less dramatic. Since the post-meal rise in glucose contributes to elevated glycosylated hemoglobin, Acarbose use may reduce the risks of long-term complications of diabetes. Acarbose may cause intestinal discomfort and flatulence, by causing carbohydrates to linger and ferment in the intestinal tract. This is less likely to occur if initial doses are kept low, then slowly raised as tolerance is gauged. Acarbose should not be used by people with serious intestinal or liver disease.

■ **Miglitol (Glyset).** This medication, just introduced, is in the same family as acarbose (the alpha-glucosidase inhibitors) and works similarly, by slowing the breakdown and absorption of carbohydrates from the intestine. As with acarbose, the primary side effect is flatulence. Miglitol is not safe for use by people with kidney damage.

■ **Metformin (Glucophage).** This drug's action in the body is not completely understood. It seems to lower blood-sugar levels indirectly, by influencing the liver not to break down and release glycogen (stored glucose) so that less glucose enters the bloodstream. Use of Metformin at higher doses also appears to slightly increase muscle tissue's sensitivity to insulin, thus decreasing insulin resistance.

Unofficially...
Although sulfonylureas work by stimulating the pancreas to release insulin, they may have an indirect effect on insulin resistance as well. Research suggests that improved blood-sugar control lowers insulin resistance. Lower insulin resistance is an important result of sulfonylurea treatment.

The main side effect of metformin is gastrointestinal disturbance such as nausea or diarrhea. It may also cause mild weight loss—a less unpleasant effect! Metformin can lower blood lipids (cholesterol and triglycerides), another beneficial effect. It is usually not prescribed for people with significant kidney, liver, or heart disease, in whom it can increase the risk for a serious complication called *lactic acidosis* of the blood. Metformin should not be used by people who abuse alcohol. And metformin treatment must be temporarily stopped if you are having a medical procedure that requires the use of intravenous contrast dye.

The use of metformin as a means to prevent diabetes is being studied in people with impaired glucose tolerance, and in women who have a condition called polycystic ovary syndrome, which often includes insulin resistance.

■ **Troglitazone (Rezulin).** This oral medication was introduced in 1996. It acts directly on muscle and fat cells to enhance the effect of insulin inside these cells (known as a *post-receptor* effect). Troglitazone reduces insulin resistance, the fundamental culprit in type 2 diabetes. It is a powerful new addition to the anti-diabetes arsenal. By increasing insulin's action, it may allow some people who do take insulin to lower their daily dose.

The main side effects noted so far in the use of this drug are fluid retention and weight gain. If you have heart or liver disease, your doctor may not prescribe troglitazone or may modify your dose. The drug has not yet been studied in people who have serious (class 3 or 4) heart disease. If you have serious heart disease, your doctor may not prescribe troglitazone, or may modify your dose. If you begin taking troglitazone, you will need to have a monthly liver function test for eight months and periodic testing afterwards. It takes several weeks for troglitazone to take effect, during which time your doctor may prescribe insulin or another medication.

Watch Out!
In women with type 2 diabetes, coronary heart disease occurs at the same age and as frequently as in men.

As with metformin, troglitazone is being studied as a treatment for insulin resistance.

Some people with type 2 diabetes can control blood sugar (glucose) through meal planning, diet, and exercise. But sometimes that's not enough and, in addition to diet, you may need diabetes pills. This doesn't mean your diabetes is getting worse. It just means you need some extra help to control your high blood sugar.

Your health care team will decide which medication is best for you based on your age, your lifestyle, your health, and your blood-sugar levels throughout the day. Table 6.3 summarizes all the oral medications and how they work.

Before you begin taking an oral medication, it's important to talk with your health care team about

- How much to take
- When and how often to take the medication
- When and how often to test your blood sugar
- What to do if you forget a dose
- Any other drugs you may be taking
- Possible side effects

While all medications can cause side effects, many are temporary. If you have side effects with your medication, talk to your health-care team.

TABLE 6.3   HOW ORAL MEDICATIONS WORK

Type of oral medication	Where it works in the body	How it works	Common brand names	Generic names
Alpha-glucosidase inhibitor	**A** Small intestine blood sugar from	Slows the digestion of some carbohy-drates and prevents going too high after meals	Precose* Glyset	Acarbose Miglitol
Biguanides	**B** Liver	Keeps the liver from releasing too much sugar	Glucophage	Metformin
Meglitinides	**C** Pancreas	Causes the pancreas to make insulin	Prandin	Repaglinide
Sulfonylurea(s)	**C** Pancreas	Causes the pancreas to release more insulin	Orinase, Diabinase, Toblinase, Dymelor, Glucotrol, Diabeta, Micronase, Glynase, PresTab, Amaryl	Tolbutamide, Chlorpro-pamide, Tolazamide, Acetohexa-mide, Glipizide, Glyburide, Glimepiride
Thiazolidinediones	**D** Muscle	Helps the muscle cells to use insulin better	Rezulin	Troglitizone

Never stop taking the medication on your own. Your
health-care team may want to adjust the dose of
your medication or try a new medication.

Oral medication and your treatment plan

Oral diabetes medications have much to offer in the
battle to control high blood sugar. There is no pill,
however, that can replace good dietary practice and
regular exercise. These form the bedrock of type 2
diabetes management, and they are still your first
line of defense.

Most oral medications are taken one to two or
two to three times daily, except troglitazone, which
is taken once a day with breakfast. Acarbose, which
directly affects digestion, is taken with meals, as is
repaglinide. Oral medications should be taken consistently on a regular basis for best results. They are
available in a wide variety of doses, so your doctor is
able to make changes that can enhance your medication's effectiveness.

A warning

If you begin taking sulfonylureas, you should know
that all of these drugs decline in effectiveness over
time. They are more effective in people who have
had diabetes for less than ten years. It is likely that
this decline is due to progressive weakening of the
pancreas and decreased insulin secretion.
(Remember that sulfonylureas work by stimulating
the pancreas to secrete more insulin. They're ineffective in the absence of a working pancreas.) About
5 to 10 percent of patients notice decreased effects
within the first year of treatment; about 50 percent
of all users will eventually stop responding to sulfonylurea medications.

Timesaver
Your community may have a diabetes specialty store, where you can do "one-stop shopping" and gain access to lots of useful information. Check with your local American Diabetes Association, or in the Yellow Pages under "Medical Supplies" or "Diabetes." Or call the ADA at (800) 342-2383.

Fortunately, changing medications or adding a second drug may revivify the usefulness of the treatment, if only temporarily. The most common combination therapy is to pair a sulfonylurea with either metformin, troglitazone, or metformin with acarbose or repaglinide. Three-drug combinations are not yet common, but may prove to be effective for some people. Your doctor may recommend other combinations since the drugs act in different ways, they may be complimentary. Luckily, it appears that side effects do not multiply when oral medications are combined.

When oral medications are not enough: insulin therapy for type 2 diabetics

Throughout this book we've emphasized that, contrary to popular belief, many people with type 2 diabetes use insulin to control high blood sugar. Some use insulin from the time they are diagnosed.

Reasons for starting insulin therapy

If your doctor has recommended that you begin insulin therapy, it does not mean that you have suddenly developed type 1 diabetes. Perhaps what's more important, neither does it indicate some moral failing on your part, some inability or unwillingness to treat your diabetes. It means only that pancreatic weakness, insulin resistance, or both have advanced to the point that other treatments are no longer sufficient. You did not cause these fundamental, underlying causes of type 2 diabetes, and you do not ultimately have control over how far pancreatic weakness will progress. You can only control how you cope with the symptoms it creates (high blood sugar and associated health problems).

Failure of oral medication is one reason for starting insulin treatment. You may need insulin, however, even if you have never used oral medications. And you will need insulin if your glucose levels are too high but you are not able to take oral medications, as, for example:

- If you are pregnant or breast-feeding,

- If you have kidney or liver disease,

- If you cannot tolerate the oral medications, or

- If you have suffered an acute injury or surgery, are fighting an infection, taking glucocorticoids (steroids), or are under unusual stress, all of which can increase insulin resistance and raise your insulin needs.

How do people with type 2 diabetes use insulin?

Insulin comes in rapid-acting, short-acting, intermediate-acting, and long-acting forms.

As long as they have some pancreatic function, people with type 2 diabetes have less difficulty stabilizing their glucose levels than do people with type 1 diabetes. Unless beta cell production virtually stops, type 2 diabetics usually do not need the more complicated, multiple-injection treatment followed by type 1 diabetics (except during pregnancy, when tight glucose control is essential to the fetus's health; see Chapter 12). People with type 2 diabetes may also use smaller daily doses of insulin; injections of as little as twenty to forty U are frequently enough. Type 2 diabetics who are obese, however, and who have high insulin resistance, may need large insulin doses, as high as 100 to 200 U per injection.

Combining oral medication and insulin

If you are starting insulin because oral medications are no longer enough to control your blood-sugar levels, you may begin with a combination of insulin and a sulfonylurea. This is sometimes called *BIDS* therapy, which stands for "bedtime insulin, daytime sulfonylurea." The bedtime insulin is typically one injection of intermediate- or long-acting insulin. The goal is to prevent rebound elevations in blood sugar that can occur following nocturnal fasting, when the liver responds by secreting stored glucose in the early morning hours when cortisol and growth hormone levels peak. During the day, the sulfonylurea drug controls glucose levels, with help from the remainder of the bedtime insulin's action.

If you have severe insulin resistance and are well established on an insulin injection program, your doctor may want to add metformin, acarbose, or troglitizone to your treatment (usually after discontinuing sulfonylureas) because these drugs make it possible to control your blood sugar with less insulin. You may be able to decrease your daily insulin dose, sometimes by as much as 50 percent.

Insulin-only treatment

Eventually, combined insulin/oral medication treatment will no longer be effective as beta cell production continues to wane. This generally happens by fifteen to twenty years after the onset of type 2 diabetes. If you reach this point, your need for injected insulin will increase and your doctor will likely advise you to discontinue sulfonylureas. After all, sulfonylureas require functioning beta cells in order to work. Or, your kidney functioning may have deteriorated, making it risky for you to use certain oral medications.

At this stage, you may increase your injections from one at bedtime to two a day, at breakfast and bedtime. Both injections are usually mixes of short-acting and intermediate-acting insulin. The short-acting insulin will cover the rise in glucose that follows a meal, while the intermediate-acting insulin provides background coverage.

You may need more injections than this, or you may eventually need to add more. (See Chapter 5 for information on multiple daily injection schedules.)

Type 2 diabetes and self-monitoring of blood glucose (SMBG)

SMBG is a critical component of both type 1 and type 2 diabetes management. It is discussed in greater detail in Chapter 5. Here, we'll emphasize again that you won't be able to achieve your blood-sugar goals without knowing what is happening in your bloodstream. No matter what tools or medications you are using to control your blood-sugar levels—diet, exercise, oral medication, and/or insulin—you will need to track the impact of specific foods, physical activity, the timing of meals, and insulin or oral medication on your glucose levels. No two people will have the same responses to foods, exercise, and treatment. SMBG is your most reliable tool for understanding your own diabetes and how best to manage it.

SMBG: how frequently?

We know that people with type 1 diabetes must be vigilant against hypoglycemia, and they routinely time SMBG to correspond to insulin and meal schedules. Medical opinion varies widely, however, as to how often people with type 2 diabetes should perform SMBG. Frequency of SMBG should be matched to your individual treatment plan, goals, and capacities.

Bright Idea
Trying to lose weight as part of your treatment plan? Remember that "eat less" really means "eat less calories." The simplest way to accomplish this is to cut out some of the saturated fat in your diet—it's the most concentrated source of calories, and the least healthy form of fat.

Guidelines for using SMBG

There are several guidelines for using SMBG to best advantage. In general, SMBG is done before or after activities that affect blood-sugar levels, for instance, eating, exercise, and sleep (blood sugar may drop during the night). Useful times to perform SMBG include

- Before any or all meals
- One to two hours after a meal, to assess the impact of eating or of specific foods
- Before or after exercise, to make sure that blood sugar is not too low, or to assess the effects of exercise on your blood sugar
- Before bed

Other factors influencing the frequency of SMBG

Here are some other issues to consider when you self-monitor your blood glucose level:

- If you have achieved stable blood-sugar levels over time, you may be asked to do SMBG only three or four times a week, usually following a meal.
- If you are started on oral medication, your team will probably ask you to monitor yourself at least once a day, perhaps before a meal or bedtime, and to test whenever you feel symptoms of hypoglycemia.
- If you have started taking insulin, you will probably need to monitor your blood glucose as often as four or more times a day to guard against hypoglycemia and to evaluate your insulin needs.
- SMBG is usually increased under other circumstances, for instance, if you are ill, undergoing

unusual stress, taking steroid medication, are pregnant, or are planning to become pregnant.

SMBG is a valuable tool: You should discuss your team's recommendation for SMBG frequency and make sure you thoroughly understand their rationale. It is a very good idea to record your glucose readings in a log book or store them in a computer file. Check your log regularly for patterns, and communicate SMBG results to your team at least once a month. This can be as simple as faxing log pages to your doctor's office.

The glycosylated hemoglobin test (hemoglobin A1c or glycated hemoglobin)

This blood test is taken at your doctor's office, usually twice yearly if you are not on insulin and four times yearly if you are. It measures average glucose control over a three-month period. It is a necessary adjunct to SMBG because it shows how well you are controlling your blood sugar on average, not just day to day or hour to hour. Your average blood-sugar control is more important than your hourly blood-sugar control when it comes to preventing the serious complications of diabetes. (See Chapter 5 for more information on the glycosylated hemoglobin test.)

Just the facts

- Treatment for type 2 diabetes targets inadequate insulin production and insulin resistance, not the complete absence of insulin.

- Proper nutrition, exercise, and achieving your target weight are the foundations of treatment for type 2 diabetes.

Timesaver
Be aware that some glucose meters take up to two minutes to provide a reading, while others provide one in as little as twelve seconds. (If you're always in a hurry, the time saved can be a big advantage.)

- If changes in diet, exercise, and weight fail to control blood sugar, oral medications, insulin, or both, may be prescribed.
- Oral medications are not oral insulin. They work by stimulating the pancreas to secrete more insulin, by reducing insulin resistance, by reducing the ability of the liver to produce glucose, or by modifying carbohydrate digestion.
- Using oral medications may increase your chances of having hypoglycemia.
- Sulfonylureas typically lose effectiveness over time as the pancreas weakens. Different medications or insulin treatment may then be introduced.
- Self-monitoring of blood glucose and logging of the results are crucial components of diabetes self-care.

GET THE SCOOP ON...
Who provides your treatment, and why ▪ Which
credentials to look for in diabetes professionals
▪ What you can learn from your certified
diabetes educator ▪ Finding a doctor ▪ Your
role as a team player ▪ Evaluating your
insurance coverage

You're Not Alone: The Diabetes Treatment Team

Chapter 7

Diabetes is a self-managed disease: No one but you can take responsibility for managing your blood-sugar levels on a day-to-day basis. But it is also a complicated disease that affects all parts of the body and can seriously damage the eyes, kidneys, nervous system, feet, and the cardiovascular system. It's no wonder treating diabetes requires a team approach. Most people with diabetes can expect to meet regularly with an array of health-care professionals, each of whom offers different expertise.

Here's a breakdown of the different health-care professionals. We'll begin by defining the core team members, and we'll identify additional professionals whom you'll see less frequently or only as needed. Then we'll tell you what professional credentials and training to look for in your health-care team, and follow with some suggestions on how to locate qualified health-care professionals.

185

Members of the team

Your diabetes care team will have a central and a supporting cast. The central, or core, team members are

- You
- Your diabetes doctor
- Your certified diabetes educator
- Your registered dietitian

These professionals will have the most significant input into what your diabetes management plan will be, and they will teach you the skills you need to follow your plan, like self-monitoring of blood glucose, meal planning, and the proper use of insulin or oral medications.

Supporting team members include

- Your eye doctor
- Your dentist
- A mental health professional
- An exercise specialist
- A podiatrist
- Your pharmacist

By *supporting*, we do not mean "less important." We mean that you may not see these professionals as often as you see your core team members, or you may see them only if special needs or problems arise. For example, if you have diabetes, it is very important to have your eyes and teeth examined once or twice a year. Your doctor and dentist are critical team members, but they don't determine your diabetes care plan.

Not every person with diabetes must see an exercise or mental health specialist, or a podiatrist, unless the specific need arises. Perhaps you are

already an exerciser, or your primary-care physician
has given you the green light to start a walking
program. Perhaps you don't feel the need to see a
mental health counselor, or maybe you are seeing
one already. Perhaps you aren't having any problems with your feet, such as corns, calluses, sore
spots, or ingrown toenails. We include these professionals, however, because exercise is an important
part of diabetes management, and it affects blood-
sugar levels; because coping with diabetes can cause
emotional distress for many people; and because
foot problems in people with diabetes must be
promptly dealt with by a professional.

You, your diabetes doctor, your diabetes educator, and your dietitian are central to your diabetes
care. Other specialists, like your eye doctor and your
dentist, are important and necessary, but not central. And other professionals we'll talk about, like
mental health or exercise specialists, are necessary
to some people with diabetes, but not to all, or not
all of the time.

The best qualifications

Now you know that you need to find a qualified core
team—a diabetes doctor, a diabetes educator, and a
registered dietitian—as well as qualified supporting
players. In order to determine who is qualified, you
need to know what credentials to look for and what
kind of special training the professionals should
have.

The diabetes physician

Ideally, your diabetes doctor (who may or may not
be your primary-care physician) is a medical doctor
(M.D.) or osteopathic doctor (D.O.) who is a board-
certified endocrinologist (an expert in disorders of
the hormones and metabolism). Endocrinologists

Bright Idea
There's a lot to
learn about dia-
betes. You may
want to partici-
pate in a dia-
betes education
program to sup-
plement what
you're learning
from your dia-
betes educator.
Your local
American
Diabetes
Association chap-
ter can refer you
to a program
that meets
national stan-
dards for dia-
betes education.
Or call the
ADA at (800)
342-2383.

are usually certified by The American Board of Internal Medicine, in both Internal Medicine and Endocrinology and Metabolism. Your diabetes doctor may also be an internist or family medicine practitioner who specializes in treating diabetes.

Medical doctors who specialize in treating diabetes are sometimes called *diabetologists*. Most diabetes physicians are endocrinologists.

Your diabetes physician will make the primary decisions about the form of treatment you should undertake, based on your diagnosis, condition, and lifestyle. He or she will monitor your overall response to prescribed treatment, and will adjust it so that it remains effective and appropriate for your case over time.

Your physician will monitor you for signs of long-term complications and will make treatment decisions if emergencies arise. He or she should check your eyes and bare feet at each visit, as well as conduct a complete physical upon first becoming your doctor and at least once each year after that. (We describe what should be included in that first exam below, under "The doctor's first examination: what to expect.")

Should your diabetes doctor be your primary-care physician?

You will need medical advice to decide this question. One factor to consider is whether or not diabetes is your primary medical problem. If, for example, you have type 1 diabetes, but you are young, of normal weight and blood pressure, with no micro- or macrovascular complications and no other major illnesses, then your primary-care physician should probably be a diabetes specialist. If, on the other hand, you have many health problems, like heart

Watch Out!
The most qualified doctors are board certified in their specialty and subspecialty areas. However, not all doctors are board certified. To find out, you can ask the doctor whether he or she is board certified or you can call the American Board of Medical Specialties at (800) 776-2378.

disease, obesity, or high blood pressure, you may
need an internist who oversees all of your care but
who arranges for you to consult a diabetes specialist
on a regular basis. You can also ask your diabetes
doctor whether he or she can fulfill your primary-
care needs.

Children and adolescents who have diabetes
may have a primary-care physician (a pediatrician
or a family medicine doctor) who takes care of their
general medical needs, such as immunizations,
colds and illnesses and routine checkups. In addition, they should see a diabetes specialist (usually a
pediatric endocrinologist) and have a diabetes
team.

If you develop complications such as kidney disease or neuropathy, or if you are at high risk for
developing specific complications, your diabetes
doctor may refer you for consultation with another
medical doctor, such as:

■ A nephrologist (kidney doctor)

■ A cardiologist (heart doctor)

■ A neurologist (brain and nervous system
  doctor)

■ A dermatologist (skin doctor)

■ A vascular surgeon (circulatory system surgeon)

■ An orthopedic surgeon (bone and joint
  surgeon)

The certified diabetes educator

The certified diabetes educator is usually a
registered nurse who has had special training and
certification by the National Board for Diabetes
Educators in educating people with diabetes about
their self-care. The certified diabetes educator

credential is *C.D.E.*; look for it following the nursing credentials *R.N.*, or registered nurse; *B.S.N.*, or bachelor of science degree in nursing; or *M.S.N.*, a master of science degree in nursing. A C.D.E. may also be someone who is not a nurse, such as a registered dietitian, a pharmacist, or a physician.

Your C.D.E. plays a very important role in helping you to adjust to having diabetes and teaching you how to treat it. Your diabetes educator will teach you the principles of diabetes self-care, such as how to: prepare and administer insulin injections; take blood and urine tests; balance insulin or medication with blood tests, meals, and exercise; deal with illnesses; and more. He or she is knowledgeable about the biology and progress of diabetes, and can help you understand the disease. The C.D.E. can counsel you on questions or concerns as they arise while you are adjusting to new treatment or to a treatment change.

Bright Idea
For guidance in putting together your diabetes health-care team, read *How To Get Great Diabetes Care*, by Irl B. Hirsch, M.D., published by the American Diabetes Association (1996). To order, call the ADA at (800) 342-2383.

The registered dietitian

The registered dietitian, or R.D., has training and expertise in the field of nutrition. The R.D. credential indicates that the professional has passed a national credentials examination. Look also for an L.D., which means that he or she is licensed by the state to practice as a dietitian. (Not all states require licensure, however.) Many registered dietitians are also certified diabetes educators.

You will probably need to meet with an R.D. once or twice as you are first learning about diabetes and self-care, then once or twice a year after that. The registered dietitian will help you develop or make changes in an appropriate nutritional plan, taking into account insulin or oral medication regimens. A good R.D. is knowledgeable about diabetes and the different meal plan approaches (such as exchange diets and carbohydrate counting), and is interested in your preferences and lifestyle. He or she will have practical suggestions about how to stick to your meal plan, at home and socially.

The eye doctor

Eye care is a top priority for all people with diabetes. Your eye care professional should be an ophthalmologist, a medical doctor who has special training and is board certified in diagnosing and treating eye disease. If you develop diabetic complications of the eye (retinopathy), you may need to see a doctor who specializes in diseases of the retina if your doctor does not.

You should have a professional eye examination—one that includes dilation of the pupil for inner-eye examination—at least once a year and more frequently if you are pregnant or on your doctor's recommendation. People who have had diabetes for more than ten years are at higher risk for developing eye disease.

Remember that your eye professional should be an ophthalmologist, a medical doctor. An optometrist is not a medical doctor. Although trained to evaluate vision and prescribe and dispense corrective lenses, he or she is not an expert diagnostician and cannot prescribe medication or treat eye disease.

The dentist

It's not fair, but people with diabetes are at greater risk for developing gingivitis (gum disease). The bacteria that cause gingivitis flourish on the high levels of sugar in your body fluids. Gum disease can progress rapidly and spread widely within your mouth, and infections within the mouth and

Moneysaver
Having trouble getting health insurance coverage for appointments with your dietitian? Try including a written referral from your doctor with your claim. Ask that it specify "medical nutritional therapy for diabetes," and list ways in which it is a cost-effective treatment.

Watch Out!
Some people who
bill themselves
as nutritionists
have no profes-
sional training or
certification to
back this up. It's
best to get nutri-
tion advice from
a registered
dietitian (R.D.).

around the teeth can occur. People with diabetes can also develop an unpleasant yeast infection of the mouth, called *thrush*. You should have your mouth and teeth examined and cleaned by a dentist (a D.D.S.) every six months. Make sure you always brush your teeth after eating and floss between them at least once a day. You should also brush your tongue daily, as part of brushing your teeth. Ask your dentist to recommend an antiseptic oral hygiene mouthwash.

The mental health professional

Having diabetes doesn't necessarily mean you need the help of a mental health professional. But diabetes is a chronic disease, and many people with diabetes and their families experience periods of depression, anger, fear, and other problems coping with the daily demands of having diabetes. These feelings and problems, if unaddressed, can wreak havoc on diabetes management plans.

In Chapter 14, we discuss some of the common emotional problems people with diabetes and their loved ones sometimes face, and we offer some guidelines for deciding when it is necessary to consult a mental health professional. If you decide to consult such a person, here is the information you need to know about the different mental health credentials.

The three basic mental health professions are:

Psychiatrist

The psychiatrist is a medical doctor with advanced training in diagnosing and treating psychological disorders. As with all medical specialists, the best-qualified psychiatrist is board certified in psychiatry. The psychiatrist can prescribe medications for psychological disorders, for example, antianxiety medications or antidepressants. Psychiatrists' fees tend to be high, from about $80 to $200 per session.

Psychologist

The psychologist is not a medical doctor and cannot prescribe medication. He or she holds an advanced university degree in the field of psychology, either a doctor of philosophy degree (Ph.D.) or a master's degree (M.A. or M.S.). There are a number of different fields of psychology, like social psychology, child or developmental psychology, and experimental psychology. The best preparation for the psychologist mental health counselor is the study of clinical psychology, which focuses on psychological disorders and training in psychotherapy. Fees for Ph.D. psychologists can be as high or almost as high as those of psychiatrists, depending upon the experience level of the psychologist. Master's level psychologists tend to charge lower fees.

Social worker

The social worker holds a master's degree in social work (*M.S.W.*) from an accredited university. It's best to see clinical social workers, who have received special training in evaluating and treating emotional disorders. Look for the credential *C.S.W.* (clinical social worker); *A.C.S.W.*, indicating that the social worker has been admitted to the Academy of Clinical Social Workers; or *L.C.S.W.*, licensed clinical social worker. The social worker is not a medical doctor and cannot prescribe medications. Social workers' fees tend to be somewhat lower than those of psychiatrists and psychologists, although some highly experienced social workers charge more.

There are a variety of other certified mental health counselors, most of whom hold master's

Timesaver
If your health-care professionals do not work in the same office, provide each member of your team with a typewritten list of all members' office phone numbers, pager numbers, fax numbers, and e-mail addresses. Include your medications and doses. This will expedite communication between team members when necessary.

degrees in an area of psychology (such as marriage
and family counseling), education (Ed.D. or M.Ed.),
or religious counseling. In Chapter 14, we give some
tips on finding a qualified mental health counselor.

The exercise specialist

The exercise specialist should be consulted on the
recommendation of your primary-care physician or
your diabetes physician. Not all people with diabetes
will need to meet with an exercise specialist. Very
few insurance plans will cover this consultation,
which could cost $50 or more an hour. Talk to your
doctor. If you have never exercised regularly, are in
very poor physical condition, are obese, or if diabetes complications (heart, kidney, or eye disease)
require you to make a change in your exercise program, it may be worth the expense to consult with
an exercise specialist about developing a safe, beneficial program.

Before you begin an exercise program, your doctor may recommend that you have a cardiac stress
test, or that you be examined by another medical
specialist, such as a cardiologist, ophthalmologist,
or obstetrician. And you may need continued monitoring by this specialist as you follow your exercise
program.

Ideally, an exercise specialist is experienced in
working with people with diabetes and may even be
a certified diabetes educator (C.D.E.). He or she
holds a bachelor's, master's, or Ph.D. in exercise
physiology, may be a registered nurse with specialized training in fitness and exercise, or may have a
degree in sports medicine, fitness, or kinesiology.
Look for a professional certified by the American
College of Sports Medicine (call [317] 637-9200 for
answers to questions about appropriate qualifications and how to find specialists in your area).

The podiatrist (foot doctor)

Foot care is another top priority for people with diabetes. Look for the credential Doctor of Podiatric Medicine (D.P.M.), or for an orthopedist (a medical doctor) who specializes in foot care. Remember, if you are diabetic, no foot problem is too small to be attended to by a professional. A D.P.M. can safely treat corns, calluses, and sores, helping to prevent dangerous foot ulcers. (Never attempt to cut or remove corns, calluses, or ingrown toenails on your own! As a diabetic, you are prone to skin and wound infections that can develop rapidly and become ulcers that are difficult to treat.) The podiatrist can also teach you proper daily foot care and how to spot symptoms of complications. Finally, the podiatrist can help you to find shoes that fit well—a must for proper foot care.

The pharmacist

Don't forget this important team player. A good pharmacist is a gold mine of information on how medications work, how they interact, how to store and use them, and what the most cost-effective choices are. Try to establish an ongoing relationship with a pharmacist you trust. It's not always easy in today's "drive-through" world, but if you have diabetes, it's well worth the effort. Even if you buy most of your diabetes supplies from a mail-order pharmacy, you will still benefit from a personal relationship with a local pharmacist.

How often will you meet with each health-care professional?

The box below contains a summary of standard recommendations for how often you should have specific medical examinations.

Watch Out!
People with diabetes can develop persistently dry, itchy skin, caused by dehydration. Cracking and scratching can lead to infection. Consider seeing a dermatologist if you have persistently dry, cracked skin.

Diabetes Care Schedule

Every 3 months:
- Regular visit to your doctor
- Glycosylated hemoglobin test
- Bare feet examined by doctor

Every 6 months:
- Dental exam (All people with diabetes)
- Kidneys: Microalbumin test

Every year:
- Cholesterol/triglycerides (More often if your levels are abnormal or to check the effects of treatment for high levels)
- Eyes: Dilated pupil examination by opthalmologist (More often if pregnant or if last exam was abnormal)

Finding a qualified doctor and other team members

This process can be as simple as looking in the telephone book (which we don't recommend) or as time-consuming as asking other people for referrals, making appointments to interview prospective team members, and interviewing several candidates for each position (a better approach). A lot depends on how much time and energy you want to invest in assembling a team.

Your health insurance coverage

Another important factor in choosing health professionals is your health insurance coverage:

- Is your health insurance plan a "preferred provider" plan or an HMO? Are you restricted to consulting doctors and other professionals who participate in the plan? You will be limited to those professionals if you want your insurance company to pay for visits. In order to consult a diabetes doctor who participates in your plan, you may need to meet first with a

primary care physician on the plan, who will
formally refer you to the diabetes doctor.

- Which diabetes specialists does your insurance
  cover? Will it pay for sessions with a diabetes
  educator? A registered dietitian? Many policies
  will cover one introductory session with both.
  What about mental health and exercise specialists? Mental health coverage varies widely, but
  fully covered appointments are frequently
  limited to six to twelve sessions per year.
  Consultations with exercise specialists are rarely
  covered.

- How many appointments a year with each professional will your insurance cover?

Make sure you know what your insurance cover-
age is before you begin looking for team members.
(For more on diabetes and insurance coverage, see
"Know your health insurance coverage, below.)

Assembling your team: first steps

Your first task is to find a good, board-certified
endocrinologist or other physician (such as an
internist or family practitioner) who specializes in
treating diabetes, not only because you need one,
but also because your diabetes doctor will be the
best source of referrals to other diabetes professionals. One place to begin your search is with the
doctor who diagnosed your diabetes—usually your
primary-care physician. It is natural for you to ask
your doctor for the names of reputable, experienced endocrinologists or diabetes specialists. If
your doctor gives you the name of a diabetes specialist, ask him or her:

- How do you know this doctor?

- What do you know about the care this doctor
  gives his or her patients?

Timesaver
Be sure to
double-check the
mental health
professionals
your insurance
will cover. For
instance, does
your policy reim-
burse only for
appointments
with a licensed
Ph.D. psycholo-
gist or psychia-
trist (M.D.)?
What about
social workers—
M.S.W.s, C.S.W.s,
or L.C.S.W.s?
Check this before
you make an
appointment
with a mental
health
professional.

Watch Out!
Doctor referral telephone lines give you the names of doctors who have paid a fee to be included in the list. Don't rely on these referral lines to select doctors on the basis of superior credentials or skills. If you do select a tele-phone line name, cross-check the doctor's creden-tials using resources given in this chapter.

- Have you referred other patients with diabetes to this doctor? Do you know how they did under the doctor's care?

- Do you know if this doctor works well with other health-care professionals?

If you feel comfortable with the answers you receive, and if the doctor named is reimbursable under your insurance plan, then make an appoint-ment with the specialist recommended by your primary-care physician.

If your doctor can't make a referral, or if he or she does not know a doctor who is reimbursable under your insurance plan, you may need to make use of other referral resources, some of which are provided in this chapter.

Diabetes clinics or care centers

Many communities have clinics or care centers that specialize in diabetes care. Many of these centers are run by hospitals. Some may be independently oper-ated. Your primary-care physician may be able to recommend one. They are listed in the Yellow Pages under "Diabetes," or you can look under "Hospitals" for the departmental directory of a specific hospital to see if it lists a diabetes unit or clinic. If a complete directory is not provided, call the main number and ask if the hospital has a diabetes clinic.

If you can find a diabetes clinic that is part of a reputable hospital, we recommend that you choose this over an independent clinic unless the clinic is a very well-established institution, like a Joslin Diabetes Clinic.

The usefulness of the diabetes care center is that it employs and makes referrals to a wide range of diabetes professionals. Most clinics have well-established relationships with doctors who treat

diabetes. If you are looking for a doctor, a local clinic
may be able to give you several names. If you have a
diabetes doctor, he or she can refer you to a diabetes
clinic, where you will find experienced diabetes educators and registered dietitians. While most clinics
do not employ mental health professionals or exercise specialists, they can provide referrals to these
and other professionals in your community.

Remember that, if you are restricted by your
health-care plan to specific hospitals, you'll need to
find a hospital on your plan that has a diabetes
clinic, or check to see whether your plan has
selected a participating clinic.

Bright Idea
To find out if
there is a Joslin
Diabetes Clinic in
your area, call
(800) 567-5461.

Hospitals

Another good way to find qualified doctors and
other health-care professionals is to call the department of endocrinology at a reputable local hospital.
If you can, it's a good idea to explore the diabetes
care possibilities at a university-affiliated hospital or
a hospital known for teaching and research. These
institutions draw the "best and the brightest" medical professionals, those who are involved in
research and teaching as well as providing care.

The American Diabetes Association

Your local chapter of the American Diabetes
Association can help you locate competent diabetes
doctors. You can find the phone number in the
Yellow Pages under "Diabetes" and in the White
Pages business section under "American Diabetes
Association." Or call the ADA at (800) 342-2383 for
the number of your local chapter.

Medical societies and professional associations

Many medical doctors who have special qualifications in a particular area of medicine join

professional associations. For help in finding a board-certified endocrinologist in your area, try contacting:

> The Endocrine Society
> 4350 East-West Highway
> Suite 500
> Bethesda, MD 20814
> (301) 941-0200
> www.endo-society.org

> The American Association of Clinical Endocrinologists
> 1000 Riverside Avenue
> Suite 205
> Jacksonville, FL 32204
> www.aace.com

Bright Idea
To find out if a medical doctor is board certified, call the American Board of Medical Specialties at (800) 776-2378.

Friends and family

People often ask friends or family members for names when looking for a doctor. Diabetes is a relatively common disease, and there's a chance that someone you know has diabetes or knows someone who does. It may be possible to get the name of a good diabetes doctor this way. The advantage of this approach is that a friend or relative can usually give you good information on the doctor's communication skills and friendliness. However, unless your friend or relative is a doctor or nurse, he or she can't accurately assess whether this specialist's training and skill level is right for your case.

When you don't know a medical professional who can make a recommendation, the following resources may be helpful.

"Top doctor" lists

Several magazines run annual "top doctor" or "top hospital" reports; *U.S. News & World Report* is one example. These lists can help you identify reputable medical specialists in your geographic area, but keep in mind that the source of these rankings is often interviews with other doctors, who may recommend friends or colleagues. The list may not reflect the physician's actual excellence or patients' opinions. Be wary of lists that are based on "patient satisfaction." It's not always clear what aspect of treatment the survey patients were asked about; the list might reflect satisfaction with office décor or the receptionist's pleasant phone manner.

If you use one of these lists to find a doctor, make sure you understand how the rankings were determined (an explanation should accompany the article). If you select any doctors from the list, check their credentials through other resources as well (for example, one of the professional societies listed above) before making an appointment.

The internet

Log on to the American Medical Association's Web site, www.ama-assn.org, for a listing of United States physicians in good standing. The list also includes the doctor's address, education, and board-certification status. It is not yet complete, however, so don't assume that a doctor whose name is not on the list is not a good doctor.

Published directories

Ask your reference librarian for a published directory listing doctors' names, education, board certification, and professional affiliations. Two good directories are *The Official ABMS Directory of Board Certified Medical Specialists* and *The American Medical Directory*.

Questions you should ask the doctor

Once your research is complete and you are at the stage of interviewing a doctor or doctors, remember

Watch Out!
The Public Citizen Health Research Group can give you a list of doctors in your state against whom serious complaints have been filed. Send $15 plus $4 shipping to Public Citizen, Questionable Doctors, 1600 20th St. NW, Washington, DC 20009, or call (202) 588-1000.

Bright Idea
The American Diabetes Association offers a free brochure called *Standards of Care* for diabetes patients. This brochure will tell you what medical care, examinations, and laboratory tests your doctor should perform or recommend, and how often. For a copy of the brochure, call the ADA at (800) 342-2383.

that you have a right to know certain facts about the doctor you will work with. It is also worthwhile to see how comfortable you are in asking the doctor questions, and how comfortable he or she seems in answering them.

A few valuable questions to ask a prospective doctor are:

- Are you board certified in endocrinology or internal medicine?

- How many of your patients have diabetes? What type of diabetes? Which type of diabetes do you have the most experience with?

- Do you follow the American Diabetes Association Standards of Medical Care for People with Diabetes?

- Do you have specific thoughts on how my type of diabetes ought to be treated? What do you think of new approaches or treatments?

- How do you see my role as your patient?

The questions just listed pertain more to the doctor's experience and approach than to the specifics of patient care. The following questions cover practical concerns:

- How often will I see you for regular visits?

- What tests do you conduct routinely? How often do you check my feet? Eyes? Glycosylated hemoglobin? SMBG log?

- Are you associated with other health-care providers who treat diabetes, such as a diabetes educator? Registered dietitian? Exercise specialist? What is your approach to working with other health-care professionals?

- What about coverage for you on your days off?

- What if I have an emergency?

Finally, after you have interviewed the doctor, ask yourself some questions:

- What was my general impression of the doctor?
- Did the doctor answer my questions satisfactorily?
- What is my sense of confidence in the doctor's level of experience? Does the doctor inspire confidence?
- Did he or she listen carefully, or ask me any questions?
- Did the doctor seem to be a "take charge" type of professional, or was his or her approach less directive? Which do I prefer?
- Did I feel comfortable with the doctor?

In considering the last question, also think about how the office staff treated you, whether you had to wait a long time for your appointment, and your reaction to the office atmosphere—things like cleanliness, orderliness, and availability of educational materials.

The most important question

The most important question to ask yourself about your doctor will not be relevant until you have worked with him or her for a while: "Is my prescribed treatment plan helping to keep my blood sugar within acceptable levels?" Your answer to this will have little meaning, of course, if you have not made an honest effort to stick to your doctor's recommendations.

The doctor's first examination: what to expect

Once you select a diabetes specialist, his or her first task as your diabetes physician should be to give you

Watch Out!
Most doctors charge a fee for interview appointments, and your insurance may not cover these. Ask about this when you call a doctor's office, and review your insurance coverage. See if some of your questions, especially those about insurance, fees, and office procedures, can be answered over the telephone by the doctor's staff.

Bright Idea
Be prepared to
tell your doctor
what your goals
for diabetes
management are,
and what you are
willing and able
to do to meet
these goals.

a thorough physical exam (which should be repeated annually). This will introduce the doctor to your overall health status, and it's also a way for him or her to check you carefully for signs of diabetes complications—a very important part of your diabetes doctor's job. You should know what is included in a thorough examination because it's important information and because it's one way of evaluating the level of care you may receive from this physician.

At minimum, a complete physical examination includes checking your:

- **Body weight.** Discuss any concerns about your weight with the doctor. Ask if he or she recommends a body weight for you.

- **Blood pressure and pulse.** Ask the doctor what blood pressure level is best for you.

- **Eyes.** The doctor should check your vision and ask if there have been any changes or problems.

- **Mouth and neck.** The doctor should examine your gums, teeth, mouth, and throat, and will ask how often you brush your teeth and floss. He or she will check for swollen glands in your neck. Thyroid function tests should be performed. (The thyroid is a gland in your neck that secretes hormones that affect growth and food metabolism. People with diabetes have a slightly increased risk of thyroid problems.) The doctor should check your neck for thyroid gland enlargement. The blood vessels of the neck should be examined for narrowing or obstruction.

- **Heart and lungs.** The doctor will listen to your heart and lungs through a stethoscope, and may order an electrocardiogram or a stress electro-cardiogram to detect heart disease.

- **Feet.** The doctor should check your bare feet for sores, calluses, infections, and signs of nerve damage (irregular reflexes, numbness, cold spots, and prickly sensations). He or she may order testing of the blood circulation in your legs.

- **Skin.** The doctor should examine your skin for signs of infection, diabetic skin complications, and problems at injection sites.

- **Nervous system.** The doctor will check your reflexes and your ability to feel pinpricks and the light touch of a cotton ball. Tell the doctor about any unusual sensations (prickling or burning) or numbness in your legs, feet, hands, or arms; about constipation or diarrhea; diffi-culty urinating; or problems with erection or sexual sensation.

- **Blood.** A blood sample should be taken for test-ing glucose levels, glycosylated hemoglobin, and cholesterol and triglyceride levels, as well as urea nitrogen and serum creatinine (to evalu-ate kidney function).

- **Urine.** A urine sample should be taken to test for ketones, glucose, urinary tract infection, and protein (or microalbumin—another test of kidney function).

For women, a complete physical may also includes a Pap smear (test for cancer of the cervix), gynecological and rectal exam, and a mammogram for women age forty and older or women who are at risk for developing breast cancer. Birth control should be discussed, including any problems or concerns, as well as plans for pregnancy. (If you have an obstetrician/gynecologist or a primary-care physician, the diabetes specialist may not perform these tests. However, he or she should ask whether you have had these tests within the last year, and should request copies of test results to keep in your file.)

For men, a complete physical also may include genital, prostate, and rectal exams.

The doctor should ask about your vaccination history, and may recommend a vaccination, such as for flu. (This vaccination is recommended for most people with diabetes.) The doctor should ask you if there are specific questions, concerns, or physical problems that you want to discuss. Finally, he or she should give you referrals to other medical specialists you should consult.

Knowing what should be covered in a first examination is a concrete and objective tool you can use to evaluate the thoroughness of a doctor's care.

Not you versus them: your role on the team

Having diabetes will challenge you in many ways. You will have to learn to think consciously (and frequently) about your blood-sugar levels. You will have to eat often enough to prevent your blood sugar from dropping too low. At the same time, you'll have to watch the amount of carbohydrates you eat in one meal or in one day. You will have to test your own blood, and perhaps inject yourself with insulin. You will have to take good care of your feet, and your mouth and gums, as well. Perhaps for the first time, you will be evaluating what you eat, getting regular exercise, and generally taking action to protect your health.

Watch Out!
If you arrive poorly organized and unprepared for your doctor's appointment, you really can't blame the doctor's tight schedule if your questions are not all answered!

A different relationship

Another area in which diabetes may challenge you to change and grow is communicating with health-care professionals. You may find yourself in the interesting situation of being in charge of your treatment, yet surrounded (or so it may seem) by doctors, nurses, and others wearing lab coats. Most of us are used to letting the doctor or nurse practitioner "do her thing" while we follow instructions; there is usually one right answer, and your job as a patient is simply to get the prescription filled and use all the medication.

It's different with diabetes. Yes, the patient with diabetes follows her team's prescriptions, but she also provides them with a lot of information that will be incorporated into her treatment. The person with diabetes

- Communicates lifestyle preferences to the team, which in turn, influence meal plans and exercise programs.

- Has personal goals for blood-sugar management that will affect how many insulin shots or what medication is taken, and how often blood is tested.

- Is responsible for letting the health-care team know when irregularities or serious symptoms arise.

If, like many people, you have always been somewhat intimidated by doctors and nurses, then these new responsibilities may make you feel a bit anxious. Still, it is very important to your health and well-being to learn to communicate as effectively and confidently as possible.

Unofficially...
Whether or not you have ever consciously thought about your personal self-care goals, you do have them!

Some tips

The American Diabetes Association offers these tips for establishing good communication with your health-care providers:

- Don't forget to listen! Anxiety can make it harder to pay attention. Your health-care professionals have a lot teach you. Try to give them the floor about 60 percent of the time.

- Never hesitate to ask for clarification of technical terms or jargon. Your doctor isn't trying to mystify you—to him or her, medical terms are a kind of shorthand that has become second nature, exactly as the professional lingo you use has become habitual for you. Far from thinking you stupid, a good doctor will respect your efforts to understand.

- Keep an appointment notebook in which you write down important information and keep questions you have for upcoming meetings.

- Consider bringing a friend or partner to appointments. Sometimes two sets of ears are better than one.

- Both sex and money can be tough to talk about. But don't avoid bringing up concerns about either one of them with your health-care professionals.

- If you feel you have made an honest effort to communicate effectively to your doctor or to other team members and yet you frequently feel you are not being heard, you might want to talk about this with a member of your team with whom you feel comfortable. On the other hand, you may prefer to discuss it directly with the person involved, or you may consider interviewing other professionals until you find one with whom you feel you can work.

Having diabetes, you will need to work actively as a patient to ensure that your needs are met, as well as hold up your end of the responsibilities for deciding how to treat *your* condition.

It is this active involvement in your own health care that can feel so new and difficult. It can also represent an opportunity for personal growth and empowerment.

Treatment costs

It's hard to state definitively what the monthly or annual costs of having diabetes are. The cost of treating diabetes varies widely because treatment regimens range from no insulin and relatively few blood tests (for a person with well-controlled type 2 diabetes, for example) to the use of an insulin pump and six to ten blood tests a day.

Nonetheless, diabetes is recognized as an expensive disease. The American Diabetes Association states that the yearly cost of treatment for the average person with diabetes is $2,500, or about $280 a month. This is not necessarily all out-of-pocket expense; it depends on what your health insurance covers. But the figure gives a sense of the economic burden of having diabetes. (Keep in mind, though, that good diabetes self-care costs less than treating the serious complications, such as blindness, heart disease, amputation, and end-stage kidney disease, that can occur if diabetes is poorly controlled.)

Know your health insurance coverage

The single most important thing you can do to keep diabetes costs down is to choose your health insurance policy with diabetes coverage in mind. If you are already locked into a plan, it's still essential that

Bright Idea
Bring the following items with you to each appointment with your diabetes physician or diabetes educator: Your medications, or a list of your medications, including dosages; your blood glucose log; and your questions.

Moneysaver
When shopping for glucose meters, compare the cost of the test strips required for each meter: Annual costs can differ by over $100!

you know exactly what parts of diabetes treatment your plan will cover, so that you can take the fullest possible advantage of your plan. This will determine the amount you pay out of your own pocket for diabetes care and supplies.

First, know what your basic insurance coverage is:

- What is the cost per doctor appointment (how much is your co-payment)?

- What, if any, is your policy's annual limit for covered medical expenses?

- What are your premiums and annual deductibles?

- What are the payments and restrictions pertaining to hospital stays?

- What prescriptions are covered? Is there a preferred or participating pharmacy or a mail-order program for supplies?

Second, evaluate what we call your "diabetes coverage." You need to know the answers to these questions:

- (This is important!) What medical equipment is covered? If "durable medical equipment" is included, that should include glucose meters, lancet devices, insulin injectors or syringes, and insulin pumps (with a doctor's letter of medical necessity).

- (Also important!) Are prescription drugs and medical supplies covered? These categories should include insulin, glucose meter strips, ketone test strips, and insulin pump supplies (with a doctor's letter).

- What laboratory tests are covered?

- Are visits to a certified diabetes educator covered? How many visits or how many hours of diabetes education are covered? How is diabetes education defined? What about visits to a registered dietitian?

- Are visits to the eye doctor (and eyeglass prescriptions) covered? What about appointments with other medical specialists, for example, kidney or heart specialists, neurologists, foot doctors, and surgeons? Is there a limit on coverage for referrals to specialists?

- What about mental health coverage? Exercise or fitness consultations?

Again, knowing all the details of your insurance coverage is your best chance for getting as many costs reimbursed as possible. It will also help you to evaluate and choose among future insurance policies should you make a change.

When diabetes is a "preexisting condition"

In all likelihood, as a person with diabetes you are concerned about maintaining health insurance. Please see Chapter 11 for more information on health insurance, Medicare, and disability coverage.

Some tips for containing costs

Keep the following points in mind when purchasing diabetes supplies:

- First and foremost, never buy supplies without knowing what is and isn't covered by your health insurance.

- Remember to get a doctor's prescription and, if necessary, a letter from your doctor for items covered by your insurance.

- Compare costs at several pharmacies. Prices vary.

Bright Idea
For information about specific insurance companies and their health insurance coverage, visit this Web site: www.yahoo.com/Business. Look for information on health insurance.

Unofficially...
About one-quarter of all health-care costs in the United States are the administrative expenses of over 1,000 private insurance companies.

- It's usually cheaper to purchase diabetes supplies through a mail-order company. Many advertise in diabetes-related magazines like *Diabetes Forecast* and *Diabetes Self-Management* (see the Resource Guide in Appendix B).

- Your pharmacist may offer lower prices for supplies ordered in bulk. (With insulin and meter or ketone strips, always check expiration dates and plan to use supplies before they expire.)

- Look for bargains each fall in the American Diabetes Association's annual *Buyer's Guide to Diabetes Supplies*, published in *Diabetes Forecast*. Or order a separate copy of the *Buyer's Guide* by calling the ADA at (800) 342-2383.

- See if there is a diabetes specialty store in your community. Your local American Diabetes Association has that information.

- Find out if you can use generic strips in your glucose meter. Most meter manufacturers have an 800 number for customer inquiries.

- If you inject insulin, consider reusing syringes. There is no reason not to if you follow proper procedures. Ask your diabetes educator or call your local American Diabetes Association for information about how to do this. Proper cleaning technique is especially important if you mix insulins yourself; don't risk contaminating short-acting insulin with the additives left in the syringe by longer-acting insulin.

- Finally, take good care of all equipment. You'll save money in the long run.

Home health care

If for any reason you become bedridden or housebound, you may need to consider home health care.

In most communities, there are a number of
agencies that provide home health care:

- **The Visiting Nurse Association.** This nonprofit,
  nationwide agency has provided home health
  care for over 100 years. You'll find a telephone
  number in the White Pages under "Visiting
  Nurse Association," or in the Yellow Pages
  under "Home Health Care Services." For general information, visit their Web site at
  www.vnahc.org.

- **The Veterans Administration (if you are an
  eligible veteran of the United States Armed
  Forces).** Check the blue government listings in
  your phone book under "United States
  Government, Veterans Affairs: Medical Care,"
  call (800) 827-1000, or visit the VA's Web site:
  www.va.gov.

- **Nonprofit public programs administered by
  county health departments.** Look in the blue
  government listings of your phone book under
  your county, then look for "Social Services" or
  "Human Services." See if there is a telephone
  number listed for services for the aging, seniors,
  the elderly, or the disabled.

- **Private for-profit home health-care businesses.**
  Check your Yellow Pages under "Home Health
  Care." You should find a number of businesses
  providing home health care.

Which home health-care provider you choose
will depend upon what your health insurance will
cover, what you can afford to pay out of pocket, and
which home health-care provider in your community is well recommended.

Timesaver
Now is the time
to review your
health insurance
coverage for in-
home health
care. What ser-
vices are cov-
ered? What is
the limit on cov-
erage? It will
save valuable
time should the
need for home
care arise unex-
pectedly.

Bright Idea
For free information about how to choose a home-care agency, write or call the National Association for Home Care, 519 C Street NE, Washington, DC 20002-5809, (202) 547-7424. Or visit their Web site at www.nahc.org.

For home health-care recommendations, ask your diabetes physician or diabetes educator, a local senior citizen center, your church or synagogue, your county Human Services or Social Services department, the United Way, or your local American Diabetes Association chapter.

If you contact an agency that provides in-home care, be sure to ask about

- *Fees for services.* The average rate is $86 a day. (It sounds like a lot, until you compare it to the average cost of a day in the hospital—$1,810.)

- *The professional qualifications of the care providers.* Are they registered nurses? Licensed practical nurses? Nursing assistants? Before calling, ask your doctor's advice about what in-home care professional will best meet your needs.

- Whether you may interview potential in-home care providers or request a change in provider.

- Whether you must commit to a minimum number of in-home care hours.

- What the agency's billing procedures are. It is more convenient for you if the agency will bill your insurance company directly instead of requiring you to pay and submit a claim to your insurance company.

Just the facts

- Diabetes treatment demands a team approach.

- The diabetes patient plays an active role in his or her treatment.

- It's important to give some thought to what your goals are for managing your diabetes, and what you are willing and able to do to meet these goals.

- Diabetes affects the whole body. Know how often to have specialists examine your eyes, feet, and teeth, and see that this is done.

- Make sure you know exactly what your health insurance does and does not cover.

Better Than Ever: Lifestyle Choices That Promote Health

PART III

GET THE SCOOP ON...
Do people with diabetes eat sugar? ▪ What
makes up a healthy meal plan? ▪
How much fat should you eat, and what kinds?
▪ What really raises your cholesterol level? ▪
"Happy hour" hazards ▪ Traveling with diabetes

Everybody's Doing It: The Right Way to Eat

Chapter 8

The connection between diabetes and food has long been the subject of misunderstanding and old wives' tales:

"People get diabetes from eating too many sweets."

"People with diabetes are allergic to sugar."

"If you have diabetes, eating sugar will kill you."

"Doctors make all people with diabetes follow the same rigid diet plan—no ifs, ands, or buts."

Everybody knows that diabetes is "sugar in the blood," so doesn't it stand to reason that sugar is poison to people with diabetes, a horrible dietary villain? Especially since eating sweets is so much fun? It can't be good.

Well, the truth is that, yes, people with diabetes do need to keep an eye on the amount of sugar they eat. But did you know that they also keep an eye on the amount of peas, corn, and beans they eat—those humble do-gooders of the edible world? Keep reading, and we'll try to shed some light on the relationship between diabetes and food, and dispel a few myths along the way.

A look at food and blood-sugar management today

Everybody is more aware of good nutrition today. Perhaps the handiest summing-up of the new wisdom on nutrition is the U.S. Department of Agriculture's Food Guide Pyramid. (See the figure below.)

Note! ➜
The Food Guide
Pyramid

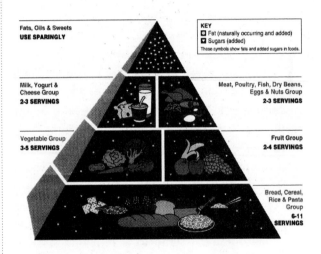

The Food Guide Pyramid embodies the USDA's recommendations for healthy eating:

- Eat a variety of foods for enhanced enjoyment and adequate intake of vitamins, minerals, and fiber.

- Avoid too much fat, saturated fat, and cholesterol. Eat smaller, leaner servings of meat; choose poultry and fish more often than red meat or pork. Avoid fried foods, fatty cold cuts, rich sauces, and whole-milk dairy products.

- Avoid too much sodium (salt). Do not bring the salt shaker to the table! Eat fewer high-sodium, processed, and canned foods.

- Eat foods with starch and fiber. Eat less refined sugar and more fruits and vegetables.

- Drink alcohol in moderation only.

Many of us are familiar with recommendations to cut back on fat and to increase complex carbohydrates (unrefined grains and vegetables). Whether we've learned how to read food labels or are eating oatmeal for breakfast, many of us are giving more thought to what we're putting into our mouths; witness the impressive array of low-fat, nonfat, salt-free, and "natural" foods that manufacturers have eagerly made available to us in recent years.

Meanwhile, our eternal fascination with weight control grows as baby boomers enter middle age and beyond. Many of us are inspired by the mirror, perhaps for the first time, to really get serious about portion control and exercise.

So if you have diabetes and are getting serious about food, you are in good company. What's good for people with diabetes, it turns out, is good for all of us. Gone are the days when eating for diabetes meant eating differently from everybody else.

Meal plans and nutritional therapy

It's true that healthy eating and eating for diabetes are beginning to look a lot alike. Diabetic or not, no one achieves optimal health by eating mostly unhealthy foods. But there is no overlooking the fact that, for people with diabetes, the consequences of poor eating habits loom larger and are scarier and more immediate. The fact is that people with diabetes are required to think in a very serious

Unofficially...
Ray Kroc, founder of the McDonald's fast-food restaurants, was a person with diabetes who lived to be over 80 years old.

way about what they eat. Meals have an immediate, daily impact on their blood-sugar levels and, therefore, on their health.

This is why diabetic meal plans are also referred to as *nutritional therapy*. Healthy eating is an integral part of diabetes management.

Diabetes health-care providers recognize that meal plans must be tailored to the individual. If not, it is much harder for people to follow meal plans. It's crucial to your management goals that your meal plan reflect your tastes and habits as much as possible. Your diagnosis, physical condition, and whether you take insulin or medication will also affect your meal plan.

Meal plans may vary, but they share some common principles:

- Your meal plan should make it easier for you to maintain stable blood-sugar levels.

- It should accommodate your daily schedule and activities as much as possible.

- It should reflect your food preferences. (Speak up!)

- It should have some flexibility.

- It should help lower the risk of high blood pressure, heart disease, and kidney disease, especially since people with diabetes face greater risks for developing these disorders.

- A meal plan for people with type 2 diabetes may be designed to encourage weight loss or to prevent weight gain; less body fat equals less insulin resistance. It may call for smaller, more frequent meals to help keep blood-sugar levels stable.

- A meal plan for people with type 1 diabetes will take into account the insulin injection schedule

Bright Idea
Don't think of your meal plan as a "diet." That implies a temporary arrangement, something you might go off. Why not call it your "healthy eating plan" or your "nutritional action plan"?

in order to maximize insulin effectiveness while avoiding hypoglycemia.

Let's look at the way meal plans contribute to stable blood-sugar levels, and how eating interacts with insulin injections or the use of oral medications. In order to understand the way meal plans work, you must first know how foods work in the body. In the next section, we will look at the effect on the body of the different elements in a balanced diet—carbohydrates, fats, protein, and fiber—especially their effect on blood glucose. With this information in mind, we'll then discuss some standard approaches to diabetic meal plans.

Carbohydrates, complex and otherwise

Of all the foods you eat, carbohydrates have the greatest post-meal effect on your blood glucose level. This is true for all people and is normal and healthy as long as there is enough insulin available to handle the increase in blood sugar.

In achieving control of blood sugar, then, it helps if

- Your total daily intake of carbohydrates is not too high or too low, and

- The post-meal glucose release into your blood is not too rapid.

These two principles are fundamental to diabetic meal plans. But let's return for the moment to carbohydrates.

Carbohydrates are starches and sugars, such as grain products, cereals, bread, pasta, potatoes, corn, beans, fruit, fructose (fruit sugar), lactose (milk sugar), corn syrup, other syrups, refined sugar, and honey.

Watch Out!
The National Cancer Institute estimates that diets lacking in fresh fruits and vegetables may contribute to as much as 35 percent of cancers in the U.S. population.

Complex carbohydrates are starchy carbohydrates that do not taste sweet, such as potatoes, beans, pasta, rice, and other grains. These are "complex" carbohydrates because the molecules forming them are linked together in long chains. It takes time for complex carbohydrates to break down during digestion, and they are not fully absorbed until they have reached the intestine.

Simple sugars, in contrast, consist of only a few molecules and are rapidly broken down and absorbed after eating. These are the sugars that are noticeably sweet, like sucrose (table sugar and candy), honey, molasses, and corn syrup. Fructose, or fruit sugar, is a simple sugar, but it is digested more slowly than sucrose. People with diabetes should eat two or three servings of fruit each day, but should avoid fruit juice, which contains no fiber.

Carbohydrates are measured in grams, each of which contains four calories, as does a gram of protein. In contrast, a gram of fat contains nine calories. Obviously, for the same amount of calories and energy, you can eat twice as many grams of carbohydrate as you can of fat. The body finds it easier to extract energy from carbohydrates than from fat or protein. What's more, complex carbohydrates are usually filling and are packed with fiber, vitamins, and minerals. In Appendix D, you'll find a list of the carbohydrate gram and calorie content of many common foods.

Lots of carbohydrates?

These factors make carbohydrates our premier source of energy. Today, we are urged by many nutrition experts to eat diets that are 50 to 60 percent carbohydrates. While this suggestion may be useful for the general population, it may not be appropriate for all people with diabetes. Remember that carbohydrates are the main source of blood glucose. Some people may need to lower the proportion of carbohydrates in their diet in order to maintain healthy glucose levels. It can take time and repeated blood tests before an individual's best nutritional plan comes to light. (See "An important message," later in the chapter for more on whether high-carbohydrate diets are always healthy for people with diabetes.)

Complex good, simple bad? Carbohydrate effects on blood glucose

All the carbohydrates you eat, whether simple or complex, are broken down into glucose. (Protein and fat contribute to glucose, too, but the majority of fat is stored or burned for energy and the majority of protein is used for tissue repair or is excreted.) It has long been believed that simple sugars cause a faster, higher spiking of glucose in the blood, and that this is why sweets and desserts traditionally have been considered forbidden for diabetics.

Modern research has provided a different picture, however. Gram for gram, both complex and simple carbohydrates cause the same rise in blood sugar. (High-fiber carbohydrates, such as beans and bran cereal, are digested more slowly and may cause slower rises in blood sugar.)

Notice that we said gram for gram. One pure gram of pasta, for instance, will have about the same effect on your blood sugar as one pure gram of sparkling white table sugar. The problem is that real life and real food are a little more complicated.

Factors affecting carbohydrate absorption

A number of factors effect how your body absorbs carbohydrates:

■ **The amount of carbohydrate in a serving.** You can't just tell yourself that chocolate pudding has no more effect on your blood sugar than whole-grain bread, so you may as well skip the bread and eat two servings of pudding. Why can't you? Because a serving of pudding has twenty-two grams of carbohydrate, while a slice of bread has eleven. More carbohydrates are packed into some foods, or, rather, some servings of food, especially those high in refined sugar or other simple carbohydrates. You must keep an eye on portion size and total carbohydrate intake.

Consider also what you are getting with your carbohydrates. What is the nutritional content of a given serving? A slice of whole-wheat bread contains lots of fiber and vitamin E, less fat, and fewer calories than chocolate pudding. Is chocolate pudding therefore a forbidden food? Not at all. It simply provides more carbohydrates per serving. And more carbohydrates mean more blood sugar. Adjusting your diet to include carbohydrate-dense foods is a part of meal planning, as discussed later in this chapter.

■ **The presence of other foods.** Carbohydrates combined with fat, fiber, or both are digested more slowly. This somewhat moderates the rise of blood glucose. That's why ice cream is not a good emergency sugar for treating hypoglycemia; the fat in it slows down the absorption of much-needed sugar.

■ **Fiber content.** Fiber is the indigestible part of grains, fruits, and vegetables, what your great-aunt Sadie called "roughage." Fiber is classified as *soluble* and *insoluble* (referring to whether it

Bright Idea
Beans and legumes (such as navy beans, kidney beans, black beans, and lentils) contain gelatin-like fiber that can help lower blood cholesterol and slow the release of glucose into the blood. They are a great food choice!

dissolves in water). Both are good for you and important for maintaining the health of the intestines and bowel. Insoluble fiber is present in wheat bran, whole grains, fruits, vegetables, nuts, and seeds.

Soluble fiber is of special interest to people with diabetes because carbohydrates containing soluble fiber are more slowly digested and release glucose more slowly. Foods containing soluble fiber are oats, fruits, vegetables, and seeds.

- **Food preparation.** Anything that makes a complex carbohydrate easier to digest will speed up the release of glucose into the blood. Imagine the difference between digesting a raw potato and a baked potato. If you take it a step further and mash the potato, it is even easier to digest. In general, the more broken down, processed, refined, or liquid a carbohydrate is—that is, the further it is from its natural state—the quicker its digestion and glucose release.

This is not to say that you shouldn't cook foods. It is simply more information about how carbohydrates work.

Simple sugars are absorbed easily whether they are in a natural state or not. Honey and raw sugar, for example, are as rapidly absorbed as table sugar. See "The Dessert Diet" in Chapter 10 for additional information on fiber and blood sugar.

About artificial sweeteners

Artificial sweeteners that contain calories, called *nutritive sweeteners*, will affect blood sugar, but may do so slowly. Examples are sorbitol, mannitol, and xylitol. These nutritive sweeteners are high in calories and must be counted as carbohydrates in the meal plan, and eating large amounts may cause the

Watch Out!
Check nonfat, low-fat, and sugar-free foods for emulsifiers or bulking agents that are digested as carbohydrates and can affect blood glucose. One common example is maltodextrin.

blood-sugar level to rise, and may also cause diarrhea or cramping.

Nonnutritive sweeteners, like saccharin, aspartame (NutraSweet), and sucralose, contain no calories and do not affect blood-sugar levels. Always check food labels for calorie amounts. Calories may be supplied by other ingredients. The table below provides information about nutritive and non-nutritive sweeteners.

Sweetener	Raises Blood Sugar?
Artificial:	
■ Saccharine (Sweet 'n Low)	No
■ Aspartame (NutraSweet, Equal)	No
■ Sucralose (Splenda)	No
■ Acesulfame potassium (Sunett, Sweet One, DiabetiSweet)	No
■ Stevia (Stevioside)	No
■ D-tagatose	No
■ Sorbitol	Yes
■ Mannitol	Yes
■ Xylitol	Yes
Natural:	
■ Fructose, High Fructose	Yes
■ Dextrose	Yes
■ Maltose	Yes
■ Honey	Yes
■ Corn Syrup	Yes
■ Molasses	Yes

You should be aware of problems that are sometimes associated with artificial sweeteners:

- They can stimulate your "sweet tooth," making you crave sugar.
- They can cause headaches in some people.

- People with a condition called *phenylketonuria* (*PKU*) should not consume aspartame (NutraSweet or Equal).

- Although the Food and Drug Administration does not recommend against pregnant women using aspartame (NutraSweet or Equal), some doctors recommend that pregnant women not use it.

Protein

Most of us grew up believing that lots of protein is essential to strong bodies and good health. And today many diet books still promise quick and easy weight loss through high-protein diets. Others argue that this approach is as archaic as Fred Flintstone's car-toppling side of dinosaur ribs. The majority of nutritionists today promote a balanced diet, one in which protein definitely has its place, but no longer commands center stage.

Sources of protein

Protein comes to us in foods such as beef and pork, poultry, fish, egg whites, milk, and cheese. Beans and legumes are rich sources of protein; grains and vegetables also provide some protein. Our bodies use protein to grow and repair tissue and to make essential enzymes. Growing children and teens, pregnant women, and people recovering from illness or injury all have higher protein needs.

Average protein requirements

What is the average protein requirement for adults? Today's standard recommendation is that protein should make up 10 to 20 percent of our daily caloric intake. For most people, this requirement is easily met by eating three to five ounces, or 60 to 150 grams, of lean protein a day. A four-ounce,

Bright Idea
Tofu (soybean curd) is a high-fiber, mineral-rich, inexpensive source of high-quality protein that is low in saturated fat. It's available at larger grocery stores, often near the produce section. Tofu is an excellent replacement for meat if you are trying to cut down on saturated fats.

120-gram serving of chicken, for example, is about the size of a deck of playing cards. One-third cup of cooked kidney beans provides three grams of protein; one cup of cooked carrots, broccoli, or zucchini gives you four grams. You can see that it does not take huge amounts of meat or other food to meet your daily protein requirements. Indeed, the traditional, red-blooded American serving of meat well exceeds daily needs. Your registered dietitian can provide many more examples of appropriate protein sources and serving sizes.

Unused protein is excreted from the body, and excessive protein can burden the kidneys. People with diabetes must keep kidney health in mind and avoid eating too much protein. People with kidney damage (nephropathy) may need to modestly reduce their protein intake, say, from 10 to 7 percent of daily intake. It is rarely advisable to go lower than this; muscle wasting may result. There is some evidence that protein from vegetable sources is less stressful to kidneys. Ask your registered dietitian or doctor.

Protein's effects on blood glucose

About 30 to 60 percent of the protein you eat is converted to glucose (as compared to roughly 90 percent of carbohydrates and less than 10 percent of fat). Protein is digested more slowly than carbohydrates. When eaten in large amounts with carbohydrates, it can slow the absorption of sugar into the blood stream. When eaten alone, protein usually produces only a small, slow rise in blood glucose.

Fats and cholesterol

Fat is on everybody's lips these days, in more ways than one. Most of us eat a lot of fat, and most of us talk a lot about eating less.

Timesaver
Ask your pharmacist or dietitian about convenient snack bars that are specially prepared for people with diabetes. They're made from slow-acting carbohydrates and can help reduce the risk for hypoglycemia, especially through the night. (They cannot be used to treat hypoglycemia once it occurs, however.)

Gram for gram, fat contains over twice the calories of carbohydrates or protein. Too much dietary fat is a prime culprit in obesity and cardiovascular disease. It's hazardous to your health not to have a basic understanding of dietary fats, especially if you are overweight and have type 2 diabetes.

Major sources of fat in the typical American diet are fried foods, whole-milk products, meats, nuts, mayonnaise, salad dressings, other rich sauces, baked goods, and desserts.

Types of dietary fats

There is a lot of confusion about the different dietary fats and the role of cholesterol. To begin with, how much fat should you eat? Total fat intake should add up to no more than 30 percent of total daily calories. In the average American diet, about half of all calories are from fat.

Some nutritional advisors (such as Dr. Dean Ornish and the Pritikin programs) recommend that fat should constitute as little as 10 percent of daily calories. Most people would have a difficult time following such a restrictive diet. A goal of 20 to 30 percent is widely accepted as practical while providing definite health benefits. It's especially important for people with high cholesterol and triglyceride levels to follow this guideline. High cholesterol and triglyceride levels greatly increase the risk of heart disease, especially for people with diabetes.

We refer to total fat because there are different kinds of fat:

- **Saturated fats.** These are fats that stay solid at room temperature, such as butter, lard, and fat in meats.

- **Polyunsaturated fats.** These fats are at the opposite end of the spectrum from saturated fats;

> **❝**
> To lengthen thy life, lessen thy meals.
> —Benjamin Franklin
> **❞**

they stay liquid even when refrigerated. A good example is safflower oil.

- **Trans-fatty acids, or TFAs (also called *hydrogenated fats*).** These are polyunsaturated fats that have undergone a high-temperature process that transforms them into artificial saturated fats. TFAs are found in margarine, solid vegetable shortening, and partially hydrogenated vegetable oils, which are widely used in commercial baked goods.

- **Monounsaturated fats.** These are in the middle of the saturation spectrum. They show varying degrees of hardening when refrigerated, but don't become solid. Examples include canola oil, olive oil, and peanut oil.

Until recently, doctors and nutritionists recommended polyunsaturated fats as the healthiest. This has changed as evidence has emerged suggesting that polyunsaturated fats may lower the body's levels of the so-called "good" cholesterol (discussed below). These days, monounsaturated fats are recommended as the best dietary choice because they lower only the "bad" cholesterol.

Follow these guidelines, then, in choosing dietary fats:

- *Total fat:* No more than 20 to 30 percent of total daily calories.

- *Saturated fat:* Less than 10 percent of total calories.

- *Polyunsaturated fat:* 5 to 10 percent—no more—of total calories.

- *Monounsaturated fat:* 10 to 15 percent of total calories (that is, close to half of all fat intake; it can make up a higher percentage of daily fat intake if desired).

Timesaver
A quick way to figure out how many grams of fat equals 30 percent of your total daily calories is to take your total—say, 1,200 calories— drop the final digit (making it 120), and divide by three. Voilà! This number is your daily fat gram allowance.

Cholesterol

Cholesterol can be a confusing topic because it's in some foods we eat (those from animal sources only) but it is also produced in our bodies by the liver. The body uses the cholesterol it makes in digestive processes and in making certain sex and adrenal gland hormones.

If we have high cholesterol (200 mg/dl or more), is it because of the cholesterol we eat or because of what our livers produce? The answer is that all saturated fats in our diet tend to raise blood cholesterol whether or not the fatty food we eat contains cholesterol. Most sources of saturated fat also contain cholesterol, like meat, butter, and cheese, but the saturated fat in these foods will do more harm to your cholesterol level than the actual cholesterol in them.

It's an important point because you may make the mistake of avoiding foods with cholesterol while assuming that too many other foods are safe. A convenience food, for instance, may sport a label proudly proclaiming that the food is "Cholesterol-Free!" And indeed it may be. But is it chock-full of partially hydrogenated vegetable oils? These are saturated fats, and they will raise your cholesterol level as surely as will bacon and eggs.

You should limit dietary cholesterol to less than 300 mg per day. But to control your cholesterol level, it is just as important, if not more important, to limit your intake of saturated fats. This means animal fats (in butter, whole milk, meats, eggs, and cheese) as well as these saturated vegetable fats:

- Hydrogenated or partially hydrogenated vegetable oils
- Palm or palm kernel oil

- Coconut oil
- Vegetable shortening
- Cocoa butter

Good and bad cholesterol

These terms do not refer to the cholesterol found in foods. "Good" and "bad" cholesterol are produced in our bodies and circulate in the bloodstream.

- **"Bad" cholesterol** is *LDL*, or *low-density lipoprotein*, cholesterol. It is bad because it accumulates on the inside of blood vessel walls and promotes hardening of the arteries.

- **"Good" cholesterol** is *HDL*, or *high-density lipoprotein*, cholesterol. It is good because it can reduce hardening of the arteries, probably by removing residues from the inner arterial walls.

When you get your cholesterol levels checked, the result will indicate not only your total cholesterol, but also the ratio of LDL to HDL. The higher the amount of HDL, the better.

Replacing saturated fats with monounsaturated fats can help promote "good" cholesterol. Regular exercise can raise your HDL level, and estrogen therapy for women can as well.

Triglycerides: also a risk

Triglycerides are an important part of your blood profile. Like cholesterol, triglycerides are a lipid, or fat, found in the body and the bloodstream. In fact, the majority of fat we eat and the fat in our bodies are triglycerides. All of the dietary fats discussed above are triglycerides, except cholesterol. Triglycerides are also made from the carbohydrates we eat that are not used for blood sugar.

Unofficially...
Some people keep the distinction between "good" HDL and "bad" LDL cholesterol clear in their minds by thinking of *LD* as standing for "Little Devil."

High levels of triglycerides in the blood are considered a risk factor for heart disease. They are also associated with insulin resistance.

The National Cholesterol Education Program lists 200 milligrams as a normal blood level of triglycerides. Levels of 200 to 400 are considered borderline high and call for changes in diet to lower them. Recently, however, research conducted at the University of Maryland Medical Center found significant cardiac risks in people with triglyceride levels from 100 to 200 milligrams—long considered normal, safe levels.

Lowering triglycerides

Triglyceride levels can be lowered by lowering total fat intake. But remember: The body can make triglycerides out of carbohydrates and alcohol, as well. Excessive amounts of sugar, starches, and alcohol can raise triglycerides in the bloodstream. Fortunately, diabetic meal plans help you to manage your intake of these substances.

If you have type 2 diabetes and are insulin resistant, please see "An Important Message," below.

Ways to cut down on fat and cholesterol in your diet

You can reduce the amount of fat you eat by making these changes:

- Avoid fried foods.

- Before cooking, trim fat from meats and remove skin from poultry.

- Choose lean meats, such as beef that is not heavily marbled (loin, round, or flank), low-fat hamburger, and white poultry meat.

- Broil meats without adding fat.

Watch Out!
Beware of hidden fat in foods that are mostly carbohydrate, for instance, hydrogenated fats in biscuit, pancake, and cake mixes, and in commercially prepared granola, cookies, crackers, and chips. Always check ingredients and fat grams per serving!

- Choose reduced-fat cold cuts, and eat them in moderation.

- Choose fish. Broil it without adding fat.

- Eat only low-fat, skim, or nonfat milk, cheeses, and yogurt. (Don't overdo it, or you may exceed your protein limit.)

- Reduce or eliminate butter, margarine, and mayonnaise. All contain large amounts of fat and are easy to eat too much of.

- Use vinegar or lemon juice instead of salad dressing.

- Use nonfat cooking sprays instead of butter or oils.

- Take advantage of the ever-increasing number of reduced-fat and nonfat food items now available. But don't overindulge; these foods are not calorie-free and many contain extra carbohydrates.

Effects of fat on glucose levels

Eating fat does not cause a rise in blood-sugar levels. Fat combined with other foods tends to slow down the digestion of those foods, causing a somewhat slower peaking of glucose. For example, the fat and protein contained in the cheese on a pizza will slow down the digestion of the carbohydrate in the crust.

An important message

Today, the majority of nutrition experts recommend a well-balanced, moderate-carbohydrate, low-fat diet. However, a diet too rich in carbohydrates may increase triglyceride levels and lower "good" cholesterol levels in some people, especially some people with type 2 diabetes who are insulin resistant. Eating more carbohydrates can lead to higher blood-sugar levels and higher insulin levels, which in some people causes triglyceride and cholesterol levels to rise as well.

For some people, blood sugar and blood lipids are better controlled with a diet in which total fat intake is about 45 percent of total calories, instead of the usually recommended 20 to 30 percent, and in which carbohydrates make up about 40 percent of calories, as opposed to 50 to 60 percent.

On such a plan, it is important to remember that saturated fat still must not exceed 10 percent of total daily calories. The increase in fat calories must come from healthy monounsaturated sources, primarily olive and canola oils. Nuts, olives, and avocados may also be used in moderation.

If you are frustrated by persistently high blood sugar and blood lipids despite your best efforts, you may want to discuss the lower-carbohydrate dietary approach with your doctor. It's controversial; medical opinion varies on this approach. But we think you should know that it has proponents. Do not begin a lower-carbohydrate, higher-fat diet without the help and consent of your health-care team. A higher-fat diet requires careful planning to prevent weight gain and higher cardiovascular risks. Follow-up monitoring is extremely important to make sure that the diet is having the desired effect on glucose levels and blood lipids.

One source of information and opinion about the lower-carbohydrate diet is *Dr. Bernstein's Diabetes Solution*, by Richard Bernstein, M.D., and Timothy Aubert (Little Brown, 1997). Another is *Sugar Busters!*, by H. Leighton Steward, M.D. (Random House, 1998).

> **❝**
> We're not pushing the low-carb diet, we're simply explaining it as an alternative. But we confess that we are enthusiastic about this diet approach, both because of our own success with it and because of numerous reports from others telling us how it lifted them out of the despair of never achieving blood-sugar control or weight loss.
> —Editorial, *The Diabetic Reader*, Fall/Winter 1997/8
> **❞**

Alcohol

In its guidelines for doctors who treat diabetes, the American Diabetes Association states that "strict abstinence from alcohol is not necessary for patients with diabetes mellitus." People with diabetes may drink alcohol as everyone who drinks ought to: in moderation, and never if one is driving.

"Moderate" alcohol consumption is usually defined as one drink a day for women and two drinks a day for men. A drink is twelve ounces of regular beer, five ounces of wine, or one-and-one-half ounces of 80-proof liquor or distilled spirits.

The person with diabetes who chooses to drink alcohol should keep the following facts in mind:

> **❝**
> My dietitian explained that one alcoholic drink a day for me is OK, as long as I count it as a food exchange. I don't have a drink every day, but it sure is nice being able to have a beer with friends if I feel like it.
> —Robert, age forty, with type 1 diabetes
> **❞**

- Alcohol is high in calories. One gram of alcohol has almost as many calories (seven) as one gram of fat (nine). In your meal plan, an alcoholic drink may count for ninety calories or two fat exchanges. (We discuss exchange plans below.)

- Alcohol is a simple carbohydrate that is quickly converted into glucose. It can raise your blood-sugar level.

- Alcohol can increase your risk for hypoglycemia (low blood sugar). It interferes with the liver's normal response to low glucose levels, which is to make new glucose. The risk is especially high if you use insulin or oral diabetes medications. In that case, drink alcohol only with meals, never on an empty stomach.

- If you drink excessively (especially if you are a binge drinker), it is unsafe for you to take sulfonylurea oral diabetes medications or the oral medication metformin.

- Drinking alcohol may cause or aggravate hypoglycemic unawareness—the inability to perceive symptoms of hypoglycemia (see Chapter 5).

  If you have been drinking and have hypoglycemia, your judgement may be impaired and you may not be able to help yourself or ask others for help. What's more, people may assume that you are inebriated and not give you the necessary help.

- If you are pregnant, obese, have a history of gastritis, pancreatitis, or liver disease, or have high triglyceride levels, your doctor may well advise you not to drink any alcohol at all.

Meal plans

"Meal plan," "diabetes diet," "nutritional therapy," or "the stuff I eat"—whatever you call it, it is a crucial component of your diabetes management.

What you eat has a direct effect on your blood-sugar levels. You can learn to adjust your diet to optimize your blood-sugar results. This is a major goal of meal plans.

With meal plans, the focus is on good nutrition, but also on managing your carbohydrate intake. Carbohydrates, after all, have the greatest impact on blood sugar. Most meal plans are designed to help you stay within a given range of carbohydrate consumption and to coordinate the effect of carbohydrate intake with that of insulin activity (whether the insulin is natural or injected).

Exchange plans

Exchange plans have been in use for many years. They work by allowing a set number per day of servings from each exchange list, or category of food.

Bright Idea
For help with meal planning, check out one of these software packages: for PCs, Sasquatch Software Inc.'s *Food Smart* ([604] 984-9691, www.food-smart. com) or Nutri-Genie's *Diabetes Meal Planner* ([800] 242-4775, www.users.aol. com/nutrigenie). For Macintosh computers, try Diabetes Educators Inc.'s *Meals 'n Carbs* (888) 302-2727, www.mealsncarbs. com.

You and your dietitian determine your dietary goals and decide on appropriate numbers of servings per meal from each food category.

Usually, seven food categories are used: starch and bread, fruit, other carbohydrates, vegetables, meat or meat substitute (such as beans or cottage cheese), milk, and fat.

Each meal contains one or two servings from several categories. For example, lunch may include one starch, one meat or meat substitute, one vegetable, and one fat. As long as you follow recommended serving sizes, you will be eating a predictable amount of each food type, and not overindulging in one area.

Where does the "exchange" come in? Within each category of foods there are many possible choices, and each one is the nutritional equivalent of and may be exchanged for one of the others. For instance, in the starch category, a serving of bread (one one-ounce slice) is the same as half an English muffin or one-half cup Shredded Wheat cereal. To fulfill a starch exchange for breakfast, you could choose any of these or any other equivalent on the starch list.

In the meat category, one serving (one ounce) of lean beef is the same as one serving (one ounce) of salmon or one-forth cup of low-fat cottage cheese.

Each major category contains many exchanges and is subdivided for thoroughness. For example, the starch list subdivisions include Starch Vegetables; Beans, Peas, and Lentils; and Starchy Foods Prepared with Fat, among others.

Exchange plans allow great variety and choice while keeping overall amounts balanced and consistent. Since portion sizes are built into the plan, there's little need to count grams.

Many foods combine categories. Pepperoni pizza, for instance, combines starch, meat, and fat servings. One piece of pizza could equal three or more separate servings. You get to decide how you use up your allowed exchanges.

Your dietitian or diabetes educator has complete exchange lists. He or she can explain in detail how to follow an exchange plan, as well as work with you to develop a good plan for you. A thirty-two-page exchange list is also available from the American Diabetes Association.

It may take some time at first, but eventually you will become adept at knowing what foods, and what portion sizes, fit into your exchange plan and your daily dietary limits. Your reward should be improved blood-sugar control!

Carbohydrate counting

Another, newer way to control your carbohydrate consumption is by counting the grams of carbohydrate in each serving. With your registered dietitian, you pick a daily number of carbohydrate grams for each day. The total number of carbohydrate grams is distributed among meals and snacks for the day, which helps to keep blood-sugar levels stable.

You'll need to learn the gram content of average portions of many foods. Your dietitian can provide examples to get you started on this, and there are many pocket-sized booklets available that list the carbohydrate grams of hundreds of foods. You will probably be surprised at how quickly you develop a feel for gauging grams.

As long as you familiarize yourself with the gram content of carbohydrate in foods, you have freedom to choose foods and portion sizes. Your goal is to stay within your gram limits. Of course, you also

Watch Out!
Some breads may look like they're made from whole-wheat flour. Check the label: They may be made from refined white flour and have been colored with caramel coloring.

want to make nutritious choices. You could conceivably stay within your limits if the only carbohydrate you ate were refined sugar, but this would not add up to healthy eating.

Balancing carbohydrate counting with insulin use

Carbohydrate counting puts a quantitative value on foods. This can be an advantage for people using multiple daily injections of insulin. You may be able to adjust insulin doses up or down, by one unit or so, based on the number of carbohydrate grams in a meal. So carbohydrate counting could be a tool to help fine-tune your insulin coverage and glucose control.

This use of carbohydrate counting must be tailored to each individual, and should not be undertaken without your doctor's approval.

The glycemic index

The glycemic index was developed in the early 1980s by researchers at the University of Toronto. The index shows how much a serving of a given food will raise blood sugar, which is the glycemic index of that food. The glycemic index of all the foods are compared to the glycemic index of bread. Fifteen grams of bread has a medium glycemic index. If fifteen grams of another carbohydrate causes a higher rise in glucose than bread, it is considered to have a high glycemic index. If its impact is lower than that of bread, it is considered to have a moderate or low glycemic index.

Each food is given glycemic ratings based on different conditions, for instance, whether the food is eaten raw or cooked, cut up or whole, its fiber content, and whether it is eaten alone or in combination with other foods.

> **"**
> Who eats just one cup of "lite" popcorn? For most people, a typical serving size is closer to one bagful than one cupful. Adjust your calories, carbohydrate, and fat count to the serving sizes you normally eat. "Lite" does not mean "free."
> —Patti Bazel Geil, M.S., R.D., C.D.E., writing in *Diabetes Self-Management* magazine, March/April 1998
> **"**

One difficulty in using the glycemic index is that each person's response to foods is different. A potato, for instance, may have a very different glycemic effect in your body than in your best friend's. The glycemic index is also extensive and may be cumbersome to use. Some people with diabetes, however, find it to be very useful in helping to control blood-sugar levels. Another way to use the glycemic index is to perform SMBG after eating certain foods in order to establish your own personal glycemic index, one that is focused on foods you like or have questions about.

The book *Sugar Busters!*, mentioned earlier, contains information on the glycemic index, as well as an abbreviated index. Information on the glycemic index can also be found on the Web site www. mendosa.com.

Away from home: restaurants, parties, and travel

Having diabetes isn't always easy, but no one's saying you have to sit home all day. With just a little extra planning, you're free to hit the road and join the fun.

Dining out

If you take insulin or oral medication, your first priority in dining out is eating on time. A delayed meal could lead to hypoglycemia.

▪ Do not leave the house without your "pocket glucose" or snack. Remember that getting caught in traffic is always a possibility. You may also want to carry an emergency glucagon syringe.

▪ Give some thought to which restaurant hours might be busier than others. Try to avoid long

> 66
> I learned a long time ago that I just don't respond well to 'forbidding' myself certain foods. I just want them more, and then I overdo it! Now I eat what I want. I'm just careful about portions, or how often I have treats.
> —Donna, age thirty-six, with type 2 diabetes
> 99

waits for a table, perhaps by eating earlier or on weekday evenings. If possible, make reservations before dining out.

- Beware the happy hour! It's very dangerous to drink alcohol on an empty stomach. Your risk for hypoglycemia skyrockets under these conditions. Cocktail snacks are little help; they're usually high in fat and loaded with salt. Eat something within your meal plan before drinking, and always drink moderately.

Who said you have to drink alcohol to be happy, anyway?

Once you are safely at your table, here are some tips for healthier restaurant eating:

- Don't hesitate to ask about ingredients used in dishes.

- Most restaurants give large servings. Ask for a doggie bag before you start eating, and immediately halve your portion.

- Ask that your fish or meat be broiled, baked, poached, or grilled without butter or oil.

- Ask that all rich sauces, dressings, gravies, or condiments be served on the side.

- Dip your fork into your side dish of salad dressing before spearing some salad. The dressing on the fork will flavor the salad bite.

- Substitute extra vegetables, salad, tomato slices, or a baked potato for those ubiquitous french fries.

- Remove skin from poultry and breading from breaded foods.

- Don't choose menu items listed as fried, hollandaise, creamy, scalloped, crispy, breaded, in gravy, marinated, or stuffed.

At the salad bar, pass up

- Cheese (except low-fat or skim cottage cheese)
- Egg yolks
- Bacon bits
- Macaroni and potato salads
- Salad dressings that are not low in fat

Parties and social situations

Along with dining in restaurants, parties and get-togethers can challenge even the best-laid meal plan. Your meal plan should leave room for variety, enjoyment, and change, and you will learn to make adjustments that accommodate treats. But, inevitably, there will be times when food is offered that is not in your plan for that day. How will you handle it?

Unfortunately, there is no one set of guidelines that will cover every social situation. So much depends upon the social function and the relationships involved, as well as your own meal plan and treatment goals.

Perhaps the most common difficulty is when someone urges you to eat something that is not in your plan for that day. Now, it won't destroy your treatment plan to eat, say, a piece of Marge's blue-ribbon blueberry pie. But it's not practical or healthy simply to eat whatever is offered all the time. You need to strike a balance between being polite and sticking to your treatment plan.

In some situations, you may be perfectly comfortable telling the truth: "I have diabetes, and I watch what I eat pretty carefully." This can be easy enough, if you're comfortable. For those times when you're not, but need to stick to your plan, it helps to have a few responses in mind:

Bright Idea
During holidays or when friends visit, try eating smaller meals more often throughout the day. You can spread out your daily intake and join in the fun.

Bright Idea
If you're worried
about overeating
at a social func-
tion, have a
healthy, substan-
tial snack before
you go. That
puts you in
charge.

- Ask for "just a bite."

- Ask for a small serving to take with you "for
  later."

- Accept the portion offered, but eat only a bite
  or two.

Remember that it's not at all unusual today to be
improving your diet or watching your weight.

And if you show genuine interest in other people, they will probably never notice what you do or
don't eat.

Travel

The cardinal rule for traveling with diabetes is that
you never leave home without a source of sugar to
fend off or treat hypoglycemia. Glucose tablets or
gel glucose in a tube are ideal for this purpose.
(Some people take emergency glucagon injection
kits with them on longer trips.)

That's sufficient advice for traveling across town.
Here are some tips for longer trips:

- Ask your doctor or nurse educator to provide a
  letter detailing your medication, dosages, any
  allergies you may have, any medicines you
  should not take, whether you use syringes, and
  any other significant issues pertaining to your
  care. Keep this on hand in case of medical
  emergencies while traveling.

- If you will be traveling for an extended period,
  get a physical exam before you go.

- Have current prescriptions on hand in case you
  need refills while traveling.

- Call the American Diabetes Association in the
  area where you will be traveling (if it is in the
  United States). They can give you names and

phone numbers of health-care clinics or providers in that area.

- Wear a medical identification bracelet or necklace indicating that you have diabetes, one that provides a phone number to call in case of a medical emergency.

If you are traveling overseas

Traveling overseas may present special nutritional challenges for people with diabetes. Here are a few suggestions to keep in mind:

- You may want to contact the International Diabetes Federation for information on diabetes resources in the country you are visiting. You may also want to contact the International Association for Medical Assistance to Travelers for a list of English-speaking doctors in other countries. (See the Resource Guide in Appendix B for information on how to contact these organizations.)

- The American Diabetes Association recommends that you learn how to say, "I have diabetes" and "Sugar or orange juice, please," in the language of the country you will be visiting. If you have trouble pronouncing these phrases, write them clearly on a piece of paper to show to people if necessary.

- Carry and wear your diabetes information.

- Stay as close as you can to your usual meal, exercise, and medication routines.

- Keep medications, insulin, syringes, glucagon, and blood-testing equipment handy in your carry-on luggage if you're traveling by plane.

- Carry at least one week of extra supplies and a prescription for each item.

- Protect test strips from extremes of heat or cold. Room temperature (59 to 86°F is fine.

- Keep food and some form of fast-acting sugar handy, if meals are delayed for reasons you can't control.

- Plan ahead for changes in mealtimes (especially when you are crossing two or more time zones). Plan times for testing your blood sugar.

- Ask your doctor about medicine for nausea, vomiting, or diarrhea.

- Find out how and where to obtain emergency medical help where you will be traveling.

Packing supplies and insulin

Packing your insulin and other medical supplies requires special care. Here are some guidelines:

- Always pack twice as much medication and supplies as you think you will need.

- Keep half of your supplies in a bag that you keep with you at all times.

- Insulin must always be protected from extreme heat or cold. Special insulated travel packs for diabetes supplies are advertised by mail-order companies in the pages of magazines like *Diabetes Forecast* and *Diabetes Self-Management* (see the Resource Guide in Appendix B).

- Insulin sold overseas may not be U-100 strength; it may be U-40 or U-80. You must have or buy syringes that match the insulin strength.

- Insulin should be stored in a refrigerator, but not in the freezer.

- If refrigeration is not possible, the bottle of insulin you are currently using can be kept unrefrigerated, as long as it is kept as cool as possible (below 86°F).
- Keep insulin away from heat and light.
- Keep extra bottles of insulin in the refrigerator.
- Never let your insulin freeze.
- Keep the bottle(s) of insulin you're currently using in the refrigerator whenever possible.
- Keep unrefrigerated insulin as cool as possible (below 86°F) and away from heat and light.
- Handle insulin gently. Insulin that is handled roughly is more likely to clump or frost.

  When you travel
- Protect insulin from becoming too hot or too cold (don't leave it in a parked car).
- Keep your insulin with you so it doesn't get lost (When traveling by plane, keep insulin and syringes in a carry-on bag, not in checked luggage).

Adjusting to time zone changes

If you use insulin, you may need to make some adjustments in your insulin schedule on days during which you cross time zones. You may want to discuss your travel plans in detail with your physician or diabetes educator before leaving. Your meal schedule, sleep, and how active you will be while traveling will all affect your insulin use.

  In general, remember that

- Traveling eastward results in a shorter day, so you may need less intermediate-acting insulin.

> **"**
> Once, after a strenuous day of walking in the Peruvian Andes, I grew progressively sweaty, irritable, and weak as my blood sugar plunged. In rudimentary Spanish, I tried desperately to explain to a hotel clerk why I needed orange juice, pronto!
> —Mark Schapiro, a person with type 1 diabetes, writing in *Health* magazine
> **"**

- Traveling westward extends your day, so you may need more insulin.

- To reduce travel-day confusion, keep your watch set on your home time until your first morning in the new time zone.

- Check your glucose level more frequently while traveling.

There's a whole world out there. Enjoy!

Just the facts

- People with diabetes can and do eat sugar.

- In controlling blood sugar, it is the total amount of carbohydrate in the diet that matters most, not the type or source of carbohydrate.

- Most people with diabetes can and do drink alcohol in moderation.

- Saturated fats of all kinds raise cholesterol levels.

- When dining out, the main concerns of the person with diabetes are to eat on time, watch portion size, and watch fat content.

- Insulin sold overseas is often U-40 or U-80 strength, not U-100. Make sure you have the right syringes.

Chapter 9

GET THE SCOOP ON...
The benefits of exercise ▪ How much to exercise
▪ How exercise affects blood sugar ▪ Insulin and
exercise ▪ Endurance exercise and diabetes ▪
Strength training and "middle-age spread"

Everybody Should Be Doing It: Exercise

B y now we've all gotten the message: Just do it! Get out there and get moving. Exercise—frequent aerobic exercise—is the closest thing we have to an all-purpose preventive medicine and, many say, a fountain of youth.

By exercise, we mean aerobic exercise, or steady, rhythmic movements of the large muscles of the lower body, resulting in a slightly elevated heart rate, slightly heavier breathing, and a bit of perspiration—that exercise glow. Examples of aerobic activities are brisk walking, jogging, bicycling, dancing, stair climbing, aerobics classes, hiking, and cross-country skiing.

Health specialists recommend that most of us should aim to get twenty to sixty minutes of aerobic exercise three to five times a week. You should always warm up and stretch your muscles (without bouncing) for five to ten minutes before exercising, and take five to ten minutes to cool down, slowing the heart rate gradually and stretching muscles gently to discourage stiffness.

251

In recent years, that recommendation has come to include regular strength training as well (building muscle strength by using light weights or calisthenics, like push-ups). Healthy muscle is our most metabolically active tissue. Muscles burn more calories than other tissue, particularly fat tissue, which can only store calories. Our muscle mass tends to shrink with age, with the result that we become more and more efficient at storing calories as fat instead of burning them. Both aerobic exercise and light strength training help to keep our bodies healthier, stronger, more efficient, and more youthful. (See the discussion of strength training, below.)

If you are a newcomer to exercise, it is important that you have some instruction in the basics of safe exercising before beginning. If you have access to a certified exercise specialist, you can start with that person. Your registered dietitian or diabetes educator may be able to recommend a specialist who has experience in designing exercise programs for people with diabetes (this is ideal). Many health or sports clubs offer classes for beginners, as do many community recreational centers and schools. Be sure to investigate the credentials of exercise instructors. Look for those who hold college or advanced degrees in exercise physiology or sports medicine, and who are professionally certified, for instance, by the American College of Sports Medicine.

> **"**
> It doesn't feel like a chore anymore. It feels like time for me. I get all my best thinking done when I'm walking, stuff I just don't have time to think about the rest of the day.
> —Donna, age thirty-five, with type 2 diabetes
> **"**

The benefits of exercise

Exercise has long been a pillar of diabetes treatment, as important as diet, blood-sugar monitoring, and pharmacological treatment. This makes perfect sense when we consider that exercise undeniably offers such benefits as

- Improved cardiovascular health and reduced risk for cardiovascular disease.

- Improved cholesterol and triglyceride levels, and increased HDL, or "good," cholesterol.

- Lower blood pressure.

- Easier weight loss.

- Improved bone health and reduced risk for osteoporosis.

- Reduced stress and enhanced sense of well-being.

  Exercise can also

- Lower blood glucose.

- Improve insulin sensitivity.

Timesaver
On days when you can't spare half an hour or more for exercise, try to compensate by getting "bytes" of exercise. Climb stairs, take a walk during your lunch hour, sweep your sidewalk, park further away from the office or store. Some activity is better than none.

Because of its particular benefits, exercise is especially important in the treatment of type 2 diabetes, which is typified by excess weight, inactivity, and insulin resistance. Exercise is also very beneficial for type 1 diabetics, but all people with diabetes need to keep certain precautions in mind in designing and implementing their personal exercise regimens.

Exercising with diabetes: what you should know

We will begin with a perhaps familiar caveat: Never start an exercise program without the advice of your medical doctor. This is especially true for people with diabetes, who should be examined for hypertension and heart disease, eye disease, nerve damage, and foot problems before undertaking exercise. In general, men age forty or older and women age fifty or older should also have a complete physical examination before starting an exercise program.

Watch Out!
If your doctor
has not recom-
mended exercise,
ask why. The
benefits of exer-
cise are too
great to just let
the issue drop.

Many doctors recommend an exercise tolerance or "stress test" for all people with diabetes over the age of 35. There are several tests that evaluate the functioning of your heart as you exercise. Many people with type 2 diabetes are older and have led sedentary lives prior to their diagnosis, and they are also more likely to have had diabetes for some time before being diagnosed. During that time complications may have developed. But whether your diabetes is type 1 or type 2, you should discuss your plans for exercise with your health-care team—if they haven't beaten you to it with a strong recommendation to exercise! And if you haven't been exercising, plan to increase your activity gradually.

Exercise and insulin resistance

As we mentioned above, exercise increases insulin sensitivity, or reduces insulin resistance. This is a major boon to type 2 diabetics. When you exercise, your muscles need more energy. They need to absorb more glucose from the bloodstream. If you exercise consistently, your muscle cells become more accustomed to responding to insulin, so that the muscles can absorb enough glucose. It may be, in fact, that regular exercise stimulates your muscle cells to increase the number of their insulin receptors.

Furthermore, if you lose fat from your body— that is, if your body mass decreases—the amount of insulin you need decreases as well. Exercise promotes fat loss and enhances the action of insulin.

The effects of exercise on blood-sugar levels

In general, exercise lowers the amount of sugar in the bloodstream, because during exercise the body uses this source of energy. The lowering effect is noticeable up to twenty-four hours following exercise, because the body continues to absorb glucose from the blood in order to replenish it in muscle and liver cells, where it is stored as glycogen.

Be aware, however, that exercise can raise blood-sugar levels under certain conditions. Both hypo- and hyperglycemia can occur during or as a result of exercise, depending upon the interaction of a number of factors.

Let's take a look at the "highs and lows" of exercise.

Exercise and hypoglycemia

How does hypoglycemia occur as a result of exercise? Again, exercise calls on the body's stores of glycogen, and also uses the glucose circulating in the blood. The greater demand for energy leads to a decrease in blood sugar.

What's more, exercise can speed up the absorption of injected insulin by increasing the flow of blood throughout the body. This effect is heightened if insulin is injected into a part of the body that is active during exercise, like the thigh or buttock.

When insulin levels are high, the liver tends not to release its stored glucose, again increasing the risk of hypoglycemia.

If insulin circulates and is absorbed more quickly at the same time that blood glucose is being burned for fuel, it's easy to see how low blood sugar could occur—especially if the person exercising has not eaten for some time and has injected insulin not long before exercising.

Taking a sulfonylurea medication can also increase your chances for developing hypoglycemia during exercise, although the risk is greater for

Unofficially...
People with dia-
betes who use
insulin and who
consistently fol-
low fitness pro-
grams over time
often find that
they can reduce
their total daily
insulin dose by
as much as 15 to
20 percent.

insulin users. Sulfonylureas increase the chance that there will be too much insulin in the bloodstream relative to the amount of glucose.

Exercise and hyperglycemia

In some cases, exercise can lead to elevated blood sugar, and even to diabetic ketoacidosis in type 1 diabetics. (Diabetic ketoacidosis [DKA] is discussed in Chapter 5.)

High blood sugar can occur when a person's insulin levels are low at a time when he or she engages in moderate to vigorous exercise, prompting the liver to release stored glucose. Under these conditions, blood glucose rapidly rises. In people whose insulin levels are low, the blood glucose level often is high before exercise is begun, which further increases the odds for hyperglycemia.

Exercise-induced hyperglycemia can persist for hours after exercise.

Avoiding highs and lows

Don't let the specter of ups and downs stop you from pursuing an appropriate, personalized exercise program. It's true that several factors need to be balanced to ensure successful exercise, such as:

- Your blood-sugar level before exercising.

- How long it's been since you ate.

- When you last injected insulin.

- How vigorously you exercise, and for how long.

Remember that these are all factors over which you have some measure of control. The box on the following page provides tips for coordinating them.

Adjusting your insulin

Adjusting your insulin treatment for exercise is something you will have to discuss with your doctor.

> ### Strategies to Avoid Hypoglycemia and Hyperglycemia with Exercise
>
> 1. Eat a meal 1 to 3 hours before exercise.
> 2. Take supplemental carbohydrate feedings at least every 30 minutes during exercise if exercise is vigorous and of long duration.
> 3. Increase food intake for up to 24 hours after exercise, depending on intensity and duration of exercise.
> 4. Take insulin at least 1 hour before exercise. If less than 1 hour before exercise, inject in a non-exercising area.
> 5. Decrease insulin dose before exercise.
> 6. Alter daily insulin schedule.
> 7. Monitor blood glucose before, during, and after exercise.
> 8. Delay exercise if blood glucose is more than 250 mg/dl (more than 14 mmol/l) or ketones are present.
> 9. Learn individual glucose responses to different types of exercise.
>
> Source: *Therapy For Diabetes Mellitus And Related Disorders,* 3rd ed., American Diabetes Association, 1998, reprinted with permission.

It is also something that you will tailor based on the blood glucose monitoring you do as a part of exercising. Here are some general guidelines on insulin adjustment:

- Avoid injecting insulin into active limbs.
- Moderate exercise lasting less than thirty minutes rarely requires insulin adjustment. A snack before exercise may be all that is needed to keep blood sugar from dropping too low.
- For most people doing moderate exercise for no longer than forty-five to sixty minutes, the

insulin dose covering that period of the day usually need not be reduced by more than about 20 percent. Check with your diabetes team for specific dose adjustments.

■ For prolonged, vigorous exercise, it may be necessary to decrease total daily insulin by as much as one-third to one-half. This means making coordinated reductions in both longer- and shorter-acting insulins.

Recommendations will vary from person to person and with individual insulin therapy regimens. If you use an insulin pump, talk to your doctor about removing the pump during exercise. Follow your doctor's recommendation. There will be more discussion of intense exercise later in the chapter.

Adjusting your oral diabetes medication

If you are not taking insulin, your blood-sugar levels are not as likely to swing dramatically up or down with exercise. You will still need to be on the lookout for glucose highs and lows, however. Ask your doctor if you should make any adjustments in the amount of medication you take on days when you exercise. Some general guidelines are to exercise:

■ One to three hours after eating a meal or snack to help avoid hypoglycemia.

■ Only if your blood glucose level is under 200 mg/dl to avoid hyperglycemia. (If it is 200 mg/dl or higher, check your urine for ketones.)

■ During times when your oral medications are not at their peak action.

Blood glucose monitoring and exercise

Blood glucose monitoring is as indispensable to your exercise program as it is to the rest of your

> **❝**
> I started to realize that another good reason to avoid 'going low' is that you have to eat to get back up! That doesn't make a whole lot of sense if you're trying to lose weight.
> —Angela, age forty-six, with type 2 diabetes
> **❞**

diabetes management plan. Frequent SMBG will help you know what to do to keep glucose levels stable and sustain your performance. Follow these American Diabetes Association guidelines for SMBG:

- Check your glucose about thirty minutes before exercising.

- If your level is less than 100 mg/dl, eat a snack to bring it up, wait fifteen to thirty minutes, and test again before exercising.

- If your level is 100 to 250 mg/dl, you should be able to exercise.

- If your level is 250 mg/dl or higher, check your urine for ketones. If the test is negative, you may exercise. If it is positive, take insulin or follow the plan recommended by your health-care team. Do not exercise until ketones are negative and blood sugar is stable. Be sure to test your blood again following exercise.

You should perform SMBG during exercise if

- You suspect you are becoming hypoglycemic.

- You are exercising for more than one hour (monitor every thirty minutes).

- You want to know how a particular exercise is affecting your glucose.

- You are pregnant.

Always perform SMBG after you are finished exercising. Adjust food intake or insulin use as needed, based on your recommended treatment plan. Check for effects of exercise later—at night and the day after exercising.

Watch Out!
If you use insulin, your risk for developing exercise-induced hypoglycemia is increased if you exercise sporadically or spontaneously without adjusting your insulin dose. Stick to a consistent exercise program, and always make the recommended insulin adjustments.

Choosing an exercise

There is no type of exercise that is especially beneficial to people with diabetes. In general, health professionals recommend that each of us engage in moderate-intensity aerobic exercise for twenty to sixty minutes at a time, three to five days a week. Whether you jog, walk, swim, dance, play sports or take aerobics classes, your body will benefit from regular aerobic conditioning. The exercise you choose is largely a matter of personal preference.

Risks from diabetic complications: unsafe exercise

However, don't forget that your overall physical condition must be professionally evaluated and taken into consideration in choosing your aerobic activities. Certain activities may be off-limits if you have any of the following conditions:

- **Volatile or difficult-to-control blood glucose.** Your health-care team may recommend against very strenuous or prolonged physical activity.

- **Cardiovascular disease.** Your exercise program must be carefully developed by your doctor or by a cardiac rehabilitation specialist to avoid overstressing the heart. Your response to a personal conditioning program must be carefully and regularly monitored. In some cases, heart disease may be present without noticeable symptoms, especially in people with diabetes. Consider getting a stress test before beginning an exercise program.

- **Proliferative retinopathy.** Exercise that increases blood pressure, even briefly, can cause a worsening of this eye disorder. Heavy lifting or straining should be avoided, as well as exercises that put pressure on the abdomen. Also dangerous is rapid head movement or any exercise that might jar the head. This may include jumping rope or high-impact aerobics classes. Body-contact sports are not advised.

- **Peripheral neuropathy.** Numbness in your feet or legs makes you more vulnerable to tissue and joint injuries. Your doctor may advise you to limit running or jogging. High-quality footwear is essential.

- **Pregnancy.** Your physician should approve any exercise you do. Avoid strenuous exercise like running or high-impact aerobics; walking, swimming, and low-impact or upper-body aerobics are safest.

Mild, moderate, or intense exercise?

Is walking enough? How about folk dancing? Or do I have to run a marathon in order to be truly fit?

Here again, the answer depends upon your overall physical condition, your personal preferences, and your personal goals. What may be a moderately intense aerobic exercise for you may be high or low intensity for someone else. You may need to begin with five or ten minutes of walking, and build up to longer time periods, or you may already be jogging for forty-five minutes and thinking about intensifying your exercise to train for a ten kilometer race. In either case, the exercise you are doing is providing physical benefits.

Above all, pick a type or types of exercise you enjoy and can stick with.

Gauging exercise intensity: checking your pulse

How do you gauge the intensity of your exercise so that you know it is providing aerobic benefits? Back in the early days of the aerobics movement, in the

Bright Idea
Make one, some, or all of your exercise sessions a regular appointment with a buddy. You'll be more motivated to stick to your plan if you know that a friend is expecting you.

> **❝** Moderate exercise gives you most of the physiological and psychological health benefits of more intensive forms of exercise while minimizing the risks of injury, both to your musculoskeletal system and to your heart.
> —Dean Ornish, M.D., in his best-selling book, *Eat More, Weigh Less* (HarperCollins, 1993) **❞**

1970s, fitness experts stressed the heart rate, counseling exercisers to determine their maximal heart rates (the number 220 minus your age) and check their pulse rates during exercise. (Find your pulse by placing your fingertips on your wrist or on the side of your neck.) Using this method, the intensity of exercise is based upon the percentage of the maximal heart rate attained:

- An example of low-intensity exercise would be twenty minutes at 60 percent of your maximal heart rate.

- Moderately intense exercise lasts for twenty to forty-five minutes at 65 to 80 percent of your maximal heart rate.

- High-intensity exercise lasts for forty-five to sixty minutes at 80 to 90 percent of your maximal heart rate.

To calculate what your heart rate should be for moderate exercise, subtract your age from 220. Multiply this number by .65 and by .8. These two numbers give you the higher and lower ends of the heart rate range in which effective, moderate-intensity exercise occurs. Divide both numbers by six to get a heart rate number that can be determined by a ten-second check of your pulse rate.

For example, say you are forty-five years old:

Maximum heart rate: $220 - 45 = 175$

For low-intensity heart rate: $175 \times .65 = 113$ beats per minute

For high-intensity heart rate: $175 \times .8 = 140$ beats per minute

Take 113 and 140 and divide each by 6 to find heart rates for a ten-second check:

$$113 \div 6 = 19$$
$$140 \div 6 = 23$$

Now you know that to achieve moderate-intensity exercise, your heart rate during a ten-second pulse check should be somewhere between nineteen and twenty-three beats.

Perceived exertion

Today, many people still use pulse check methods. Many others, however, have learned to gauge the intensity of their exercise based on their own perceived level of exertion, a commonsense approach endorsed by many exercise specialists. How hard you feel you are working during exercise tells you whether the exercise intensity is low, moderate, or high. Generally speaking,

- If you are sweating somewhat and your breathing is somewhat labored—that is, you are able to keep up a conversation, but not without taking a breath every few words or so—then you are probably performing moderately intense exercise and are experiencing aerobic conditioning.

- If you are gasping for breath and unable to speak, you are exercising too hard for optimal benefits. This is *anaerobic* ("without oxygen") exercise.

- If you can talk easily while exercising, you are probably not exercising vigorously enough.

Some people recommend singing as the test. If you can sing uninterruptedly while exercising, it's time to step up the pace. While exercising, you should be thinking "Hmm. This pace pushes me a bit. I notice I am working a bit."

Moneysaver
Many people invest in expensive exercise equipment or a year-long health-club membership, hoping this will inspire them to begin an exercise program. Don't make major purchases until exercise is a habit, a part of your life. You don't need expensive equipment to start a walking program!

Should you monitor your heart rate?

It is imperative that you discuss this with your health-care team. It should come up when you are examined before beginning an exercise program. People with diabetes are at higher risk for cardio-vascular disease, kidney disease, and eye disease, all of which are aggravated by high blood pressure. Your doctor may want to evaluate your heart rate and blood pressure response during exercise. Generally, your doctor will want to make sure that your systolic blood pressure never exceeds 180 during exercise. He or she may ask you to monitor your heart rate during exercise to make sure you stay within moderate levels of intensity.

Furthermore, if you have autonomic neuropathy that is affecting your heartbeat, your doctor may need to determine your actual maximal heart rate through tests. A simple formula will not be accurate.

Unofficially...
Have you heard of the International Diabetic Athlete's Association? The IDAA can be reached at 1647-B West Bethany Home Road, Phoenix, AZ 85015, or call (800) 898-4322.

Stop!

Always stop exercising and seek medical consultation if

- You experience difficulty breathing or shortness of breath.

- You experience pain, pressure, or aching in the chest, arm, back, or jaw.

- You feel lightheaded or faint.

- Your heartbeat is unusually rapid, slow, or irregular.

- You have persistent pain anywhere, especially in your joints.

- You experience any symptoms of hypoglycemia. Check your blood and take appropriate action.

Strength training

You may be thinking, "Look, I put in my three to five aerobic sessions a week. Now you tell me I need to start lifting weights, too?"

Well, it's your decision. Make it an informed one. Consider these benefits of adding a light muscle-building component to your fitness regime:

- Well-toned, larger muscles burn more calories, even at rest.

- Toning your muscles can reduce calcium loss from bones.

- Stronger muscles can help protect joints from strain.

- Stronger muscles make everyday chores and activities easier to do.

- Strength training may help prevent "middle age spread." As we age, we tend to lose muscle mass, which is slowly replaced by fat. As that happens, our bodies burn fewer and fewer calories. Eventually the fat starts to win.

We're not talking here about attaining the bulging, 0 percent body fat, I-live-in-the-gym-and-maybe-take-steroids physiques you see on the covers of bodybuilding magazines. Like aerobic exercise, strength training need not be intense in order to provide benefits. It's mostly a matter of recognizing that you do have muscles, and that they play a role in your metabolism and fitness. They're not just along for the ride.

Ask your doctor or health-care team

Let your doctor know you would like to begin a light weight-training or floor-exercise (calisthenics such as push-ups, squats, and lunges) program to tone

Watch Out!
Beware of post-exercise hypo-glycemia, which can occur six to twenty-four hours after pro-longed exercise, while the body uses blood glu-cose to replenish the muscle glycogen burned during exercise. Post-exercise hypoglycemia can occur during the night or on the day following exercise.

your muscles. Ask him or her to examine you for any reason why you should not begin such a program. Ask for your doctor's recommendations about beginning strength training.

Proper technique matters

You can start an aerobics program with a good pair of walking shoes and the great outdoors. Unfortunately, starting a strength training program is not as simple as that. You will need training in safe and correct ways to perform muscle building exercise. Lifting weights or stressing muscles improperly is not only dangerous, it is ineffective and a waste of your time.

Here are some suggestions for getting instruction in strength training:

- Check your library or book store for books on weight training. Look for a recently published book that is written for the average person. Check out strength-training sections in good exercise or fitness books.

- Check your local YMCA, community recreation center, community college, or other centers of adult education for introductory courses on weight lifting or strength training.

- Look for videos on strength training that you can rent or buy. Before choosing one, you might want to find an article in a consumers' guide magazine or book that rates exercise videos. Health and fitness magazines also periodically rate exercise equipment and videos.

- Check out fitness shows on television.

- Join a health club. If you belong to a club, ask about strength-training classes for beginners.

■ Hire a personal trainer. Even one or two sessions can get you off on the right foot.

It's not necessary to invest in expensive home machines. Done properly, lifting small weights (even soup cans!) or doing floor exercises is just as effective.

Of course, if you know you'll use a fancy machine and you want to splurge . . . .

For all you ironfolk: diabetes and intensive exercise

One look at television coverage of the New York and Boston marathons tells the story: Today, many, many people are attracted to the challenge of pursuing intensive, "elite" athletic and fitness goals. People who aren't running marathons may be found bicycling across America, trekking in the Himalayas, kayaking, windsurfing, or scaling mountain peaks in national parks from coast to coast.

Unless your doctor has told you otherwise, having diabetes should not stop you from pursuing endurance activities.

For people with diabetes, a challenge

Managing prolonged, strenuous exercise can be difficult, however. It is a challenge that people with diabetes should not take lightly, especially those who use insulin. You must discuss your goals and plans with your health-care team. Don't fail to get their approval before plunging into more intensive activities. You and your team will need to review your treatment plan and make any changes necessary to safeguard your health.

The insulin pump can be a boon to people who engage in prolonged exercise because it eliminates the need to stop for injections. Very athletic people

Bright Idea
When exercising
outside the
home, always
carry personal
identification
and a medical-
alert bracelet,
necklace, or tag
that indicates
you have dia-
betes and gives
a phone number
to call in case
of a medical
emergency.

who use insulin may want to discuss this option with their physicians.

General guidelines for prolonged exercise

Keeping your blood glucose stable during prolonged exercise requires balancing your meal content, meal timing, and insulin use. It also calls for glucose tests during the period of exercise. Some commonly recommended guidelines are

- Do SMBG one hour before exercising, and again thirty minutes before. This will tell you if you are heading "up" or "down" so that you can take steps to correct the situation before committing to a lengthy and demanding activity.

- Test your glucose periodically during the exercise period. How often you do this will depend upon your glucose control patterns, your experience with this type of exercise, and your doctor's recommendation.

- Eat a snack containing twenty to twenty-five grams of carbohydrate every thirty minutes during prolonged exercise. Discuss with your dietitian or doctor appropriate snacks for your needs.

Insulin use and prolonged exercise

Engaging in prolonged exercise can significantly change your insulin needs on the days you exercise. This is why it is very important to perform SMBG frequently when you are beginning a new type of exercise or when you are increasing the duration or intensity of your exercise. You need to know how your personal insulin needs are affected.

You also need to consult your health-care team about the right way to change your insulin treatment on exercise days. Do not attempt to make these changes yourself.

To give you a sense of how your insulin regimen might possibly be affected, here are some ways in which your doctor might alter your regimen:

- Remember that it is usually best not to inject insulin within one hour of exercising and to avoid injecting into active limbs.

- If you take a single morning dose of intermediate-acting insulin, this may be reduced by 30 to 35 percent on the day of exercise.

- A single morning dose may be changed on the day of exercise to a split dose, taking 65 percent of the usual dose in the morning and 35 percent before dinner.

- If you take a mixed dose of short- and intermediate-acting insulin, the short-acting insulin may be decreased by 50 percent.

- Short-acting insulin may be omitted altogether.

- Intermediate-acting insulin may be decreased prior to exercise, with supplemental doses of short-acting insulin to be taken later if needed.

- Post-exercise insulin doses need to be adjusted based upon SMBG and previous experience with hypoglycemia following exercise.

These examples show that your insulin needs can really change with prolonged exercise. Again, you should closely monitor your exercise response and work with your team to develop the best care plan for you.

Keep an eye on your feet

Proper foot care is essential for all people with diabetes, but especially for those who exercise. Follow these guidelines:

Unofficially...
Peter Powers, M.D., has type 1 diabetes and ran the Boston Marathon in two hours and thirty-eight minutes in 1979, one of the fastest times on record for a person with diabetes (and a fast time for anyone!).

Bright Idea
Planning to participate in a marathon? Call the race sponsors beforehand to find out whether blood-sugar testing booths and medical personnel will be available along the course (they often are). Make sure you know where on the course the booths are located.

- Stop problems before they start: Invest in well-fitted sports shoes that are designed for the activity you choose and that "breathe" (leather or natural fabric canvas).

- If you have numbness in your feet, you may need to have a podiatrist (foot doctor) check your shoes for proper fit.

- Always test shoes for comfort before buying. Don't try to break in painful, uncomfortable shoes.

- Wear well-padded, seamless sports socks designed to keep perspiration away from your skin.

- Check your feet daily for redness, irritation, blisters, areas of heat, areas of numbness, ingrown toenails, or toenails that are separating from the toe. Don't delay if you spot a problem; get proper treatment right away.

Just the facts

- People with diabetes benefit from regular exercise.

- "The exercise prescription" has long been a central component of diabetes treatment.

- Exercise can cause both hypoglycemia (low blood sugar) and hyperglycemia (high blood sugar). It must be balanced with food intake, insulin adjustments, and glucose monitoring.

- Some forms of exercise are harmful for people with diabetes-related complications. You should have a complete physical examination before beginning an exercise program.

- Men age forty and older and women age fifty and older should always have a complete physical before beginning an exercise program, whether or not they have diabetes-related complications.

- Aerobic exercise need not be intensive to be beneficial.

- Foot care is essential for all people with diabetes, but especially those who exercise.

GET THE SCOOP ON...
Different types of alternative medicine ▪ The
five centers and the six factors ▪
Doshas, ch'i, and meridians ▪ The desert diet ▪
Herbal remedies and diabetes ▪ Alternative
medicine and doing your homework

A New Age? Diabetes and Alternative Medicine

Chapter 10

In 1990, Americans spent $13.7 billion on alternative medical treatments, according to a 1993 survey published in the *New England Journal of Medicine*. Most of that huge sum came directly out of pocket.

In 1992, the National Institutes of Health established the Office of Alternative Medicine, dedicated to supporting and researching holistic and alternative medical treatments and practices. Today, the OAM supports research being conducted at such top-drawer institutions as Harvard Medical School, Columbia University, and Stanford University.

In 1996, Oxford Health Plans (a large HMO) offered some of its 1.4 million health insurance consumers "complementary therapy" coverage, providing for acupuncture, massage therapy, nutrition counseling, naturopathy, yoga, and chiropractic treatments.

Watch Out!
The majority of treatments and approaches classified as "alternative medicine" have not yet been subjected to extensive scientific research. Don't be swayed by jargon or personal testimonials. At your library or bookstore, ask for help in locating information on clinical studies conducted by reputable scholars or institutions.

These signs of the times suggest that we are entering a new age of medical treatment. Not a time in which standard or conventional medical treatments will be overturned—that is both unlikely and unnecessary—but one in which standard treatments may be supported or enhanced by alternative measures.

The very fact that alternative medicine is being scientifically researched brings it closer to the mainstream of traditional American medicine (sometimes called *allopathic medicine*). *Alternative medicine* is usually defined as a body of healing practices that are not taught or performed in the United States. A second characteristic of alternative medicine is that many of its practices, such as acupuncture, chiropractic, homeopathy, and naturopathy, have not been subjected to the rigorous scientific investigation that is the cornerstone of traditional (and modern) Western medicine. Even though our reliance on science and technology is greater than ever, alternative medicine is growing in popularity. Many people, especially those who suffer from chronic diseases, feel that traditional medicine fails to take the whole person—body, soul, and emotions— into consideration. They argue that standard medical treatment is cold and less effective as a result. And adherents of alternative medicine point out that the practices some people call "new age," "holistic," or just plain "weird" have ancient and venerated histories in other countries, such as China and India.

For now, the fate of alternative medicine in America is unclear. Research into what works and what doesn't work is underway, but it is far from conclusive. In the meantime, more people are choosing alternative treatments. It makes sense to educate

ourselves about what is being offered, and to carefully research the scientific status of any alternative
medicine that we might choose for ourselves.

Types of alternative medicine: sorting it out

The term *alternative medicine* is a broad one. It covers
certain philosophical attitudes toward medical practice (such as holistic medicine, homeopathy, and
naturopathy) as well as specific treatments and techniques (such as acupuncture, biofeedback, and
herbal remedies).

Holistic medicine

This is an umbrella term that is often used inter-
changeably with the term *alternative medicine*. It does
not refer to one specific type of treatment. *Holistic
medicine* is medical practice that treats diseases by
focusing on the whole person, not just the illness.
Holistic medicine also

- Focuses on treating the causes of disease, not
  just the symptoms, and looks at the patient's
  whole lifestyle, including nutrition, stress, and
  personal relationships.

- Emphasizes prevention of disease and maintaining optimal health, as opposed to treating
  disease only.

- Holds that the interrelationship between mind
  and body is a crucial component of physical
  health, and that emotional, mental, and spiritual factors affect health.

Any health-care practitioner can adopt a holistic
approach if he or she chooses. There are medical
doctors who have had traditional medical training
but consider themselves to be holistic practitioners

> **"**
> Responsible prac-
> titioners of
> alternative medi-
> cine do not
> claim, for exam-
> ple, that they
> can cure cancer
> or multiple
> sclerosis. Rather,
> they believe their
> methods can
> marshal forces in
> the body that
> may help to
> combat illness in
> concert with
> conventional
> medicine.
> —Jane E. Brody,
> health writer, in
> the *New York
> Times*
> **"**

because of their philosophical approach to health care. Many such doctors have received additional training or certification in an area of alternative medicine.

Homeopathy

This controversial school of medical thought emerged in Germany in the 1700s and was developed by a doctor named Samuel Hahnemann. Hahnemann sought an alternative to the brutal medical practices of his time, such as bloodletting and purging (both of which were used to treat diabetes!).

The word *homeopathy* is from the Greek words for "like" (as in *similar*) and "disease." This reflects the core premise of homeopathy, which is that the symptoms of illness indicate that healing is occurring. Symptoms should not be suppressed; they are a sign that the body is healing itself. Therefore, if symptoms can be induced or exaggerated, the body will heal. Homeopathic health care makes use of mild dilutions of minerals and herbal substances that are thought to induce symptoms of the illness being treated.

There have been no studies that conclusively support the homeopathic philosophy.

Naturopathy

The naturopathic practitioner believes that the human body possesses the inherent ability to heal itself. This ability depends upon a state of balance and harmony with the many natural forces of health, for example, air, light, healthy food, emotional well-being, relaxation, sound sleep, and exercise. The ill person is experiencing an imbalance of these forces or is disconnected from some or all of them.

Watch Out!
If you have diabetes and are considering adding some form of alternative medicine to your regular treatment, talk to your doctor first. An alternative treatment could interact with your standard care, or even interfere with it. Some herbs, vitamins, and supplements can be toxic, alone or in combination with prescription drugs.

The naturopathic practitioner is holistic in approach and does not rely solely on drugs to treat disease. He or she examines many areas of the patient's life, and recommends such measures as nutritional change, herbal remedies, stress reduction, meditation, massage, and breath control to complement any traditional treatments used.

Ayurvedic medicine

Ayurvedic medicine, or *Ayurveda,* is another holistic system of healing that evolved in India 3,000 to 5,000 years ago. This ancient tradition holds that health comes from the balancing and nurturing of basic life energies within the body. Ayurveda focuses not on treating specific symptoms, but on enhancing life energy, which is within us and around us. Ayurvedic medicine views each person as having one of several distinct body types, or doshas. A person's dosha, or basic physical constitution, helps to determine what course of treatment is best.

The Ayurvedic practitioner typically relies on herbal treatments, meditation, and massage to encourage the body's natural healing tendencies. He or she believes that our life experiences and our emotional and spiritual development play an important role in our health, and may make recommendations for changes in these areas.

Traditional Chinese medicine

The basic tenets of Chinese medicine have been recorded in documents dating from the 2nd century BC. This ancient holistic tradition sees the body as having five centers of vital activity: the heart or mind, the lungs, the liver, the spleen, and the kidneys. It also identifies six factors that can cause disease in the body: wind, cold, heat, moisture, dryness, and fever. Finally, traditional Chinese

Watch Out!
If you consult a naturopath, make sure he or she has a Naturopathic Doctor (N.D.) degree from one of the three accredited universities of naturopathy: John Bastyr College of Naturopathic Medicine in Seattle, WA; The National College of Naturopathic Medicine in Portland, OR; or Southwest College of Naturopathic Medicine in Scottsdale, AZ.

medicine identifies moods or emotions that will harm health if they are too extreme, including worry, anger, and grief, as well as surprise and extreme happiness. In Chinese medicine, disease is caused by imbalances in any or all of these factors and by interactions between them. A practitioner of Chinese medicine might look not only at the patient's physical symptoms, but also his food preferences, personal relationships, language, facial expressions, mood, and gestures. The prescription for treatment might include suggestions for improvements in diet, relationships, or outlook.

Another basic principle of Chinese medicine is that health is affected by the flow of energy, or *chi* (pronounced *chee*), through the body. Treatments such as acupuncture, acupressure (a form of massage), and certain forms of healing touch are meant to redirect, release, or balance the flow of *chi* within the body. Martial art and other techniques for disciplined body movement, like tai c*hi*, are also believed to enhance the body's use of c*hi*.

Along with acupuncture and other manipulations of c*hi*, herbal remedies, or "botanical medicines," are central to traditional Chinese medicine. Ginseng, mint, bear's gall, safflower, and Chinese ephedra (*mahuang*) are just a few of the hundreds of plants and herbs that have been used for centuries by Chinese practitioners.

Common specific treatments

Some treatment modalities that fall under the general category of alternative medicine are more widely available than others.

Acupuncture

This "alternative" treatment is rapidly becoming part of mainstream medicine in the United States.

Bright Idea
Contact the National Institutes of Health's Office of Alternative Medicine for help in evaluating alternative medical practices. The telephone number is (888) 644-6226, or visit the NIH's Web site at www.nih.gov.

Acupuncture is the ancient Chinese practice of inserting very fine needles into specific points in the body. The purpose is to unblock or free up the flow of *ch'i* (life energy) into that part of the body, restoring it to health.

Unofficially...
4,000 of America's 10,000 licensed acupuncturists are medical doctors (M.D.s).

The acupuncture needle may not be inserted into the area that is actually painful or ill. The practitioner chooses the insertion site based on his or her understanding and training regarding nerve or *ch'i* pathways.

Practitioners of traditional Chinese medicine believe that *ch'i* flows through the body along certain set pathways, or *meridians*. They believe that *ch'i* must flow freely through all meridians for optimal health. Acupuncture improves health and clears up specific symptoms by unblocking the flow of *ch'i*. The meridians are said to come into contact with the body's surface at about 360 different acupuncture points. Needles are inserted at select points to influence the flow of *ch'i*.

Western practitioners of acupuncture (and its allied treatments, acupressure and electrostimulation) are more likely to believe that acupuncture is effective because it stimulates the nervous system to release endorphins, the body's natural "feel good" hormones. Endorphins can reduce pain and improve mood.

Acupuncture is used to provide local anesthesia during medical procedures. It is also used to treat pain, nausea, and nerve damage.

Acupuncturists should be licensed by the American Academy of Medical Acupuncture or by the American Association of Acupuncture and Oriental Medicine.

Never allow an acupuncturist to insert a needle into your abdomen if you are pregnant or into any

Bright Idea
When it is done correctly, acupuncture is not painful. But if you don't want to be treated with needles, consider acupressure. In this treatment, pressure is applied to the same areas where an acupuncturist would insert a needle.

growth that may be cancerous. All acupuncture needles should be sterile (germ free). Ask the practitioner how he or she sterilizes needles.

Chiropractic

Chiropractic, or spinal manipulation, is perhaps the most familiar alternative treatment in America. It has been widely available for over 100 years, and has long been controversial. Over time, evidence has shown that some chiropractic treatment may offer certain benefits.

For example, in 1994 the United States Department of Health and Human Services conducted a large study comparing chiropractic with bed rest, surgery, and drugs for the treatment of lower back pain. Chiropractic was shown to be the most effective technique.

The chiropractor (or D.C., doctor of chiropractic) believes that pain is the result of misalignments of the vertebrae and major joints. He or she will treat your pain through "adjustments," manipulations of the back, neck, or legs, that aim to put the spine into proper alignment. The practitioner believes that proper alignment will stop painful nerve pressure and correct imbalances of posture that can damage muscles and joints.

Chiropractors also offer massage for painful muscles, as well as ultrasound treatments and electrical stimulation of the muscles. They may give advice on physical therapy or exercise.

Be skeptical and ask questions if a chiropractor tells you that you require many X-rays and a lengthy treatment to correct spinal misalignment. Also beware of the chiropractor who tells you that chiropractic can cure allergies, cancer, indigestion, or other disorders that do not involve the musculoskeletal system.

Biofeedback

Biofeedback therapy is a method of teaching patients how to enter a state of relaxation in which they concentrate on controlling physiological functions that are usually automatic.

This method allows people to influence negative or harmful processes in their bodies. For example, a woman who gets tension headaches can learn through biofeedback how to relax the neck and scalp, improving circulation in the head. A patient with heart disease may learn to slow his heart rate, slow his breathing, and reduce harmful physical stress. Other examples of biofeedback use are pain management through relaxation and visualization; management and prevention of panic attacks; improving bladder control; help for stuttering and asthma through breath control; and help for hyperactive children through learning how to enter states of relaxed concentration.

Biofeedback treatment is usually performed by a professional mental health practitioner—a psychiatrist, psychologist, or social worker trained in the techniques of focused relaxation and visualization. Biofeedback requires that the patient be hooked up to an instrument capable of showing the patient's physiological state, such as a heart monitor or thermometer. The instrument or machine used depends upon the condition being treated. The goal of biofeedback treatment is to teach the patient to enter a relaxed state and to focus on influencing the troublesome physiological process.

The instrument used gives tangible feedback to the patient about his or her success in lowering heart rate, for example, or relaxing a muscle spasm. In this way, the patient can learn what a healthier, more relaxed state feels like, and how to go about

66
It is preferable to diagnose and treat patients as unique individuals than as members of a disease category.
—From *Principles of Holistic Medical Practice*, by the American Holistic Medicine Association
99

Unofficially...
The March/April 1997 issue of *Diabetes Self-Management* reports that a study presented at the American Association of Diabetes Educators in 1996 showed that subjects using biofeedback in the treatment of chronic foot ulcers experienced faster healing.

achieving it. Eventually he or she no longer needs the instrument to help identify this state.

Herbal medicine

The medicinal use of herbs and plants is a major component of many alternative treatments. It is an ancient practice; documentation of herbal treatments date back to early civilizations in China, India, and Egypt. People in Western countries have also relied on herbal remedies for centuries.

A booming business

In America, herbal medicine has long been considered thoroughly unorthodox. Today, however, we are witnessing an explosion in botanical medicine. Herbal and botanical preparations can be found at the corner drugstore or the pharmacies in large grocery stores. Health-food stores boast row upon row of herbal teas, capsules, and tinctures (plant extracts in alcohol solutions). Echinacea for colds, garlic for cholesterol, gingko for mental sharpness, and St. John's wort for depression are just a few examples of now-mainstream herbal offerings.

Although the volume of research on botanical remedies—and their popularity—is increasing, they have not been scientifically proved to cure medical conditions, at least not yet. These preparations are offered as dietary supplements, not drugs, which means that manufacturers can sell them without testing and approval by the Food and Drug Administration (FDA). If the FDA gets reports of harmful effects from a supplement, however, it can impose safety requirements, like warnings or dosage changes, or even seize or ban products.

Read the label

The companies that sell herbal preparations are responsible for guaranteeing the purity and safety of these products. The manufacturer is also responsible for any claims made about the product's effectiveness.

Read the label on a jar or box containing an herbal remedy. The content is significant. Most describe the product as a "dietary supplement," not a drug or medicine. Some warn that the product and its claims have not been evaluated by the FDA, or that the product is not intended to diagnose, cure, treat, or prevent disease. Most labels instruct the consumer to take the product in conjunction with a healthy diet or healthy lifestyle, which begs the question of what will be the true cause of any improvement in health.

These provisos indicate that the majority of herbal remedies lack rigorous scientific evidence to support claims made about whether they work. This does not necessarily mean that herbal remedies are harmful or ineffective. Millions of people through the ages, and today, would argue otherwise, based on their personal experiences. But it is a fact, nonetheless, for the savvy consumer to keep in mind.

Do your homework

You need to do your homework if you plan to use medicinal herbs (or any other alternative treatment, for that matter). This does not mean talking to the health-food store salesperson or the holistic practitioner who is already convinced of the usefulness and safety of herbal remedies, or who stands to make a profit by recommending them. Nor does it mean reading a book touting a "miracle cure" or a "cure-all" remedy. Instead, learn which remedies claim to treat which ailments, and look for scientific research, preferably clinical studies, demonstrating the effectiveness of a specific herb or plant.

Watch Out!
In September of 1998, the *New England Journal of Medicine* published six reports of serious illness caused by dietary supplements. Robert DiPaola, M.D., warns that "there is no such thing as a safe agent just because the word 'natural' is attached to it. Patients need to be warned and careful."

The goal is to find scientific research or evidence that is not linked to the selling or promotion of a product. At your library or on the Internet, check current or past issues of respected medical and scientific journals like *Science, Nature,* the *Medical Letter,* the *Journal of the American Medical Association,* the *New England Journal of Medicine, The Lancet* (a British publication), or the *Harvard Health Letter.* Other major universities or hospitals may publish health letters for the general public. *Prevention* magazine is a good source of balanced information on new and alternative treatments. It is widely available, including in grocery store magazine sections. (See Appendix B, "The Resource Guide" in for information on how to find these publications.)

Another option is to read books or articles by established health writers, such as Jane E. Brody or Dr. Isadore Rosenfeld. You might also explore the archives of major newspapers for recent articles on a particular remedy.

Recently, Harvard-trained botanist and physician Andrew Weil, M.D., a best-selling author on the topic of holistic health care, inaugurated a scientific journal called *Integrative Medicine.* According to Weil, *Integrative Medicine* will contain high-quality scientific research that "neither rejects conventional medicine nor embraces alternative medicine uncritically." The journal certainly fills a gap, and may be a valuable aid in furthering public and professional understanding of holistic medicine. (See the Resource Guide in Appendix B for information on how to find *Integrative Medicine.*)

While medical science continues its explorations, remember that herbs can be toxic, cause allergic reactions, or interact with prescribed drugs.

> "
> The herb industry is booming today. A great deal of its promotional efforts are pure baloney. In response, the medical profession likes to issue dire warnings of the dangers of self-care in general and herbal medicine in particular.
> —Andrew Weil, M.D., writing in *Natural Health, Natural Medicine*
> "

For example, Chinese ephedra (mahuang) can raise the blood pressure and heart rate, which can be dangerous for some people. And some forms of ginseng can also act as a potentially dangerous heart stimulant. Always talk to your doctor before trying an herbal remedy.

Diabetes and alternative medicine

Long before the era of modern treatment, healers have recognized and grappled with diabetes. For centuries, traditional or folk medicine has recommended certain plants for controlling blood sugar.

In Europe, for example, blueberry leaf tea has been used to lower blood sugar. In India, Ayurvedic healers use a plant called *gurmar* (*Gymnema sylvestre*), the "sugar destroyer." In Jamaica, diabetes has been treated with ackee fruit. In America today, some tout the nutritional supplement chromium picolinate as a treatment for diabetes.

Yet none of these substances, nor any other non-pharmaceutical substance, has been shown to lower blood glucose enough to replace conventional treatment for diabetes, namely insulin and oral diabetes medications.

The desert diet

It's possible that a diet rich in certain foods may be a natural complement to diabetes treatment. Research underway in the American southwest has demonstrated that certain starchy foods may markedly slow down the rise of glucose following a meal. Botanist Gary Paul Nabham of the Tucson, Arizona–based organization Native Seeds/SEARCH, along with University of Australia nutritionist Janette C. Brand, have found that diets high in "desert foods," which are plants containing

Moneysaver
If you decide to purchase an herbal remedy, try to buy freeze-dried herbs or herbal tinctures. These are usually the purest, most cost-effective forms.

amylose (a starch) and soluble fibers called *gums* and *mucilages,* produce lower glucose peaks after meals.

Nabham and Brand's research has focused on foods traditionally eaten by a tribe of Native American people called the O'odham, who have long cultivated specific desert crops. Since about 1940, the O'odham people have experienced one of the highest incidences of type 2 diabetes in the world. Around 1940, the O'odham began to eat less of their traditional desert foods, replacing them with processed and refined mainstream foods. Researchers speculate that the physical constitution of the O'odham, and their previous diet, made it difficult for them to handle large amounts of fat and refined carbohydrates, leading to an epidemic of obesity and type 2 diabetes.

Ms. Brand has documented similar patterns in dietary change and increases in type 2 diabetes in Micronesia and New Zealand.

This research suggests that people with diabetes may benefit from eating foods that, like the desert foods, contain amylose, gums, and mucilages. The O'odham people get these nutrients from Emory oak acorns, prickly pear pads, mesquite bean pods, and tepary beans. But the same beneficial fibers and starches are in beans and legumes commonly found in grocery stores, such as pinto, navy, lima, and garbanzo beans, and lentils.

There is no alternative to insulin

Certain natural substances may, indeed, affect blood-sugar control. But it would be very dangerous for any person with diabetes who uses insulin or oral medications to attempt to stop using these medications in favor of using herbal or other "natural" remedies. People with diabetes who wish to

experiment with the hypoglycemic effects of alternative remedies should never do so without first
consulting their doctor.

A new old-fashioned approach

It is interesting to note that conventional diabetes
treatment has long included a "holistic" emphasis
on diet and exercise. You may not know your gingko
from your garbanzo, but you may be using a "whole
person" approach to managing diabetes.

Exercise and diet have proven to be powerful
natural techniques for improving blood-sugar levels
and protecting against complications. Indeed, exercise combined with the proper diet is the only treatment prescribed for some type 2 diabetics. The role
of exercise and diet in diabetes care is an example
of how lifestyle factors and the health of the whole
person can enhance a course of treatment that is
focused on individual symptoms.

A thin line? Mind and body

As public and scientific interest in holistic medicine
grows, patients and practitioners alike are asking
whether the state of your mind can affect the state
of your health? Answers to the question range from
a flat-out "That's ridiculous" to the belief that our
thoughts literally determine everything about our
physical reality.

We can't hope to settle this profound and fascinating question here. However, we can take a look
at two emotions that definitely seem to affect the
body and are relevant to the management of diabetes: stress and depression.

Stressed out

Renowned stress researcher Hans Selye has defined
stress as "a[ny] bodily change produced as a

Bright Idea
Exercise is one of
the most effec-
tive stress
busters we know
of. Exercise regu-
larly to help keep
stress under
control.

response to a perceived demand placed upon the individual." Stress can result from both real and imagined demands, and from both positive and negative events—anything that inspires anxiety or that requires change and adjustment. Stress can also be caused by strong emotions, especially anger.

The hallmark symptoms of stress include increased heart rate, high blood pressure, muscular tension, rapid, shallow breathing, and the release of the so-called "fight or flight" hormones like adrenaline and cortisol.

During our days as cave dwellers, the fight or flight response made sense. It helped to save us from immediate and very real emergencies, such as escaping the attacks of wild animals. Today, our stressors—demanding jobs, horrendous traffic, and juggling work and family, to name but a few—tend to be everyday experiences. This chronic stress can lead to lower back pain, digestive disorders, headache, bruxism (teeth grinding), and its often associated disorder, TMJ (temporomandibular joint) syndrome, a painful condition of the jaw.

Chronic stress and high blood pressure may also contribute to heart disease. Stress may increase cholesterol and promote the buildup of harmful plaque in the arteries, leading to blockages. Frequent and prolonged bouts of high blood pressure may damage the insides of arteries, making it easier for plaque to collect.

Stress and diabetes

Stress is known to be a cause of both hypo- and hyperglycemia in people with diabetes. One of the body's reactions to stress hormones is to release stored glucose, providing extra energy as you "fight or flee." This raises blood-sugar levels. On the other hand, if stress occurs when there are high levels of insulin in the blood, the liver may be inhibited from releasing stored glucose and low blood sugar can occur.

Not all people with diabetes experience these responses to stress. Stress usually interacts with other individual factors in affecting blood-sugar control. One of the most significant elements is how well controlled blood sugar is before the onset of stress. People on tight glucose control regimens may be especially vulnerable to highs and lows caused by stress. Other factors include the person's overall coping ability, his or her usual degree of anxiety, and the amount of social support available.

Another way that stress can affect blood-sugar control is its impact on your self-care behavior. Distracted, worried, stressed-out people may be less careful in following their treatment programs.

Depression and diabetes

So far, research into whether or not depression is more common among people with diabetes is inconclusive. According to the American Diabetes Association, some research shows that, indeed, depression is more common, recurs more often, and lasts longer among people with diabetes than in the general population. Common sense suggests, though, that the person who lives with a chronic and serious disease—especially one that, like diabetes, demands daily management—might easily feel some depression.

Depression can be a serious health problem in and of itself, one requiring medical treatment. (See Chapter 14 for information on recognizing and treating serious depression.) The state of being depressed can also lead to other health problems,

Watch Out!
Beware of attempting to escape stress with such unhealthy "coping" techniques as overeating, cigarette smoking, and excessive alcohol or drug use.

which makes it especially significant in people with diabetes. People who are chronically depressed

- Tend to have higher levels of stress hormones, with all the hazards this can entail.

- Tend to have a higher incidence of high blood pressure and heart disease (if other risk factors are present).

- Tend to take less than good care of themselves.

- May be more likely to take up unhealthy habits such as smoking, drinking, or overeating in hopes of alleviating their depression.

What's more, poorly controlled blood-sugar levels can aggravate depression by causing fatigue and sleeplessness. Lack of energy can disrupt participation in enjoyable activities, and can also disrupt healthy patterns of self-care.

Some tips for coping

66

Prevention is preferable to treatment and is usually more cost-effective. —From the *Principles of Holistic Medical Practice*, by the American Holistic Medicine Association

99

All told, depression can indeed affect the physical well-being of the person with diabetes. He or she will probably need to give some thought to emotional health care, whether that takes the form of professional counseling, healthy stress management techniques, or some combination of these. Some people may turn to holistic practitioners for help in coping with the interaction of mind and body, emotions and health. Others may not need to do so.

Whatever your choice, here are some well-established methods for taking the edge off stress and "the blues":

- Learn and use a basic relaxation technique, for example, simple breathing exercises, muscle relaxation, meditative techniques, yoga, or prayer.

- Engage in regular, enjoyable physical activity.

- Stay socially connected to positive people.

- Accept the fact that life will always include some stress and some emotional pain. Keep stressful events or situations in perspective, as in "This too shall pass," or "I've survived worse!"

- Identify factors that are out of your control, and let go of them.

- Identify factors that you can control, and take an active approach toward them.

- Break your goals down into realistic, short-term steps, and think only about the step at hand.

- Get a pet! Research shows that pet owners experience less depression and stress.

- Read a good book.

- Discipline your mind against negative thought patterns.

- Develop a hobby.

- Volunteer.

Just the facts

- More Americans are choosing alternative medicine techniques to help manage their diabetes than ever before.

- Scientific research into the efficacy of alternative medicine techniques is increasing, but it is inconclusive so far.

- In considering an alternative medical technique, it is important to examine the best available scientific evidence for that approach.

- There are no alternatives to injected insulin or oral diabetes medications, at least not yet.

- Always talk to your doctor before using alternative medicine. Let your doctor know if you are using any herbal remedies or alternative treatments.

Special Concerns

GET THE SCOOP ON...
Telling your employer you have diabetes ▪
Your rights as an employee ▪ ADA, FMLA,
HIPAA, and COBRA ▪ Maintaining your health
insurance coverage ▪ The rights of children with
diabetes in school

PART IV

I've Got a Life:
Diabetes at Work
and School

Chapter 11

Monitoring your blood. Giving yourself injections. Examining your feet. Noticing the shakiness or perspiration brought on by low blood sugar, and digging into your briefcase for a few hard candies . . . .

Managing diabetes is mostly a very personal affair. But what about the public aspects of having diabetes? You have a full and active life out there in the real world. A huge part of that life is work. Whether you love your job, hate it, or simply tolerate it, work can suddenly seem scary. At least three tough questions will rear their heads:

- Should I tell employers or potential employers that I have diabetes?

- How do I deal with discrimination, if it occurs?

- What about maintaining my health insurance coverage?

Bright Idea
Never let having
diabetes domi-
nate your view of
yourself or your
career prospects.
The important
issue is not
whether you
have diabetes,
but whether you
can do the job.

It's time to fill in these knowledge gaps. First,
let's look at employment rights under the law for
people with diabetes.

Job interviews: questions and answers

Here's the nitty-gritty:

- It is illegal for a potential employer to ask a job
  candidate about whether he or she has any medical conditions, unless:

- The employer has made a job offer to the candidate, and

- The employer asks this of all persons receiving
  offers.

If a job candidate who has been offered a position is asked about medical conditions and answers
that he has a medical condition, the employer

- Is required to make reasonable accommodations for the medical condition at the place of
  employment (e.g., wheelchair ramps), and

- Can withdraw the job offer only if the person
  cannot perform the essential duties of the job,
  even with reasonable accommodations in place.

"Reasonable accommodations" for a person with
diabetes might include such provisions as work
breaks for checking glucose levels, permission to
keep diabetes supplies and snacks in the workplace
or to eat snacks at one's desk, more frequent bathroom breaks, or regular hours.

If the employer has offered a job, has been told
about the candidate's diabetes, and is completely
and genuinely unable to make reasonable accommodations for the diabetes, then that employer may
have the legal right to withdraw the offer.

But the employer who can make such accommodations and who withdraws the offer is probably

breaking the law. The employer who hires a less qualified candidate who does not have diabetes may also be skating on thin ice.

What law is this employer breaking? Several laws have been passed that protect people with medical conditions in the workplace.

The Americans with Disabilities Act

This was signed into law in 1990. One of its specific aims is to protect against employment discrimination. The Disabilities Act complements an earlier piece of legislation, the Federal Rehabilitation Act of 1973.

The Rehabilitation Act applies to employees of the federal government or employees of companies that receive federal funding. The Disabilities Act applies to all civilian employees who work for companies employing fifteen or more people. (See the Resource Guide in Appendix B for information on how to get or see a copy of the Americans with Disabilities Act.)

Both of these laws make it illegal for employers to discriminate against you if you are qualified for the job and are able to perform it with reasonable accommodations provided at the workplace.

Perhaps most people with diabetes do not identify themselves as "disabled." But the law protects all people who may be regarded as disabled. Under the Disabilities Act, the disabled person is defined as one who

- Has a physical or mental impairment that substantially limits one or more major life activities,

- Has a record of such impairment, or

- Is regarded as having such an impairment.

This protects people with diabetes who do not view themselves as disabled. If a potential employer

Unofficially...
Until 1989, if you had a parent with diabetes, you were not allowed to enlist in the armed forces regardless of your health status.

decides that a person with diabetes is disabled, in the sense of being unable to work, then that employer automatically must treat the person with diabetes in a lawful manner, as decreed by the Americans with Disabilities Act. That means selecting employees based on their qualifications only and providing reasonable accommodations for employees with disabilities.

On the job

Once you are a working employee, your employer can inquire about your medical condition only if the questions are work related and if your employer's concerns relate to the needs of the business. The employer's inquiry must be performance based, not based on hunches, appearances, or suspicions. If you are satisfactorily performing your duties, you should not be subjected to questions about your physical health.

The Family and Medical Leave Act (FMLA)

This law, enacted in 1993, can also help you to cope with diabetes in the workplace. The FMLA allows workers up to twelve weeks of unpaid leave each year to attend either to their own serious illnesses or those of family members. It applies only to companies employing fifty or more persons who live locally (within seventy-five miles of the workplace). Leaves of twelve weeks may be taken, or much shorter leaves are allowed, for instance, one day off every week. Employers must continue to pay for the employees' health insurance coverage during medical leaves.

Employees seeking medical or family leaves must work for one employer for at least one year, and for 1,250 hours or more. It is usually necessary to give the employer thirty days' notice when requesting a leave.

Under the FMLA, you may request leave to care for

- Yourself
- Your spouse
- Parents
- Step- and foster parents
- Minor children
- Minor step- or foster children
- Adult children who are incapable of self-care

You may not request leave to care for

- Unmarried partners
- In-laws
- Siblings
- Grandchildren
- Grandparents

The FMLA legitimizes the needs of people who are living with medical conditions. It is a powerful tool for keeping people with medical conditions in the workforce. (See the Resource Guide in Appendix B for information on how to get or see a copy of the Family and Medical Leave Act.)

Closed doors: careers that exclude people with diabetes

Despite the advances made in protecting equal opportunity for people with diabetes and other medical conditions, there are still a few careers that maintain blanket exclusions against people who are insulin dependent. These are careers in which the duties are such that, if an employee were to experience an insulin reaction (severe hypoglycemia) on

Bright Idea
For answers to questions about the Americans with Disabilities Act, call the Americans with Disabilities Act Information Line at (800) 514-0383. Or try the National Institute of Disability and Rehabilitation Research, at (800) 949-4232. Or try this U.S. Department of Justice Web site: http://usdoj.gov. crt/ada.

the job, the results could be very dangerous. Today, people on insulin generally cannot work as

- FBI agents
- Commercial truckers
- Bus drivers or other commercial drivers
- Heavy machine operators
- Police officers (hiring practices vary widely)
- Commercial airplane pilots

(In December of 1996, the Federal Aviation Administration overturned a ban prohibiting insulin-treated persons from flying private and recreational planes. It's now possible to apply for special medical certification. Pilots must meet medical requirements and adhere to a strict medical protocol.)

Bright Idea
Remember that if you can live with diabetes, you can work with diabetes.

Anyone is entitled to challenge any employer in a court of law on a charge of discriminatory exclusion. Keep in mind, however, that employers in these areas have a track record of successfully defending exclusions in court. If you decide to fight a blanket exclusion, be prepared for just that: a fight. Then again, courtroom victories help to change the law!

The military

As we've noted, even a family history of diabetes (in parents) barred you from enlisting in the military in the past. Now, you cannot enlist if you have diabetes.

If you are diagnosed with diabetes while in service, your case will be reviewed on an individual basis. A medical board will summarize the specifics of your condition, and this summary will be passed on to a Physical Evaluation Board.

Much of the Board's decision will depend upon whether or not you need to take insulin or oral medication, how well controlled your blood glucose is, and the nature of your military duties. The Board will declare you either fit or unfit for military service. If you are declared unfit and are discharged, you have a right to appeal this decision.

Should you tell your employer?

You know your rights. But what's the right thing to do? Only you can make the decision about how forthright you are about having diabetes. The sad fact is that discrimination against people with diabetes exists. Not many people know a lot about diabetes—what it is and what it isn't. And most who don't understand diabetes probably don't have a burning desire to master the subject.

You don't intend to lie, but some thought and caution may be in order. What next?

If you already have a job

Presumably, if you have a job, you are performing it to the best of your abilities and have earned a reputation for doing good work. If you have recently been diagnosed with diabetes, it's your responsibility to manage the disease as well as possible so that you can keep up the good work.

Unless you are required to undergo regular physical examinations for your employer, it is entirely your choice to speak up or not.

You may wish to tell a few trusted colleagues, in case you need help during a hypoglycemic episode. You may want to instruct a colleague in the symptoms of hypoglycemia, how to administer a glucagon injection, and where you keep your emergency glucagon kit.

If you will be injecting insulin at work, you may decide that your life will be easier if at least some people know.

You will need to tell your employer if accommodations for your self-care are not in place (for instance, the flexibility to take more bathroom or snack breaks). And you will certainly need to discuss your diabetes with your employer if you wish to apply for FMLA leave.

Finally, you may wish to be open about your diabetes because you see it as an opportunity to educate people about what people with diabetes can do in the workplace.

If you are looking for a job

Admittedly, interviewing for jobs when you have diabetes can be difficult. It's hard to know what to reveal, and when, especially to someone you have probably just met.

It helps to be prepared with a consistent plan of action. Establish some guidelines for yourself that begin with the legal rights we detailed above:

- **Note the timing of questions about your health.** How seriously are you being considered for the job? Has the employer actually offered you the job? Do not volunteer information. If health questions come up, focus on your record and qualifications, and assure the interviewer that you have no health problems that would prevent you from meeting the job expectations.

- **Consider aligning yourself with the employer's worries.** The employer's main concern is probably not whether you have diabetes, but whether the work will get done. Try shifting the focus from diabetes to reliability. You might say something like, "If I were you, I think I'd be worrying about . . . ." Ask what the concerns are. Acknowledge that the employer's concerns are understandable. Come to interviews prepared to state and respond to legitimate employer worries—not to beg for a job while apologizing for the "defect" of diabetes.

■ **Emphasize the positive.** Point out that you pay close attention to your health, probably much closer attention than the average person does. Explain that managing diabetes requires self-discipline. If you don't smoke and rarely drink, say so.

■ **If a physical examination is required, provide full information about your diagnosis and treatment.** It's likely that the examining physician will not be a diabetes specialist, so be prepared to explain your self-care regimen. Discuss your methods for avoiding health emergencies, such as frequent self-monitoring, regular meals, and regular exercise.

It happens: responding to employment discrimination

It is serious business if you feel that you have been discriminated against because you have diabetes. If discrimination has occurred—if the offer of a job for which you are qualified has been withdrawn; if you have been passed over for a promotion you genuinely deserved; or if you have been discouraged from rising in your career—then your employer or prospective employer may have broken the law.

Taking steps
The American Diabetes Association recommends this sequence of actions should you feel you have been the victim of discrimination:

■ First, consult with an attorney to be clear on the merits of your case, your rights, and your legal

Watch Out!
It is illegal for an employer to fire an employee with a medical condition because company health insurance costs have risen.

course of action. State laws and procedures differ.

- Next, try to educate your employer or prospective employer about diabetes and diabetes management.

- If this does not resolve the situation, you or your attorney may need to begin negotiating with the employer. This can involve educating the employer about the Americans with Disabilities Act and pointing out the employer's legal responsibilities under the law. The employer's concerns should be heard and addressed. The goal is to achieve a mutually agreeable solution outside the courtroom.

- If negotiations fail, you may have to take legal action. You will need a lawyer's services for this. If you belong to a union or professional group, they may be helpful at this time. Find out if there is a person designated as an employment discrimination officer within your union or group.

Timesaver
If you are considering making a claim of employer discrimination, consult an attorney as soon as possible. Early legal counsel will help prevent wasted action and false starts on your part.

State laws and resources

Most states have an office or commission whose duty it is to investigate discrimination, for instance, a Human Rights Commission or an Equal Employment Opportunity Commission. These offices should provide free information on employment discrimination issues. For more information about the Equal Employment Opportunity Commission, call (800) 669-4000. This number will automatically connect you with the EEOC office nearest you.

Your state may require that you file charges with the state discrimination office prior to filing a lawsuit. In fact, you may be prohibited from filing a lawsuit unless the state has reviewed your claim and has granted you a "right to sue" letter.

If your state does not have an equal employment opportunity commission, try the state or local Department of Labor, Department of Employment, or Department of Human Resources. These offices may have staff members who specialize in investigating discrimination claims. You'll find telephone numbers under the state or county listings in the blue government pages of your phone book.

Bright Idea
For more information on employment rights, contact the Disability Rights Education and Defense Fund, Inc., 2212 6th Street, Berkeley, CA 94710, (510) 644-2555.

What you can do

Employment discrimination is notoriously hard to prove, because often the term "best qualified" can apply to different people for different reasons. You will need to gather as much strong evidence as possible if you seek to prove discrimination. Here are some suggestions:

- Get a written statement from the employer clearly stating the reasons why you weren't hired or promoted or were let go.

- Compile materials showing the employer's formal stance regarding equal opportunity, for example, the job application form, policy manuals, and equal opportunity mission statements.

- Keep copies of the specific job announcement, the job description, and job performance criteria.

- Keep copies of your job evaluations.

- Make a list of potential witnesses. Be prepared to state the relationship of these people to you and to the employer, and how these people have come by the relevant information.

- Put together a diary of events you feel pertain to the discrimination. Provide dates, places, names, and titles. List all actions you have taken to address the situation fairly, for example, talks with the employer, attempts to educate and negotiate, requests for reasonable accommodations.

Maintaining health insurance coverage

Perhaps the most frightening and frustrating part of working with diabetes is concern over keeping adequate health insurance coverage. Few of us can afford to lose the health insurance provided by employers, but most of us need and want the freedom to change companies or change careers. It's hard to make changes, to grow professionally by leaps and bounds, with the albatross of a "preexisting condition" hanging around your neck.

The Health Insurance Portability and Accountability Act of 1996

Fortunately, these worries should be lessened by the recent passage of the Health Insurance Portability and Accountability Act (HIPAA).

The HIPAA was signed by President Clinton in October of 1996. It became effective on July 1, 1997.

Originally called the *Kennedy-Kassebaum Act* after Senators Edward Kennedy of Massachusetts and Nancy Kassebaum of Kansas, who introduced it, the HIPAA is the first comprehensive federal health-care legislation enacted in many years. It was seen by some advocates for health-care reform as being the next best thing to a national health-care plan that offers coverage for all Americans.

The HIPAA makes it easier for people with diabetes to get and keep health insurance. It regulates the workings of the majority of group health-care insurers, and places new requirements on insurers

Moneysaver
Your chances for getting a reasonable rate on private life or disability insurance increase with good diabetes control, as demonstrated by good glycosylated hemoglobin results and healthy blood pressure and cholesterol levels.

selling individual plans. (See the Resource Guide in Appendix B for information on how to get or see a copy of the HIPAA.)

Under the HIPAA,

- Insurers and employers may not discriminate against workers because of their health, and

- All workers eligible for health insurance coverage (which usually means all workers with benefits) must be offered coverage at equal prices.

HIPAA further provides that

- If you have had continuous group coverage for more than six months, a new employer cannot deny you coverage due to a preexisting condition.

- If, however, you have been diagnosed with diabetes within or up to six months prior to changing jobs, your new employer may refuse or limit your health-care coverage for twelve months.

- This twelve-month waiting period can be applied to you only once.

- A twelve-month waiting period can be reduced by the number of months you had continuous coverage following your diagnosis at the previous job. For example, if you were diagnosed three months before changing jobs and had insurance coverage throughout that time, your new employer could refuse or restrict your health insurance coverage for nine months instead of twelve.

It is the responsibility of employers to know and follow HIPAA law. One of the ways they do this is to provide certificates of "creditable coverage," which certify that an employee has been under continuous group coverage for a specified time. As noted above,

Bright Idea
For answers to questions about health insurance, call the National Insurance Consumer Helpline at (800) 942-4242.

this coverage can be credited toward reducing the one-time-only waiting period for persons with a pre-existing condition. If you are leaving a job for a new one, consult with human resource personnel at both places of employment about the procedures you and your employers must follow in order to ensure your rights under HIPAA.

The HIPAA and individual coverage

Watch Out!
HIPAA preexist-ing condition laws do not pro-tect people who have never had health insurance or who have not had health insur-ance for sixty-three days or more. Avoid gaps in your coverage.

The HIPAA also protects people with diabetes who are between jobs and may want to purchase individ-ual health insurance policies. Under the HIPAA, you are eligible for an individual policy, regardless of having a preexisting condition, as long as

- You have had continuous coverage under a group plan for the previous eighteen months.
- You are not currently eligible for coverage under any group plan.
- You have used up COBRA coverage, discussed below.

Charming the COBRA

HIPAA is a tremendous boon for people with med-ical conditions who wish to change jobs. What about someone who is leaving a job that provides health insurance but does not yet have another job lined up? If you go without continuous coverage for sixty-three days or longer, then a new employer may apply preexisting condition restrictions to your health-care eligibility and coverage, even under HIPAA. It's in your best interest not to let your coverage lapse.

This is where the Consolidated Omnibus Budget Reconciliation Act (COBRA) comes to the rescue. Under COBRA, you and your covered dependents can stay on the health insurance plan provided by your previous employer (as long as that employer is not the federal government, a church, or employer of fewer than twenty people).

Some important features of COBRA are

- To maintain coverage after leaving a position, you must notify your employer in writing within sixty days after leaving. (It's probably wise to do this as soon as you know it's what you want.)

- Coverage begins on or extends back to the date you would have lost your previous insurance had you not requested a COBRA extension.

- Coverage can last up to eighteen months after you leave your job, twenty-nine months if you are disabled, and thirty-six months for your dependents.

COBRA coverage is more expensive than group coverage through an employer. Usually, you pay your premium and the employer's share, and often a service fee as well. But this is usually less expensive than an individual policy.

Between COBRA and the HIPAA, you should be able to maintain health insurance coverage through job changes and times when you are not working. Make sure that you give employers timely notification of your plans, and that you and they understand the procedures to be followed to ensure your continued coverage.

Government entitlement programs: medicare, medicaid, and social security disability insurance

The United States government provides health insurance coverage for citizens who are retired or are unable to work.

Bright Idea
The government maintains a Medicare Hot Line. Call (800) 638-6833 with your questions on Medicare insurance. For questions about Social Security Disability Insurance, call the Social Security Administration at (800) 772-1213.

Bright Idea
Always get a written statement of prescription from your health-care provider detailing your medical need for a supply or service. Always submit a copy of the statement with Medicare claims.

Medicare

Medicare is the federally funded health insurance program for people age sixty-five and older and for people of any age who cannot work because of disability.

Medicare coverage comes in two parts, Part A and Part B. Both parts have deductibles and co-payments. Most people with Medicare get Part A. Part B requires an additional monthly fee.

Part A helps to cover hospital care, medical care in a nursing home, and hospice care, while Part B helps to cover doctor's appointments and services, diagnostic tests, ambulance services, outpatient hospital services, and medical equipment and supplies.

Medicare covers some, but not all, of the expenses associated with diabetes treatment. For both type 1 and type 2 diabetes, Medicare (Part B) will help cover:

- With a doctor's prescription, your blood glucose meter, test strips, lancets, and other meter supplies. If you use insulin, coverage is for up to 100 test strips and 100 lancets each month, or more if your doctor provides a letter of medical necessity. If you do not use insulin, coverage is for up to fifty test strips and fifty lancets every two months, or more if you provide a letter of medical necessity from your doctor.

- Diabetes education and training services furnished by a certified professional, including outpatient nutritional counseling that is performed by a registered dietitian and is prescribed by your doctor.

Medicare will not cover:
- Oral diabetes pills, insulin, syringes, or insulin pumps.

Medicare may help to pay for outpatient nutritional counseling that is prescribed by your physician.

Medicaid

Medicaid is a combined state and federal assistance program for people who may or may not be disabled, but whose incomes are very low (for example, a single mother on welfare). Medicaid eligibility and coverage varies from state to state. In recent years, there has been a movement among some state governments to encourage people to get off welfare and begin working. Medicaid eligibility may be more restricted in these states.

Contact your local Social Security Administration for information on Medicaid in your state (look in the blue government listings in your telephone book).

Social Security Disability Insurance (SSDI)

This program provides health insurance and income for people younger than sixty-five who have some work history and who have contributed to Social Security, but who can no longer work due to disability. People with diabetes who have certain kinds of neuropathy, amputation, or retinopathy may be eligible for SSDI.

To qualify for SSDI, you must be medically evaluated and designated as disabled. You must also earn less than $500 a month. The SSDI evaluation and application process can be lengthy. If you are turned down for SSDI, you may re-apply.

Recent legislation affecting medicare diabetes coverage

In May of 1997, the White House and Congress reached an agreement to balance the federal budget by 2002. The budget agreement includes a bill,

> **❝**
> Medicare will pay for an amputation [but] not the education and supplies to prevent it. That's just ridiculous. Diabetes is an example of why we need to improve coverage for preventive care.
> —House Representative Elizabeth Furse, D-Oregon, mother of a daughter with diabetes
> **❞**

Unofficially...
About 25 percent
of the Medicare
budget is used to
treat people with
diabetes.

H.R. 58, that increases the Medicare budget by an unprecedented $300 million in additional funding for diabetes research, treatment, and preventive measures.

President Clinton signed the budget into law in August 1997 and it went into effect on July 1, 1998. One of the first improvements in Medicare coverage under the new law went into effect on that day. Prior to July 1, 1998, Medicare did not cover glucose meters and related supplies for people with diabetes not on insulin (which is the majority of people with type 2 diabetes), nor did it cover non-hospital-based diabetes education. Now, Medicare reimburses *all* of its diabetic beneficiaries for these necessary supplies and services.

The new budget's emphasis on funding for preventive care represents a significant advance and is widely applauded. It provides only a broad outline for change, however. Specific regulations for allocating Medicare's budget increase are not yet in place. It will take time to shape and realize the budget's objective of increasing preventive measures and reducing the severity and prevalence of diabetes.

Children with diabetes in school

Just as the law protects employees with diabetes against discrimination in the workplace, so it protects children with diabetes in the public schools.

Public schools receive federal funding, and under the law, all federally funded programs are required to accommodate persons with special needs. Anti-discrimination law recognizes diabetes as a chronic health condition in the category of "other health impairment."

There are two laws protecting children against discrimination in school:

- **Section 504 of the Federal Rehabilitation Act of 1973.** This section specifically recognizes the public schools as coming under Rehabilitation Act regulations.

- **The Individuals with Disability Education Act (IDEA) of 1990.** (Previously the Education for All Handicapped Children Act of 1975, it was amended and renamed in 1990.) IDEA guarantees "free appropriate public education, including special education and related service programming for all children with disabilities."

For copies of one or both of these laws, contact the nearest U.S. Government Printing Office Bookstore. Look in the blue government pages of your phone book under "Federal Government: Government Printing Office."

Your rights as a parent

Both the Rehabilitation Act and IDEA require that a school's reasonable accommodation of a child with a disability be documented in a written plan. A child's accommodation plan is either a Section 504 plan or an Individualized Education Plan (an IEP); the differences between the two are discussed below.

As a parent of a child with diabetes attending public school, you have the right to

- Request that your child receive special services or accommodations.

- Develop with school officials an IEP or a Section 504 plan.

- Include outside experts, such as your child's doctor, in developing a plan.

Bright Idea
The American Diabetes Association provides free back-to-school kits for teachers and day-care providers who have students with diabetes. The kits provide clear, concise information about diabetes and about diabetes management in children. To order a kit, call the ADA at (800) 342-2383.

Timesaver
For up-to-date,
easy-to-read
summaries of
legislation that
affects diabetes
care, read the
*Diabetes
Advocate*, pub-
lished ten times
yearly by the
American
Diabetes
Association,
www.diabetes.
org/advocate.

- Withhold your signature from a plan that does not meet your child's medical needs. The law requires that all parties agree to an accommodation plan before it is implemented.

- Be notified of any proposed changes in your child's plan, review any proposed changes, and be included in meetings held to review your child's plan.

The difference between an IEP and a Section 504 plan is that an IEP, if agreed upon and implemented, makes the school eligible for federal aid to help pay for services included in the plan. A Section 504 plan does not qualify your child's school for federal funds.

The choice of which law to invoke in making a plan, then, is based on the extent of services your child needs. If, for example, your child requires a registered nurse at the school or special transportation, you may need to request and develop an IEP under IDEA to help pay for the plan. On the other hand, a Section 504 plan should be sufficient if your child does not need accommodations that require additional funding, for example, the right to perform blood glucose monitoring any time or anywhere, or to eat snacks or meals at specific times.

If your child's needs aren't being met

See "Taking Steps," part of the discussion on dealing with employer discrimination, earlier in this chapter. The information there also applies to handling discrimination at school.

The American Diabetes Association emphasizes that the best course of action to take in dealing with discrimination is to educate, negotiate, and then litigate. We are all aware of the great costs of time, money, and goodwill that litigation exacts. Make a genuine effort to educate school personnel, and also to understand their concerns. Enlist the help of your child's health-care team in educating others and in establishing an accommodation plan that is both reasonable and safe. Document your efforts from the beginning, whether or not you anticipate a legal battle.

If education and negotiation fail, your best bet is to talk to an attorney before taking any further action.

In Appendix D, you'll find two forms that are helpful to parents of school-aged children with diabetes: a "One-Page Care Guide for Children in School," which provides diabetes care instructions for your child's teacher, and a "Before School Starts Checklist for Parents," which provides a to-do checklist. These forms are reprinted with the kind permission of their author, Jeff Hitchcock, who created and manages the excellent Internet Web site, www.childrenwithdiabetes.com, and who is the father of a young girl with type 1 diabetes.

Social aspects of diabetes at school

So far we've focused on children's rights under the law. The child whose needs are being accommodated and who is attending school often faces the curiosity and, sometimes, the resentment of classmates. Why, for example, does Tommy or Brenda get extra snacks or frequent bathroom breaks?

How parents and children deal with these concerns depends on the age of the child, the degree to which blood-sugar levels are stable, and the child's wishes regarding how much to reveal.

Parents owe it to their child and to teachers to inform teachers of their child's condition and needs. Most teachers, of course, are concerned about the welfare of students and will cooperate

Bright Idea
The American Diabetes Association publishes a brochure for parents and school-age children called *Your School and Your Rights*. Your local ADA affiliate should have one, or call the ADA at (800) 342-2383.

with parents' needs and wishes as much as they can. But it takes communication.

Theoretically, a child with diabetes could get through each school day managing the illness without ever saying that he or she has diabetes: "I just need snacks to keep my energy up," "I take these shots because my doctor wants me to for my health," and so on. After all, children have every right to keep their health concerns private as long as responsible adults are aware of their needs.

Realistically, though, it is probably easier in the long run to find a way for each child to communicate with peers about diabetes. Children from grade school on up will probably respond positively to a class presentation about diabetes, one that includes diabetic children to an extent that is comfortable for the children involved. Ask your child's health-care team for guidance or help. There is no reason for children not to have a basic awareness of diabetes and other medical conditions that might, and often do, affect their peers. Isn't it easier for a child to say, "I have diabetes," and let it go at that, then for her to come up with creative alternative explanations, which will probably only arouse more curiosity? What's more, bringing differences out into the open gives children the much-needed reassurance that adults, at least, are not afraid or ashamed.

Teachers have a responsibility to foster tolerant attitudes among students toward one another. Parents and children have a right to expect this from teachers. Thoughtful, honest, and educated communication from all parties will usually be the best method for protecting children's welfare at school.

For more on diabetes in children, see Chapter 13.

Just the facts

- Federal law requires that employers make reasonable accommodations for employees with diabetes.

- In most states, you must file a claim of discrimination with your state Equal Employment Opportunity Commission (or equivalent) before you can file a lawsuit.

- The Health Insurance Portability and Accountability Act has made it easier for persons with "preexisting conditions" to maintain health insurance coverage, as long as coverage never lapses for more than sixty-three days.

- Federal law requires public schools to make reasonable accommodations for students with diabetes.

- In public schools, reasonable accommodations must be documented in individual written accommodation plans.

GET THE SCOOP ON...
Diabetes and the pill ▪ Impotence: who, why,
and what next ▪ Depression and sex ▪ Talking to
your doctor ▪ Protecting your unborn baby

The World Goes 'Round: Diabetes and Sexuality

Chapter 12

It would be interesting to know if there is any topic under the sun that is thought about as much, read about as much, observed as often on screens big and small, yet talked about as little, as sex.

It might get more than a little exposure on sensational television talk shows. And we're used to a lot of casual "humor" about sex on prime-time TV, along with steamy dialogue and suggestive situations. But privately, sex remains one of the most sensitive, most important, and least discussed areas of our lives.

Which means that it can be very uncomfortable for people with diabetes to talk about their sex lives with health-care providers, just as it can make health-care providers uncomfortable as well. We're all human; there can be shyness and avoidance on both sides. But the medical fact is that diabetes can affect sexual functioning, and sexuality is an appropriate concern for diabetes patients and their health-care providers.

Reading this chapter won't necessarily make the uncomfortable feelings disappear. But it will at least provide an overview of the impact of diabetes on sexuality, and perhaps serve as the starting point for an informed exchange between you and your health-care team.

Avoid complications of diabetes

The more serious sexual problems associated with diabetes, such as impotence (the inability to have or keep an erection) or reduced sexual sensation, are usually the result of long-term diabetes and its associated complications, particularly vascular damage and neuropathy.

In other words, having diabetes does not necessarily sentence you to sexual dysfunction. Maintaining healthy sexual functioning is one more reason to practice good diabetes management and avoid complications.

Sex and hypoglycemia

Watch Out!
If you use an insulin pump, you may need to turn it off and detach it during sexual activity to avoid low blood sugar. (You can keep the flexible tubing inserted during sex.)

Sex is an exciting physical activity (at least, one hopes it is). It burns calories (meaning it burns glucose), and it can lower blood-sugar levels. If you take insulin or oral medications, and especially if you are not in good physical condition, be on the lookout for hypoglycemia after sex.

To avoid hypoglycemia, take the usual precautions: Check blood-sugar levels before or after sex (or at both times), and eat a snack if levels are too low. Adjust insulin dose or timing as recommended by your health-care practitioners.

It may not sound romantic, but neither is a hypoglycemic episode (a serious health problem under any circumstances).

Oral contraceptives (birth control pills)

Women with diabetes may wonder if hormones contained in birth control pills will affect their blood glucose, or even whether it is safe for them to take birth control pills. This is a decision you must make with your doctor. Research so far shows that

- Most women with diabetes who do not have complications, do not smoke, and do not have other risk factors that would make use of birth control pills unsafe can use them.

- Birth control pills can increase insulin resistance in some women with type 2 diabetes.

- Women with type 2 diabetes, or who are at risk for type 2 diabetes, can still use birth control pills, but frequent blood glucose monitoring is recommended.

One type of birth control pill, called *monophasic* because each pill taken throughout the cycle contains the same amount of estrogen and progestin, may help to keep blood-sugar levels stable throughout a woman's menstrual cycle. (See the section on the menstrual cycle and blood-sugar control in Chapter 13.) *Triphasic* pills, in which estrogen levels vary during the cycle, may aggravate swings in glucose levels.

Sexual concerns for women with diabetes

The sexual problems most commonly reported by women with diabetes are

- Vaginal yeast infections and vaginitis
- Poor vaginal lubrication

Yeast infections and vaginitis

Vaginal yeast infections are caused by an overgrowth in the vagina of a fungal organism, *Candida albicans,* which is normally present in smaller amounts in the vagina. Symptoms of a yeast infection are a thick, lumpy, white vaginal discharge and vaginal itching.

Yeast organisms thrive on excess sugar in the blood and tissues. If blood sugar is poorly controlled, yeast infections are more likely to occur. They are also more likely to occur in women who are taking antibiotic medication because the medication can kill the "good" bacteria in the vagina, creating a niche for yeast organisms.

Vaginal yeast infections are treated with vaginally applied creams or suppositories containing antifungal medication, such as *miconazole nitrate* or *nystatin.* These treatments are available without a doctor's prescription at drug stores and pharmacies, usually found near the tampons and sanitary napkins. If they don't work for you, your doctor can prescribe stronger medications.

Yeast organisms can also cause infections on the skin's surface, usually in moist skin folds, such as under the breast or around the groin. These skin infections are treated with topical creams containing the anti-fungal medications mentioned above.

Vaginitis refers to inflammation and tenderness of the vagina, usually caused by a bacterial infection. Symptoms include excessive, often thin vaginal discharge that may smell bad, and itching.

Vaginitis can be caused by imbalances in the normal vaginal bacteria brought about by douching or the use of irritating soaps in the genital area. It may also be caused by poor hygiene or by sexually transmitted diseases, such as gonorrhea and chlamydia.

Bright Idea
Eating yogurt with active bacterial cultures has been shown to reduce the incidence of vaginal yeast infections, or you can buy acidophilus preparations in liquid or capsule form, to be taken orally, at your health-food store.

As with yeast infections, vaginitis can result from high blood-sugar levels, which promote the growth of bacteria.

Vaginitis is treated with antibacterial creams or oral antibiotics that are prescribed by a doctor.

Both yeast infections and vaginitis cause discomfort that can easily interfere with sexual pleasure. Fortunately, both conditions are less common when blood sugar is well controlled.

Vaginal dryness

A lack of vaginal lubrication, or wetness, during sexual arousal is a complaint that is more common in women who have diabetes than in women who do not. (Otherwise, there is little evidence that women with diabetes experience more sexual difficulties than do other women.)

Low estrogen levels can cause the vagina to be drier than normal during sexual excitement. (Estrogen is a female hormone that helps to regulate the menstrual cycle and protects premenopausal women from bone loss and heart disease.) This can make intercourse painful. Dryness of the vagina can be treated with water-based vaginal lubricants (such as KY Jelly or Replens) that are available at pharmacies and drug stores, usually found near the tampons and sanitary napkins. Saliva is also an effective lubricant.

If you are experiencing vaginal dryness, tell your doctor so that he or she can examine you for hormonal problems. Your doctor may recommend estrogen replacement therapy, in the form of a patch, pill, or vaginal cream.

Estrogen replacement therapy can improve vaginal lubrication, and it is proven to lower the risk of heart disease in women. But hormone replacement

Watch Out!
Don't use petroleum jelly (Vaseline) or anything that is not water based or water soluble to moisten the vagina. The vaginal membranes can't clean the vagina of non-water-soluble products. Your doctor or diabetes educator can recommend a vaginal lubricant.

therapy raises other health concerns, such as a potentially increased risk of breast or endometrial cancer, that you should discuss with your doctor. (See the discussion of hormone replacement therapy in Chapter 13.)

Genital pain

Pain during sexual activity is not particularly associated with diabetes, but a higher incidence of vaginal infections may lead to persistent pain, burning, or tenderness around an area called the *vaginal vestibule* (the opening and inner opening of the vagina). Sometimes this is caused by infection of glands that are near the vaginal opening, like the Bartholin's glands. Women who experience persistent pain with sexual activity should see a gynecologist who specializes in diagnosing and treating sexual problems.

Diabetic nerve damage and reduced sexual sensation

For women with diabetes, one cause of sexual difficulties can be nerve damage, or diabetic neuropathy (see Chapter 4) that affects the genital area. Nerve damage is a long-term complication of diabetes; it doesn't occur without a long period of high blood-sugar levels. Nerve damage in the genitals, as well as poor circulation (another long-term diabetic complication) can cause reduced sensitivity to touch.

This is not especially common among women with diabetes, but it can occur. Diabetic neuropathy must be quite severe to affect sexual responsiveness. Although sensitivity to touch can be affected, it is rare that the nerves controlling orgasm are affected by neuropathy. Many women need some degree of direct clitoral stimulation to experience sexual pleasure and orgasm. Women with diabetes and neuropathy are no different. If you have nerve damage, experiment with degrees of touch. A lighter or firmer touch may make a difference. More intensive clitoral stimulation, perhaps from a vibrator or from oral sex, may also help. In the future, oral medications similar to the new impotence drug for men, Viagra, may become available to help women with decreased ability to achieve orgasm.

It's important not to jump to conclusions about what might be interfering with sexual response. There can be a number of reasons why sex may feel less pleasurable than it has before. The problems we describe above can really get in the way of enjoying sex. Emotional factors can also interfere with sexual pleasure, as discussed below. And the quality of your relationship with your sexual partner can enhance or weaken sexual enjoyment.

Discuss your sexual feelings with your partner, and discuss any sexual difficulties with your doctor so that they can be thoroughly evaluated.

Sexual concerns for men with diabetes

The primary sexual difficulty experienced by men with diabetes is impotence, or the inability to have or maintain an erection of the penis.

Impotence

Impotence certainly is not limited to men with diabetes. Impotence (called *erectile dysfunction* by physicians) affects some 10 to 20 million American men. Over half of all men between the ages of forty and seventy experience some degree of impotence.

In men with diabetes,

■ 9 percent experience impotence between the ages of twenty and twenty-nine.

■ 15 percent experience impotence between the ages of thirty and thirty-four.

Bright Idea
Sexual needs and preferences can change. Ask yourself if sexual pleasure is easier with particular types of stimulation. This can help to determine the source of any difficulties. Perhaps all that is needed is a change in lovemaking techniques. Experiment!

- 55 percent experience impotence between the ages of sixty and seventy.

- 95 percent experience impotence at age seventy and older.

Impotence varies in severity. You're not impotent if you occasionally fail to have or sustain an erection. True impotence means that this happens all the time, most of the time, or frequently, even when you feel sexual desire or interest.

Impotence also does not include premature ejaculation, delayed ejaculation, lack of ejaculation, or lack of orgasm. And it does not mean lack of sexual desire.

Causes of impotence

Unofficially...
Worry and stress can actually decrease the level of testosterone in a man's body.

Impotence can be caused by emotional factors such as depression, worry, fear of sexual "failure" (performance anxiety), and relationship difficulties. These factors are more likely to cause temporary or occasional impotence (except in the case of severe depression). When emotional factors are the cause of impotence, men typically have normal erections during sleep, sexual fantasizing, or masturbation, when psychological pressures are less intense.

In men with diabetes, impotence usually has a physical cause. The most common causes are

- Age—impotence is primarily a problem for men in their fifties and older

- Blood circulation problems

- Nerve damage

Getting older happens to everyone, but men with diabetes are especially prone to problems with blood circulation and nerve function. These can be long-term complications of diabetes (see Chapter 4).

For erection to occur, the spongy erectile tissues of the penis must have a generous supply of blood. Circulatory problems—weakened, collapsed, or blocked vessels—reduce or stop the supply of blood to the penis. And nerve damage that interferes with genital sensation, or with the automatic triggering of an erection, can also prevent normal erections.

Impotence caused by blood vessel and nerve problems tends to develop slowly and worsen over time. Usually, a man will begin to notice

- Less firm erections,

- Fewer erections, and

- Erections that don't last, with each problem slowly worsening.

Men with diabetes who wish to enjoy active, healthy sex lives have one more reason to maintain stable blood-sugar levels and to avoid or control diabetic complications.

Other causes

If you are bothered by impotence, talk to your doctor. It is important to rule out causes of impotence that are not related to diabetes. Some other culprits are

- **Medications.** Many types of medication can trigger or aggravate impotence, such as blood-pressure medication, antidepressants, antipsychotics, tranquilizers, nonsteroidal drugs for pain, swelling, or ulcers, and anticonvulsant (epilepsy) medication.

- **Cigarettes.** Smoking is a major contributor to hardening of the arteries. It can diminish blood flow to the penis. If nothing else has inspired you to quit smoking, maybe this will.

Watch Out!
Men who take nitroglycerin (ISMO, Isordil) for chest pain may experience a severe drop in blood pressure, fainting, and even death if they also take *sildenafil* (Viagra). If you take sildenafil, do not use nitro- glycerin medica- tion to treat chest pain during sexual activity.

- **Excessive alcohol.** It is widely known that alco- hol can increase sexual desire but reduce sexual performance. Intoxication can interfere with the normal physiological processes that lead to erection, and it may lower testosterone levels.

- **Marijuana and opiates (hash or opium).** These drugs can suppress sexual functioning and may lower testosterone levels in chronic users.

- **Amphetamines (speed or uppers).** These can interfere with the nervous system's control of normal erections.

Less common medical causes of impotence are abnormally low testosterone levels and *Peyronie's dis- ease*, which distorts the shape of the penis and may inhibit erections or cause painful erections.

Treating impotence

Men seeking treatment for impotence have more options today than ever before.

If medications, smoking, or drug and alcohol use are causing impotence, appropriate changes must be made first if the impotence is to improve.

If impotence is caused by other underlying phys- ical factors, the following treatments can be tried. We present them in order of treatment effectiveness and convenience, starting with the most effective and convenient:

- **Oral medication.** The newest treatment for impotence, introduced in 1998, is *sildenafil* (trade name Viagra). Sildenafil works by blocking enzymes that can interfere with the automatic erection process. Sildenafil is a very effective treatment for impotence. It is not an aphrodisiac; it will not cause an erection unless the man feels sexual interest or desire. Men who do not have erectile dysfunction will not have harder or longer-lasting erections by taking sildenafil.

Sildenafil is a very new drug, and while it looks promising, it is too soon to know what the long-term side effects, if any, might be.

- **Medicated Urethral System Erection (MUSE).** In this treatment, the man inserts into his urethra a small gel suppository containing a drug (*alprostadil*) that causes an erection. (The urethra is the tube inside the penis through which urine and semen pass). Compared to injecting drugs, this method avoids bruising and there is less chance of *priapism* (a painful, sometimes harmful condition in which the erection lasts for more than an hour and won't subside).

A gel containing alprostadil that can be applied to the surface of the penis, causing an erection, may be available by the year 2000. (The product is called *Topiglan* and is under development by the MacroChem Corporation of Lexington, Massachusetts, (781) 862-4003, www.macrochem. com.)

- **Injection therapy.** This involves self-injecting a drug (*papaverine*, *phentolamine*, or *alprostadil*) into the base of the penis, which causes an erection lasting usually from thirty minutes to an hour. Injection therapy can cause some bruising of the penis, and sometimes priapism.

- **Penile implants.** Surgeons can place within the penis a prosthetic device that can make the penis firm. There are two types of penile implants: inflatable and semi-rigid. Inflatable implants (much more expensive) are small cylinders inside the penis that are filled with

Bright Idea
For information about impotence and impotence treatments, call Medic Drugs Impotence Resources at (800) 686-8886, or visit their Web site at www.en.com./ medic/impotence.

fluid when an erection is desired. The fluid is held in a small reservoir implanted in the abdomen; a small pump within the scrotum is squeezed by hand to get fluid into the cylinders. Semi-rigid implants are flexible silicone rods that do not change in firmness.

- **Vacuum or pump devices.** These are tubular devices that are placed around the penis when an erection is desired. The device creates a vacuum pressure that draws blood into the penis. The device is removed and a special ring or band is placed around the base of the penis to help keep the blood inside it. The band can cause bruising if kept on too long.

- **Yohimbine** (trade names Yocon, Yohimex, and Aphrodyne). This is an older oral medication derived from the bark of an African tree, the yohimbe. It sounds like alternative medicine, but it is listed in the *Physician's Desk Reference* and is available only with a prescription. Research shows that it increases sexual arousal and performance in rats. It is not clear how effective it is in human beings, but it may be helpful for some. Yohimbine can cause high blood pressure, however.

- **Testosterone injections, patches, and pills.** The majority of men who are impotent do not have abnormally low testosterone levels, but it is something your doctor should rule out, especially if sex drive is low. Oral testosterone preparations are associated with a higher incidence of liver problems.

Watch Out!
Your risk for prostate cancer must be carefully assessed before you use testosterone treatments, which can increase the risk. If you begin testosterone treatment, you must be carefully monitored for complications such as breast enlargement, testicular atrophy, and liver abnormalities.

Psychological factors in sexual problems

Sigmund Freud, father of psychoanalysis, once said that sometimes a cigar is just a cigar. Even Freud recognized that not everything in life has deep psychological meaning.

Still, emotions and psychology do play a significant role in the sex lives of both men and women. Indeed, most practitioners believe that most sexual difficulties stem from emotional or relational issues. When sexual problems arise, it is important to question whether emotional factors are at work.

Depression

One of the classic symptoms of depression is the loss of interest in sex, or a loss of pleasure in having sex. (Loss of pleasure in other enjoyable activities also signals depression.) People with diabetes are at increased risk for depression, both because coping with a chronic disease can be depressing and because high blood-sugar levels can cause fatigue and a general feeling of illness. This in turn can lead to social withdrawal and to feeling sad or overwhelmed.

In some people, whether or not they have diabetes, depression is the result of chemical imbalances in the brain. In these people, lack of interest in sex can be quite pronounced.

If your sexual happiness has lessened, you may be depressed. Your doctor or a mental health specialist can help you determine what is causing the depression and whether you should take an antidepressant medication.

Watch Out!
Unfortunately, a side effect of some antidepressant medications is delayed orgasm or inability to reach orgasm. Be sure to review side effects with your doctor if he or she prescribes antidepressant medications.

Relationship and communication difficulties

Not all sex takes place between people who have close or ongoing relationships. Sex within such relationships offers many joys, but many challenges as well.

Often, the quality of a sexual relationship reflects the quality of the entire relationship. Your ability to communicate your needs to your partner can have a big effect on your sex life. Chronic anger (about sexual or other matters), unexpressed anger or hurt, and shame over sexual desires can all inhibit sexual enjoyment.

A little honest reflection should be all it takes to begin evaluating the state of communication between you and your partner. Do you feel you can trust your partner with your true feelings, sexual or otherwise? Have you kept your partner in the dark about some of your feelings? How have you responded to your partner's opening up to you?

All couples, at some time or another, struggle with hurt feelings, anger, and feelings of disappointment with a partner. Many couples find that professional counseling can help resolve persistent problems and get their communication back on track.

Ask a member of your health-care team, or a clergyman or clergywoman, for the names of reputable couples counselors. Or call the department of psychiatry at a respected hospital for the names of trustworthy mental health clinics or practitioners.

Past sexual trauma

People who have experienced rape, molestation, sex with a physically or emotionally abusive partner, or any sexual experience that was repugnant, painful, or frightening often find that these traumas affect their sexual functioning long after the fact.

It is beyond the scope of this book to provide detailed information on the impact of sexual abuse. Our objective is to point out that, if there is sexual trauma in your background, it could be the source of sexual difficulties today. Severe or repeated sexual abuse can also cause depression, self-destructive behaviors, addictions, eating disorders, and low self-esteem. (These symptoms can have other causes, however.)

Recovery from sexual abuse usually requires the help of a mental health professional who has experience in working with the symptoms and difficulties that past abuse can cause. It is essential to see a reputable, experienced professional. Do not simply pick someone out of the phonebook. Seek a referral from your doctor or a doctor who specializes in treating sexual disorders.

Your doctor's role

You and your doctor share a responsibility to bring up sexual matters. Sexual functioning is an important "window" into a person's general health and quality of life. As one who is overseeing your health care, your doctor should be willing to discuss sexual issues with you. Ideally, he or she should even bring up the topic!

If your doctor has not asked you about your sexual functioning, ask if he or she would mind discussing it. Regardless of who brings it up, you and your doctor should regularly go over these questions:

■ Have you noticed a decrease in sexual desire or interest?

■ Have you experienced vaginal dryness (if you are a woman) or problems with erections (if you are a man)?

Unofficially...
A survey of male and female doctors showed that 85 percent of doctors ask their male patients about sex but only 33 percent ask their female patients about sex.

- Do you have pain or discomfort with sexual intercourse (if you are a woman)?

- Is it more difficult for you to reach orgasm than in the past?

- Are you less satisfied with your sexual relationship than you were before?

Unofficially...
The movie *Steel Magnolias* stars actress Julia Roberts as a woman with type 1 diabetes who gets pregnant against medical advice, then dies of a stroke and kidney failure. This is Hollywood melodrama. It is not what happens to the vast majority of women with diabetes who have children!

Diabetes and pregnancy

Many people believe that women with diabetes are unable to have healthy, safe pregnancies and healthy, normal babies. This is simply not true. There was a time when diabetic women faced serious difficulties in pregnancy, such as miscarriages, stillborn babies, and birth defects. These problems are caused by uncontrolled or poorly controlled blood sugar. Today, our knowledge of tight glucose control and how to achieve it, as well as improvements in prenatal care, have greatly reduced the risks to mothers and infants.

It's your responsibility to plan ahead, practice intensive diabetes management, and get high quality prenatal care. If you do so, your chances of delivering a healthy baby are excellent.

Excellent glucose control

The woman with diabetes who wishes to have a child must understand the importance of achieving excellent glucose control. This means not just average, or OK, but excellent, near-normal blood-sugar levels. (The fasting blood-sugar level of a nondiabetic woman is actually lower during a normal pregnancy.)

Your doctor will recommend the specific glucose level goals that are best for you. Blood-sugar levels for pregnant women are lower than for women who are not pregnant. An example of typical pregnancy glucose goals would be

- Before breakfast: 60 to 90 mg/dl.

- Before lunch, supper, and bedtime snack: 60 to 105 mg/dl.

- One to two hours after meals: 120 to 130 mg/dl.

- Early morning (2 a.m. to 6 a.m.): 60 to 100 mg/dl.

Before you conceive

Preferably, the mother's glucose control is excellent at the time she conceives. Ideally, she should plan three to six months ahead for pregnancy and should meet with her health-care team to begin treatment changes.

She must also have a complete physical examination before becoming pregnant. It is very important for you and your doctors to be aware of any complications of diabetes you may have, especially kidney disease or eye disease. Severe complications can threaten a pregnancy. And pregnancy can make complications worse, especially if your diabetes is poorly controlled.

Keep in mind that it may take several months to learn the methods of intensive, or "tight," glucose control (frequent blood monitoring, using the monitoring to make adjustments in insulin dose, or other factors) and to achieve and maintain near-normal blood sugar. More important, studies show that good blood-sugar control in the three to six months *before* pregnancy improves the chances for a good outcome. (Remember that the glycated hemoglobin test is a valuable tool for evaluating your glucose control in the months before you conceive. Ask your doctor to order this test.)

Bright Idea
Studies show that starting tight glucose control before conception lowers the risk of birth defects to 1 to 5 percent, compared to 10 percent when tight control starts after conception.

Women with well-controlled type 2 diabetes who are not taking oral medications may tighten their glucose control with dietary and exercise adjustments recommended by their doctor, along with increased glucose monitoring.

Women with type 2 diabetes who take oral diabetes medications will need to stop these medications and take insulin during pregnancy. Oral diabetes medications can cause birth defects and cannot be taken by pregnant women. However, insulin needs increase during pregnancy, and so does insulin resistance. If you are not currently taking insulin, you will need time before pregnancy to learn how to use it.

Poor control and birth defects

Women with diabetes should strive for near-normal glucose levels before conceiving because the first twelve weeks (the first trimester) of pregnancy is a critical time in the baby's development. The heart, brain, spinal cord, kidneys, and bones undergo most of their development during this time. If the mother's blood-sugar levels are high, these organs (and others) can suffer serious defects. Poor glucose control at the time of conception also raises the risk for miscarriage.

During the second and third trimesters, glucose control continues to be extremely important. The risk for devastating birth defects is much smaller, but the baby may grow too large, which may result in delivery before the baby's lungs are completely mature. With poor glucose control, the woman has increased risks for high blood pressure, *preeclampsia* (very high blood pressure and fluid retention), and early labor. Any diabetic complications the woman has may worsen under the stress of pregnancy and poor control.

Oversized babies

The other major risk of poor glucose control during pregnancy is that it can lead to the development of large, obese babies, weighing ten pounds or more at birth. (In some families, this may be a genetically normal size.) The medical term for oversized babies is *macrosomia*. Large babies face greater risks at delivery, as do their mothers. Delivery may be very difficult, or may take too long. A large baby may need to be delivered by caesarean section.

How babies become oversized

The fetus developing in the womb shares its mother's blood supply. If the mother's blood sugar level is high, the baby's pancreas is stimulated to produce large amounts of insulin (which is not shared with the mother). Large amounts of blood sugar and insulin cause fat to develop.

If the mother's blood sugar is at near-normal levels, the baby usually grows to a normal size.

Risks of being oversized

First, as mentioned, deliveries of large babies can be more complicated and risky.

Second, a baby born with an overactive pancreas, one that is producing a lot of insulin, is at risk for developing hypoglycemia (low blood sugar) after birth.

Third, due to the baby's size there is a greater risk of somewhat premature delivery. Labor may start and the baby may be delivered before its internal organs are ready to take on life outside the womb. In particular, the baby's lungs may be immature.

Diabetes management during pregnancy

You want to protect the health of your baby. Your goal during pregnancy is to maintain near-normal blood glucose levels. You will need to practice intensive diabetes management. What's involved?

Generally speaking, intensive glucose control means frequent blood-sugar monitoring (usually seven or more times per day), frequent insulin injections (three to five injections per day) or insulin pump therapy, and making adjustments in meal times, meal content, and activity levels, based on blood-sugar monitoring, so that blood sugar remains stable.

Insulin use

If you plan to use an insulin pump to achieve tight glucose control during pregnancy (as is becoming increasingly common), you should begin using the pump three to six months before conceiving, so that you are familiar with pump operation and you achieve near-normal glucose levels before you become pregnant.

If you plan to use insulin injections, your doctor must decide how much insulin you need, how often to inject, and what types of insulin to use.

- Most women will need at least twice-daily injections. These might be a morning shot of a mixture of intermediate (NPH) and short (Regular) acting insulin (70/30 percent, respectively), and a pre-dinner shot of NPH and Regular (50/50 percent each).

- For most women with type 1 diabetes, three daily injections may be recommended: The 70/30 percent mixed morning dose, an injection of short-acting insulin at dinner, and an injection of intermediate-acting insulin at bedtime.

Watch Out!
For pregnant women, intensive self-care includes testing the urine for ketones every morning before breakfast, and any time that your blood-sugar level is 240 mg/dl or greater. Diabetic ketoacidosis is associated with a high risk for stillbirth.

- Some women will need an additional injection of short- or rapid-acting insulin with their lunch or a snack.

Most women need larger doses of insulin as pregnancy progresses. This is due to their increased body size and because hormones and enzymes secreted by the placenta make them more resistant to insulin.

During the first trimester, however, you may actually go through a temporary period of reduced insulin need, again probably due to hormonal shifts. This can happen around weeks eight through twelve. You are more vulnerable to hypoglycemia at this time. Your doctor will be on the lookout for this pattern.

Glucose monitoring

To guard against high blood sugar, low blood sugar, and ketoacidosis, your doctor will probably recommend that you perform glucose monitoring at least seven times per day. Usual recommended times for monitoring are

- Upon rising (a fasting level)
- One to two hours after breakfast (during pregnancy, you may notice a sharper rise in glucose following early-morning carbohydrates)
- Before lunch
- One to two hours after lunch
- One to two hours before dinner
- One to two hours after dinner
- At bedtime

Intensive treatment plans must be tailored to each individual. Your diagnosis, state of health, and previous treatment plan must all be considered. If

66

When I was pregnant, my blood sugar used to shoot up after breakfast. I was eating too many carbohydrates in the morning. My dietitian told me to spread my carbs out more through the day, and it helped.
—Pat, age thirty-three, with type 2 diabetes

you want to become pregnant, or if you have discovered you are pregnant, meet with your health-care team as soon as possible so that they can put together the right treatment plan for you, which you can begin to follow immediately, before you conceive.

Food

Doctors recommend that most pregnant women, diabetic or not, get 100 to 300 extra calories per day—which isn't exactly eating for two! A weight gain of twenty-two to thirty-five pounds is generally considered healthy, with a gain of about two to four pounds during the first trimester and one-half to one pound each week thereafter.

Seek the recommendation of your doctor or a registered dietitian on what foods to eat. Most women need to pay attention to the following nutritional needs during pregnancy:

- Protein should usually be increased by ten grams per day. Look for low-fat sources, such as skinless, broiled poultry (white meat), water-packed tuna, or low or nonfat cottage cheese.

- The need for iron, folic acid (folate), and calcium is higher during pregnancy. These micronutrients are important to the fetus's development. Eat plenty of dark-green leafy vegetables, dried beans, and whole-wheat products. You'll need at least 1,500 to 2,000 milligrams of calcium a day, which can include as much as 1,200 from a quart of milk. (Make yours skim!)

Most doctors prescribe a special, folate-rich vitamin and mineral supplement for expecting mothers.

Bright Idea
Eating small, frequent meals can be very helpful during pregnancy. This strategy can help to keep glucose levels stable and can relieve nausea. And small meals are easier to manage as the baby begins to press against your stomach.

Exercise

There are excellent reasons to exercise during pregnancy, including improved cardiovascular fitness, greater muscle strength, lower glucose levels, easier weight control, and stress reduction. After all, delivering a baby and caring for a newborn are two of the biggest physical challenges you will ever face!

If you were a regular exerciser before becoming pregnant, your doctor may recommend that you stick to your exercise routine, keeping in mind the safety guidelines we list below. If you are not an exerciser but want to reap the many health benefits of exercise while you are pregnant, it is possible for many women (not all) to begin a low-intensity exercise program during pregnancy.

Whatever your situation, you must discuss exercise with your doctor and get his or her approval and recommendations.

Here are some guidelines for safe exercise during pregnancy:

- Monitor your blood sugar before and after exercise, and during exercise if necessary.

- Limit the strenuous part of your workout to fifteen minutes.

- Keep your heart rate under 140 beats per minute (twenty-three beats per ten-second pulse count).

- Keep your body temperature under 100°F.

- To keep your workout safe yet vigorous, try fast walking or add arm movements to your walking. Upper body exercises and walking are probably the safest aerobic exercises for pregnant women.

- Stop immediately if you feel lightheaded, faint, weak, or very out of breath.

Watch Out!
Do not take large doses of unprescribed vitamins and minerals during pregnancy. The effects on the unborn baby are unclear, and could be harmful. Stick to the supplement your doctor prescribes.

Watch Out!
Uterine contractions during exercise can be a sign that you are working too hard. Your doctor can teach you how to monitor yourself for contractions.

Pregnancy and hypoglycemia

Being on a tight glucose control plan during pregnancy may make you more vulnerable to episodes of hypoglycemia. Symptoms can be different when you are pregnant; instead of shakiness and perspiration, you may be more likely to experience sudden, pronounced drowsiness or confusion.

Pregnant women can also develop hypoglycemia unawareness. For these reasons, it is very important that you monitor your blood consistently and take steps to prevent "lows." There is no evidence that hypoglycemia will directly harm your unborn baby, but it could put you in an unsafe position in which harm could result.

Always test your glucose level:

- Before driving.
- Before and after exercising.
- If you are nauseated and having a hard time eating (see Chapter 5 for tips on managing your blood sugar during illness).

Always have a snack of simple carbohydrate and a glucagon injection kit at hand, and make sure that family and colleagues know how to help if hypoglycemia occurs.

See Chapter 5 for more information on hypoglycemia.

Medical care during pregnancy

High quality, consistent prenatal care is as important to the health of your baby as glucose control is. Along with making a commitment to intensive diabetes management, you must commit to intensive obstetric care throughout pregnancy.

We've already noted that good prenatal care begins with a thorough pre-pregnancy physical exam.

Once you are pregnant, expect to see your diabetes doctor and your obstetrician at least every other week during your pregnancy, at least through the thirty-second week. After that, you will probably meet once weekly.

You should also meet with a registered dietitian. Try to do this before you conceive. Your dietitian will let you know how often you should have nutrition counseling appointments during pregnancy.

Besides regular appointments, you will need

- Screening for neural tube defects in the fetus (damage to the early brain and spinal cord). This is done at fifteen to twenty weeks. (Adequate folate during pregnancy greatly reduces the risk of neural tube defects.)

- An ultrasound examination early in the pregnancy to check for birth defects.

- Ultrasound tests every four to six weeks during the pregnancy to check the growth and size of the baby.

- A fetal echocardiogram, which tests the structure and functioning of the baby's heart, at eighteen to twenty weeks.

In addition, your doctor may order fructosamine tests, which show how well controlled your glucose is on average over two to three weeks. (See Chapter 5 under "Other Blood-Sugar Tests.")

- If you have a history of eye problems or if you have had diabetes for more than five years, you must see an ophthalmologist as soon as possible in your pregnancy, and periodically throughout your pregnancy as recommended by the opthalmologist.

Timesaver
Have you recently been diagnosed with diabetes, and know that you want to have children? Try to begin your care with an endocrinologist who has experience in caring for diabetic women who are pregnant. Or find an obstetrician-gynecologist with that experience.

Labor and delivery

Your blood sugar will be monitored closely during delivery, not only for your protection but to protect your baby's health as well.

- If your blood sugar is too high during labor and delivery, the baby will produce too much insulin and will become hypoglycemic after delivery.

- If your blood sugar is too high, you could develop ketoacidosis.

Your blood sugar should stay close to normal (60 to 100 mg/dl) while you deliver your baby.

Controlling blood sugar during delivery

The most commonly used method for keeping glucose levels stable during labor and delivery is to give the mother intravenous insulin and glucose while frequently monitoring blood glucose (usually every hour). That way, the balance between insulin and glucose can be adjusted as needed. It also provides a much-needed source of calories and energy for the mother in labor.

Your need for insulin may be much smaller during labor, because it is hard physical work and burns a lot of energy at a time when you will not be eating. You may not need any insulin at all, in fact.

Your baby

Your baby's blood glucose levels will be closely monitored in the twenty-four hours after birth. The baby will also be checked for jaundice, which is common in newborns. Jaundice is treated with blue-light therapy.

If the baby was delivered prematurely, or is very large, he or she will be watched for respiratory difficulties. The baby's lungs may not be completely mature.

Bright Idea
Be sure to keep track of any insulin you give yourself on the day of your delivery. Let your doctor know, so that any necessary adjustments can be made in your intravenous insulin.

After delivery

Your glucose levels will be followed in the days after delivery. This will determine your insulin needs.

Most women can resume their pre-pregnancy insulin program by three or four days after delivery. Keep in mind, though, that the weeks following delivery may be a time of swings in blood glucose. Your hormones are rearranging themselves, you are probably exhausted, and your appetite and eating habits may be unpredictable.

It's important to keep your follow-up appointments with your doctor for help in assessing your glucose control and in adjusting your treatment to your post-delivery state. It's a happy time, but extremely demanding. You may need more support and guidance than usual in order to stick to good self-care.

Breastfeeding

There is no reason why mothers with diabetes shouldn't breastfeed their children. Indeed, the American Diabetes Association reports that children who are breastfed for at least three months have a lower incidence of type 1 diabetes.

Remember that you cannot use oral medications if you breastfeed. They are not safe for your infant.

Breastfeeding is wonderful for your baby, but be aware that it can make glucose control more difficult. The amount of caloric energy needed to create breast milk can cause your glucose level to become low. If you use insulin, your insulin requirements may change. Your appetite may be greater, and you may have special nutritional needs.

Discuss your plans to breastfeed with your doctor. You may want to consult a registered dietitian, too, for help in balancing your nutritional needs

Unofficially...
About 50 to 60 percent of women who have gestational diabetes will develop type 2 diabetes within five to ten years, especially overweight women. An oral glucose tolerance test done six to eight weeks following delivery can help to predict your risk.

with your diabetes management. You may need to snack before breastfeeding, especially during night-time feedings, to keep glucose levels stable. You should continue to do frequent glucose monitoring for as long as you are a nursing mother.

Gestational diabetes mellitus (GDM)

This temporary form of diabetes arises during pregnancy in women who were not previously diabetic. Obstetricians routinely test all women for GDM. It usually appears around the twenty-fourth week of pregnancy. It usually disappears once the infant is delivered.

GDM occurs because hormones produced by the placenta block the action of insulin in the body, causing insulin resistance. The problem is compounded by the woman's increased body size. She needs more insulin, yet she is also more insulin resistant.

Two to 5 percent of pregnant women develop GDM. No one knows exactly why some women develop it. It is more common in women who have the risk factors for type 2 diabetes, and in older pregnant women (in their thirties and forties). Women who develop GDM have an increased risk for developing type 2 diabetes later in life. If you develop GDM, consider having a glucose tolerance test six to eight weeks after you deliver your baby. It can help to predict your risk of developing type 2 diabetes.

If you have GDM, your baby faces risks from your high blood-sugar level. Since GDM arises after the first trimester, your baby is not at grave risk for birth defects. But uncontrolled high blood sugar can cause your baby to become too large, which, as discussed earlier in this chapter, can make delivery

Bright Idea
If you have gestational diabetes, look for the book *Managing Your Gestational Diabetes*, by Lois Jovanovich-Peterson, M.D. (Chronimed Publishing, 1994). Dr. Jovanovich-Peterson has type 1 diabetes and is the mother of two.

more complicated and dangerous for both mother and child.

Treating GDM

The goal of GDM treatment is to keep the mother's glucose levels as close to normal as possible for the remainder of her pregnancy. To help you achieve this, your doctor will recommend dietary changes. He or she will also recommend that you test your blood-sugar levels frequently, usually four to six times a day.

Some women with GDM will need to start insulin injections.

Just the facts

- Sexual difficulties are a legitimate and important medical concern.

- If your doctor doesn't bring up sex, you can and should.

- Impotence is treatable.

- Women with diabetes have a higher incidence of vaginal yeast infections and vaginal dryness. Both are treatable.

- Excellent control of glucose levels and excellent prenatal care are the keys to a safe pregnancy and a healthy baby.

- Poor blood-sugar control during the first trimester increases the risk for severe birth defects and miscarriage.

- Unborn babies whose mothers have diabetes can grow to be too large if the mother's glucose levels are not well controlled.

- Gestational diabetes increases your risk for developing type 2 diabetes.

GET THE SCOOP ON...
Diabetes and your period ▪ Protecting your
heart ▪ Insulin and eating disorders ▪
Psychological issues for kids and teens ▪
Staying healthy, solo-style

You Have Diabetes and . . .

Chapter 13

D iabetes affects different lives differently. Women, children, and teens face unique challenges in coping with and treating diabetes. So do people with diabetes who live alone.

Women's hormonal cycles can cause changes in blood-sugar levels. And women are often more vulnerable to concerns over body image, weight gain or loss, and eating habits. Children must handle social pressures and the big responsibility of diabetes self-care. Teenagers struggle to reconcile their need for independence with their need to submit to the regimen of diabetes management. People living alone must take extra precautions against diabetic emergencies.

In this chapter we try to identify some of these special concerns, and we give some tips for coping with them.

Bright Idea
If you or some-
one you know is
a woman with
diabetes, you
may want to read
the American
Diabetes
Association's
publication
*Women and
Diabetes: A Life
Plan for Health
and Wellness,*
written by
Laurinda M.
Poirier and
Katharine M.
Coburn (1997).

Special concerns of women with diabetes

A woman with diabetes may be troubled by poor glucose control during the last half of her menstrual
cycle. She is at greater risk for developing heart disease than are women who do not have diabetes. She
may be overly focused on food intake and body
weight. She may be more vulnerable to feeling
stressed out, depressed, or both.

Diabetes and the menstrual cycle

It happens every month: you get your period. And
for many women with diabetes, something else happens: their blood-sugar levels become high, despite
the most conscientious self-care.

To understand how this can happen, recall that
during the menstrual cycle, the levels of two female
sex hormones, estrogen and progesterone, rise and
fall. Estrogen and progesterone interfere with the
action of insulin. When the levels of these hormones
are at their highest, the body is more insulin resistant, and blood sugar can rise.

This is true whether or not you inject insulin.
Women who treat their diabetes with diet and exercise, or with oral diabetes medications, can also
experience increased insulin resistance. When the
body is more insulin resistant, blood-sugar levels will
climb if the insulin supply is not increased. At what
point in the menstrual cycle are blood-sugar levels
likely to rise? Estrogen and progesterone levels build
to their highest point during the last half of what is
usually a twenty-eight day cycle. This is the part of
the cycle following ovulation (the release of an egg
from an ovary), which usually occurs midway
through the cycle (around the fourteenth day from
the beginning of the last menstrual period).

During the two weeks or so following ovulation, hormone levels rise. In the days just before menstruation begins, hormone levels are at their highest and insulin resistance can be high, and so, too, can blood-sugar levels. Some women find that their normal treatment regimen is not enough to control blood-sugar levels at this time.

Coping with hormonal fluctuations

If your glucose levels become higher as your period approaches, you will need to make adjustments in your self-care at that time. Two preliminary steps that could help are

- Try to determine exactly when you ovulate each month. Estrogen and progesterone begin rising following ovulation. You can check for ovulation by using a special ovulation thermometer (which measures the rise in your basal body temperature that indicates ovulation has occurred), or you can use a home ovulation predictor kit that tests your urine, which is more expensive, but more accurate. Both are available at pharmacies.

- Keep a separate record of your fasting blood glucose reading every morning. Over time this record will help you to predict monthly changes in your blood-sugar levels. In most women, these changes will be similar and predictable from month to month.

Once you know when your blood-sugar levels are likely to rise, you can make appropriate changes in your treatment. You may make dietary changes, increase your exercise, or alter your oral medication doses (with your doctor's approval). If you take insulin, you might gradually increase your dosage of longer-acting insulin (NPH, Lente, or Ultralente) in small steps so that the level of insulin in your blood is higher before your period. If you use an insulin pump, you may need to increase the basal rate.

High blood sugar and PMS

Unofficially...
A recent study shows that consuming adequate calcium can calm the symptoms of PMS. Ask your doctor or registered dietitian.

Many women experience premenstrual syndrome, or PMS, in the days just before their period begins. This may due to the high level of progesterone at that time in the cycle. Woman may experience water retention, irritability, depression, and cravings for certain foods, especially carbohydrates and fats. Giving in to these cravings can raise blood-sugar levels.

You can take several steps to help tame PMS:

- Avoid salty foods, caffeine, alcohol, and chocolate.

- Get plenty of exercise.

- Practice relaxation techniques (such as breathing exercises, meditation, visual imagery, muscle relaxation, massage, and yoga).

- Talk to your doctor. He or she may have other recommendations, or may prescribe a medication that helps relieve the symptoms of PMS.

Women and heart disease

The female sex hormone estrogen is known to protect premenopausal women from developing coronary heart disease, the leading cause of death in men and women in the United States.

But women with diabetes, unfortunately, do not enjoy this protection.

A landmark study of heart disease, carried out in Framingham, Massachusetts, showed among other things that women with diabetes are just as likely to have heart disease as men with diabetes, regardless of the women's ages. Unlike their nondiabetic sisters, women with diabetes who are still menstruating and producing estrogen seem to lose the protective effects of estrogen.

This increased risk is caused by insulin resistance, a hallmark of type 2 diabetes. Insulin resistance leads to high levels of insulin in the bloodstream. This in turn is associated with high blood pressure and high levels of cholesterol and triglycerides. What is more, most women with type 2 diabetes have central-body obesity (the apple body shape). The combination of insulin resistance, high insulin levels, high blood pressure, high levels of cholesterol and triglycerides, and central-body obesity greatly increases the odds for developing atherosclerosis (hardening of the arteries).

To improve your chances for maintaining a healthy heart, consider these steps:

- Make sure that your doctor appreciates the higher risk for heart disease that premenopausal women with diabetes face.

- If you smoke, stop.

- Get regular, moderate aerobic exercise to condition the cardiovascular system and to help elevate your "good" HDL cholesterol. Follow your doctor's recommendations for an exercise program.

- If you have reached menopause, consider hormone replacement therapy. This can reduce the risk for heart disease.

- If you are age fifty or older, consider asking your doctor to order a stress test. People with diabetes can develop silent heart disease.

- Control high blood pressure and high cholesterol.

- Maintain good blood-sugar control.

- Lose weight. Follow your doctor's recommendations for weight loss.

- Ask your doctor about taking *metformin* (Glucophage) or *troglitazone* (Rezulin). Both medicines are oral diabetes medications. Metformin can lower triglyceride levels and promote weight loss; troglitazone also lowers triglycerides and can improve blood pressure.

Stress and depression

Stress can raise blood-sugar levels. Depression can cause self-care to suffer. These emotional states can deeply affect the person with diabetes.

Women in general are more prone than men to develop mood and anxiety disorders. Women with diabetes are especially vulnerable to depression and stress, partly because high blood-sugar levels can affect physical well-being, and thus mood, and partly because living with a chronic, closely managed disease can cause stress and depression.

Women with diabetes should learn to recognize symptoms of depression and stress, as well as sources of depression and stress in their lives. (Remember that anxiety and irritability may be signs of low blood sugar.) Learn to cope with these emotions, and seek professional help if necessary. Chapters 10 and 14 provide more information about emotions and diabetes.

Eating disorders

Eating disorders grow out of a preoccupation with food intake, body weight, and body shape. This focus can have psychological roots in family dynamics, perfectionism, unexpressed anger, and the strong cultural valuing of thinness.

Unofficially... Controlling high blood pressure reduces the risk of coronary artery disease by 15 percent and reduces the risk of stroke by 40 percent.

Women account for the vast majority of eating disorder cases. Some evidence in recent years suggests that women with diabetes, especially those with type 1 diabetes, are especially at risk for developing eating disorders. Weight and food are subjects of much concern for a person with diabetes.

There are three types of eating disorders:

■ **Bulimia nervosa.** Women with bulimia engage in binge eating followed either by purging (through vomiting or the abuse of laxatives, diuretics, or enemas) or by a nonpurging behavior designed to prevent weight gain from the binge. For example, women who use insulin can omit or change doses as a means of preventing weight gain.

■ **Anorexia nervosa.** Women with anorexia have an intense fear of food and of gaining weight. They may be severely underweight, yet see themselves as fat and refuse to gain weight. Anorectic women either reduce their food intake to near-starvation levels or engage in a binge-purging cycle. They may exercise compulsively and intensively. Anorectic women who use insulin may omit or reduce their insulin dose to promote weight loss through sugar calories eliminated in the urine.

■ **Binge-eating disorder.** This refers to recurrent episodes of voracious, rapid eating to discomfort, accompanied by distress and guilt. No purging behavior follows the binge episodes.

Many women restrict calories or exercise compulsively. A full-fledged eating disorder, however, is a potentially life-threatening medical and psychological problem requiring professional treatment.

Watch Out!
Women with diabetes should be aware that diuretics (drugs that relieve bloating by causing the body to flush out excess fluid) can increase the amount of insulin your body needs. If you take diuretics, you must monitor its effects on your glucose levels.

Some other telltale symptoms of an eating disorder are

■ Weighing less than 85 percent of what is normal for your height and frame.

■ Missing three or more consecutive menstrual periods.

■ Feeling like you can't stop eating or that your eating is out of control.

Bright Idea
For help in finding a qualified therapist, contact the American Anorexia/Bulimia Association, 165 West 46th Street, Suite 1108, New York, NY 10036, (2l2) 575-6200.

Women with diabetes should keep in mind that they may be tempted to misuse insulin in order to lose weight. They should also be aware that they may, at times, feel a sense of loss of control over their bodies as they work hard to manage a chronic disease. These factors can make women with diabetes more vulnerable to eating disorders. When diabetes is present, treatment is more complicated.

Seek the help of a mental health professional if you suspect, or know, that you have an eating disorder. Let your doctor know as well. An eating disorder is not likely to get better on its own, and it can have devastating effects on your diabetes management and your health in general.

Diabetes and osteoporosis

Osteoporosis is a common disorder in which bones become thinner, weaker, more brittle, and more likely to fracture. It is most common in women who have reached menopause and who do not take estrogen supplements. Women with type 1 diabetes are at increased risk for developing osteoporosis. Women with type 2 diabetes, on the other hand, seem to have a lower-than-average risk of developing osteoporosis for reasons that are not entirely clear. It may be because more women with type 2 diabetes are overweight and that body fat protects against bone loss. Having too little insulin can affect the absorption of calcium and the growth of bone cells. People with untreated type 1 diabetes have about 10 percent less bone density than is normal for their age and sex. Bone loss stops once insulin treatment is begun, but the smaller bone mass creates a higher risk for eventual osteoporosis when bone loss increases after menopause. To guard against osteoporosis

- Consume the minimum recommended daily amounts of calcium (1500 mg) and vitamin D (500 IU).

- Get regular exercise, like walking or dancing, that forces the bones to bear some weight. This keeps bones healthy and dense.

- If you are at or near menopause, speak to your doctor about bone-density tests and, if necessary, medications for the prevention or treatment of osteoporosis.

Don't wait to have a painful, debilitating fracture before thinking about osteoporosis! For more information, contact the National Osteoporosis Foundation at 1150 17th Street NW, Suite 500, Washington, DC 20036, phone: (202) 223-2226, Web: www.nof.org.

Hormone replacement therapy

As women enter menopause (typically around age fifty), the reduction of estrogen in their bodies greatly increases their risk for heart disease and osteoporosis. Since all women with diabetes already have an increased risk for heart disease, and some (those with type 1 diabetes) are at increased risk for osteoporosis, it is important for older women who have diabetes to consider with their doctors the possibility of hormone replacement therapy (HRT).

Unofficially... At the turn of the century, most women lived for less than ten years after their last menstrual period. Today, most women live for thirty-five years after their last period. It is no wonder that medical science is increasingly interested in studying the effects of hormone treatment.

In HRT, women take estrogen in the form of pills or skin patches. Vaginally applied creams are available to treat the vaginal dryness that can come with menopause. (Vaginal dryness is also a common complaint of women with diabetes, even premenopausal women. See Chapter 12.)

Before starting HRT, each woman must weigh the potential risks and benefits. HRT reduces the risk of heart disease by 50 percent, and has been shown to prevent bone loss (osteoporosis). And HRT doesn't disrupt glucose control. On the other hand, some research indicates that HRT increases the risk of breast cancer and endometrial cancer (cancer of the uterine lining). Estrogen taken with progesterone does not increase the risk of endometrial cancer, but the effect of HRT on breast cancer risk is not clear.

Hormone replacement therapy is an option that must be thoroughly discussed with your primary-care physician.

Bladder problems

Women with diabetes may be more likely to develop bladder infections due to

- Nerve damage that affects bladder functioning and

- Higher than normal blood-sugar levels, which nourish bacteria.

Nerve damage (diabetic neuropathy) can stop you from sensing that your bladder is full or prevent your bladder from emptying properly. Either condition can predispose you to bladder infections.

Bladder infections cause a burning sensation and pain with urination. The urine may be cloudy or bloody. Bladder infections can ascend to the

Bright Idea
For more information on health and menopause, contact The North American Menopause Society, P.O. Box 94527, Cleveland, OH 44101, (216) 844-8748. Or visit their Web site at www.menopause. org.

kidneys, causing kidney damage. It is essential to treat bladder infections with doctor-prescribed antibiotics.

If you repeatedly develop bladder infections, you and your doctor should discuss referral to an urologist, preferably one with experience in treating people with diabetes. To reduce the frequency of bladder infections

- Never retain urine in your bladder. Always urinate when you feel the urge.

- Try to make sure that you completely empty your bladder when you urinate.

- Don't get dehydrated. You should drink enough water during the day that your urine is pale yellow to transparent in color. Aim for eight eight-ounce glasses each day.

- Urinate before and after sexual activity Sexual activity can cause bacteria to enter the urethra (the tube through which urine leaves the body) and the bladder.

- Always wipe from front to back after a bowel movement.

- Limit your intake of caffeine and alcohol. This may reduce irritation of the bladder and urethra.

You're a child: special concerns of children with diabetes

There is not enough space here for a detailed discussion of the medical treatment of diabetic children. Treatment varies because it is tailored to the child's age and to changes in size and maturity.

Luckily, there are many resources available to parents of newly diagnosed diabetic children. Your

Bright Idea
Young Adair Gregory has written a book called *Sugar Was My Best Food: Diabetes and Me* (published in 1998 by Alfred Whitman and Co.) for readers ages nine to twelve. Adair was diagnosed with type 1 diabetes at age nine. He recounts his fears, frustrations, and experiences at diabetes camp. He includes his e-mail address and a promise to answer all letters!

child's health-care team is a primary source of information on what to expect and on the role of parents in their children's care. The American Diabetes Association has many informational brochures and books for children and parents. Your local library and bookstores should have relevant books, or can help you get them. The magazine *Diabetes Self-Management*, published by the American Diabetes Association, regularly carries articles for parents.

The Internet is a rich resource, as well. For starters, look up the Juvenile Diabetes Foundation International at www.jdfcure.com or Children with Diabetes at www.childrenwithdiabetes.com.

Here, we identify some of the psychological and social elements of childhood diabetes. We hope this will give you a foothold in this complex terrain.

Infants and toddlers (zero to three years)

Children this young are completely dependent on their caregivers for management of their diabetes.

For children under five, repeated episodes of severe hypoglycemia may cause problems in cognitive (mental and intellectual) development. Parents must learn to recognize signs of hypoglycemia in their children, especially those who are not old enough to talk or describe their feelings.

The three most significant tasks for parents of very young children with diabetes are

- Negotiating the sharing of tasks in diabetes caretaking,

- Establishing a meal schedule that the child follows, and

- Preventing severe hypoglycemic episodes.

Caretakers need to keep in mind that the child cannot yet understand why shots and finger sticks are necessary. Children this age will also resist eating on schedule. Battles will inevitably arise, and this can be emotionally draining for parents. It is crucial for caretakers to support one another and, if possible, to have other sources of help, such as family, friends, or a support group.

Children ages four to seven
One problem affecting children this age is their tendency to interpret diabetes as something they have caused and to see their treatment as punishment for being "bad." Parents, and at this point teachers, should try to correct this misperception.

Interaction with other children with diabetes can be very helpful at this stage, as it demonstrates to children that they are not different, alone, or outcasts.

At this stage, children's motor skills and cognitive abilities allow them to take on more responsibility for their care, which can be a source of pride. But parents must be sure to keep their own expectations realistic and continue to provide close supervision and care.

Children ages eight to eleven
At this stage, children are very focused on their relationships with friends and peers. It is a time of comparing themselves to other children their age and striving hard to gain acceptance and approval. Being different can be very painful at this time.

For this reason, the parents of a child with diabetes in this age group need to support their child's

- Participation in activities, and
- Development of a positive self-image.

Although children look to one another for acceptance, they also thrive on parental approval

Bright Idea
Many children benefit from attending a diabetes camp. Ask your physician or diabetes educator or contact your local American Diabetes Association for information on the right camp for your child. Visit their Web site at www. childrenwithdiabetes.com.

Timesaver
To avoid time-consuming bat-tles, remember that giving chil-dren choices works better than prohibi-tions. Saying, "You can wear your red sweater or your green windbreaker" can be a lot more effective than saying, "You can't go outside wearing just a tee shirt."

and pride. Parents can clearly affirm these and can focus on positive behaviors, communicating their belief in the child's abilities by encouraging and sup-porting the child's activities and interests.

Active children and their parents will need to keep hypoglycemia in mind, and should review pre-vention, symptoms, and treatment of hypoglycemic episodes.

At this stage, most children can begin to do some glucose monitoring and give themselves injections with adult supervision. They can begin to identify and choose healthy foods. Also, older children can begin to understand the benefits of consistent, long-term diabetes management. Parents should begin to educate children about preserving their health—not with horror stories, but with an emphasis on teaching that good care today means better health tomorrow.

Children who have begun to perform glucose testing during the school day may find that class-mates feel special and rewarded if they are asked to help out with the testing. This helps to educate peers about diabetes while providing social support to children with diabetes and encouraging responsi-ble diabetes management.

In Appendix D, you'll find two forms that are helpful to parents of school-aged children with dia-betes: a "One-Page Care Guide for Children in School," which provides diabetes care instructions for your child's teacher, and a "Before School Starts Checklist for Parents," which provides a to-do check-list. These forms are reprinted with the kind permission of their author, Jeff Hitchcock, who created and manages the excellent Web site, www.childrenwithdiabetes.com, and who is the father of a young girl with type 1 diabetes.

Special concerns of teens with diabetes

Many adults would love to regain their teenage physiques. But their teenage psyches? That's another story!

The teenage years are an infamously rocky time. Having diabetes doesn't make it any easier.

Early adolescence: ages twelve to fifteen

This can be one of the most challenging times of life for children with diabetes and their families. The younger teen struggles with dramatic changes in size, appetite, and hormone levels that can interfere with stable glucose control.

It is also a time of heightened concern about social acceptance (young teens want desperately to fit in with peers) and when children experiment with independent actions and opinions. These things can also upset a well-established treatment plan, which the young teen may question, criticize, sabotage, or reject.

Parents of younger teens struggle with wanting to support greater independence and responsibility, especially in the area of diabetes self-care. How much independence is too much? What about young teens who insists that they are capable of completely taking over their diabetes care?

Parents walk a fine line between helping their children to grow and shifting too much responsibility onto young shoulders.

Here are some emotional difficulties facing young teens with diabetes and their parents:

- **Anger.** Younger teens may vent a lot of anger about having diabetes. They may rage at their parents, blaming the parents for giving them diabetes or "torturing" them with self-care requirements. Here, too, parents walk a fine

Watch Out!
Don't forget that complications of diabetes, like eye or kidney disease, can begin in childhood if glucose levels aren't well controlled most of the time.

line. They should not submit to abusive behavior, yet they need to respect their child's legitimate anger. More important, they need to support their teen's attempts to verbalize feelings that could otherwise be expressed in unhealthy, destructive behaviors (called *acting out* emotions).

- **The need for adult guidance and support.** No matter how loudly the young teen demands freedom and independence, he or she still craves parental guidance and attention. Parents should not overestimate their younger teen's ability to understand the disease of diabetes, its long-term complications, or the teen's ability to manage self-care without a lot of positive reinforcement from parents.

- **Concerns about body image.** Boys and girls alike can perceive themselves as weak, damaged, or unattractive because of diabetes. Especially girls' body image concerns must be taken seriously by parents and health-care providers. Many adolescent girls are preoccupied, even obsessed, with being slim. They are at risk for developing eating disorders, particularly in light of their medical need to focus on food intake. Adolescent girls may secretly omit or reduce insulin injections, causing blood sugar to soar, urination to increase, and calories to be purged. (This is a form of bulimia nervosa; see the discussion on eating disorders earlier in this chapter.)

Parents need to remain involved in their young teen's insulin treatment and glucose monitoring. Give your child some reasonable choices for greater independence, but do not withdraw your attention,

Unofficially...
The physiological changes of puberty are associated with increased insulin resistance in adolescents both with and without diabetes.

even if your teen initially resists or rejects your attempts to negotiate. Young teens want to know that parents support their growing independence but aren't going to desert them as they grow.

Later adolescence: ages sixteen to nineteen

This tends to be a calmer period than early adolescence for many teens with diabetes. Glucose control has usually become stable again, as growth and hormonal upheavals have subsided. Ideally, the older teen has eased into taking on the majority of responsibility—and, finally, total responsibility—for his or her day-to-day diabetes management.

At the same time, however, older teens face the often frightening challenge of separating from their families and living on their own.

The pressures that most teens face at this stage have to do with:

- Preparing for college or employment and
- Preparing for and mastering the skills necessary for living independently.

Older teens who feel overwhelmed by these tasks may use their diabetes to avoid greater independence. Some continue to have poor or inconsistent glucose control, either because they want to avoid independence or because they are experiencing problems, unhappiness, and neglect at home.

If poor glucose control persists in older teens, parents need to step in and help sort out what is at the root of the problem. Family counseling may be in order.

Older teenage girls who are worried about their weight should be evaluated for insulin misuse if glucose levels are not well controlled.

These girls need to understand the critical importance of planning pregnancies, of excellent

Bright Idea
One safe way to support your teen's growing independence is to encourage the teen to see doctors or other health-care professionals without you. You will not stop communicating with them, of course, but he or she may need more privacy now when meeting with doctors or diabetes educators.

Watch Out!
Teenagers with diabetes who drive or are learning to drive must be reminded that hypoglycemia and driving do not mix. They must also remember that drinking alcohol increases the risk for developing hypoglycemia.

glucose control during pregnancy, and high-quality prenatal care for diabetic women who become pregnant. The sexually active (or potentially sexually active) older teen must be aware of the serious risks for birth defects caused by high blood sugar during the first trimester of pregnancy.

It is easier for parents to anticipate the demands of independent living than it is for their older teens. Parents can help teens face the transition by encouraging young adults to make concrete plans for self-care before they have left home. An older teen may not have given any thought to planning meals around a hectic work and school schedule or instructing a roommate on how to recognize and treat hypoglycemia. (Make sure that your college-bound teen takes along a glucagon injection kit!) Parents can help with anticipatory strategies for independent diabetes management.

Special concerns when you're managing diabetes on your own

If you live alone, you need to be your own best friend when it comes to managing your diabetes. Think of your store of diabetes knowledge as your partner in keeping you safe, and support that partner! Make sure you have accurate and complete knowledge about diabetes and diabetes treatment. You will have to rely on your own judgment. Fortify it with good diabetes education.

Know your medication
It is essential that you understand how your insulin or oral medications work—when to take them, in what dosage, why you take them, and the basic facts about the way they work in your body. You also need to understand how these substances interact with

other factors that affect glucose levels, such as exercise, eating, and stress.

If you don't understand your medication or insulin, you increase your risk for both high and low glucose levels.

Safety strategies

- Don't forget your most powerful ally: frequent blood-sugar monitoring. It's tempting to rely solely on the way you feel, but this is risky. The best way to prevent dangerous highs and lows is to test your blood sugar often.

- Don't fail to check your urine for ketones if you are ill, and don't lower your insulin dosage even if it is hard to eat. Ketoacidosis can develop quickly. (See Chapter 5 for tips on managing your blood sugar when you are ill.)

- Be familiar with the symptoms of ketoacidosis, which include having a blood-sugar level of over 240 mg/dl; experiencing sleepiness, stomach pain or nausea, extreme thirst, blurred vision, or labored breathing; and having a fruity odor on your breath. Call your doctor right away if you have these symptoms.

- If you have type 2 diabetes, call your doctor if your blood sugar is higher than 350 mg/dl.

- If you are ill, ask a friend, neighbor, or relative to check in on you periodically until you are feeling better.

- Don't succumb to a constant diet of fast-food meals as a substitute for "cooking for one." Make dishes for two or three people and freeze extra portions.

- Ask your registered dietitian for help in designing a "cooking for one" meal plan.

Bright Idea
Designate one day a month to be your diabetes shopping day. Replenish your supplies of easy-to-eat carbohydrates, such as raisins, nondiet soda, crackers, hard candy, or any snacks you use to fend off hypoglycemia. This ensures that you always have the right snack on hand. Include your teenager, if he or she has diabetes, as a way of being together and promoting good self-care.

- Always keep some glucose tablets or gel and a telephone at your bedside. If possible, program your phone for one-touch speed dialing of an emergency assistance number.

- Don't be afraid to ask your health-care practitioners for guidance and help.

One question that comes up for people with diabetes who live alone is whether to keep a glucagon injection kit on hand. After all, glucagon is used to treat severe hypoglycemia, when the affected person is unable to care for him- or herself. It's preferable to eat some carbohydrate before hypoglycemia becomes severe. Glucagon can be self-injected, however, if a person cannot swallow a carbohydrate or can't keep it down.

Perhaps the best thing to do is to keep a glucagon kit on hand, with clearly posted instructions for finding and using it. Educate a few people whom you see often about how and when to administer glucagon injections.

What about insulin pumps?

Some people worry about using an insulin pump if they live alone for fear of increasing the risk of developing hypoglycemia.

However, a modern insulin pump is equipped with safety features. It cannot accidentally overdose you; you program the amount of insulin it delivers within a given period. You can also program pumps to shut off automatically if you have not touched the controls after a certain period of time. This protects against nighttime overdose and hypoglycemia. Also, the pumps beep if the flow of insulin is blocked for any reason, helping to prevent elevated glucose levels.

Watch Out!
Regular medical care is very important to people who live alone and who may not have anyone reminding them to take care of themselves. Be sure not to miss glycosylated hemoglobin tests or examinations for complications.

Overall, there is no reason why a responsible adult who lives alone cannot use an insulin pump. It is simply necessary to have a thorough understanding of how to operate the pump, and to take the same precautions against hypoglycemia that you would with any intensive insulin regimen.

Social support

Even if you love living alone, it's wise to cultivate a network of support. Become familiar with your local medical and educational resources. Besides friends and family, here are some other support resources to keep in mind:

- **Your health-care team.** Always speak to a health-care practitioner if you have any concerns about your diabetes management.

- **Your local American Diabetes Association.** The ADA is a source of information and referrals to support groups and educational classes in your area.

- **Your local hospital or Visiting Nurse Association.** These organizations may be able to provide services or refer you to services should you need someone to check in with you.

- If you are feeling lonely or isolated, consider volunteer work through the ADA or other organizations.

There is no reason why you cannot live independently with diabetes. Just be sure that you know your local resources, understand your treatment plan and are comfortable with it, and keep your store of diabetes knowledge up to date. Enjoy your freedom!

Bright Idea
Ask your diabetes-care team to put you in touch with other people who have diabetes and live alone. You can swap success stories and survival tips. Or visit a diabetes chat room through the American Diabetes Association Web site, www. diabetes.org.

Just the facts

- Just before the menstrual period begins, high levels of hormones can make it harder to control blood glucose.

- Women with diabetes are as likely to develop heart disease as men with diabetes, regardless of their age.

- Reducing or omitting insulin doses to cause weight loss is a form of eating disorder.

- Parents must remain involved in their children's diabetes management throughout the teen years.

- Parents face the challenge of balancing their involvement in their child's care with fostering independence.

- There is no reason you cannot live alone if your diabetes is well managed, your health in general is good, and you have cultivated a network of support resources.

Someone You Love: Friends, Families, and Diabetes

PART V

GET THE SCOOP ON...
Coping with diabetes as a couple ▪ How best to
help your partner who has diabetes ▪
Parenting and diabetes ▪ Diabetes etiquette ▪
Getting help from a mental health professional

In It Together: Personal Relationships and Chronic Illness

Chapter 14

Here's a paradox of chronic illness: On the one hand, you can feel utterly alone with your illness. On the other hand, your illness affects everyone who is close to you.

Both things are true. No one but you can know exactly what it is like for you to live with diabetes. Yet those who are close to you live with your diabetes, too.

Another paradox is that chronic illness can stress personal relationships, and also strengthen them. Resentments will flare; expectations will be disappointed; sadness, guilt, and anger will set in. Out of these challenges, however, new strength and greater closeness can be forged.

Having diabetes can sometimes feel like the worst thing in the world. However, knowing that you are loved and cared for when times are tough can feel better than anything.

373

Your need for social support

We all need to know that there are people in our lives who care about us. This is a simple fact of human existence, and people with diabetes are no exception.

Unofficially...
According to the American Diabetes Association, the secret of living well with diabetes is to combine self-awareness with good diabetes information.

Acknowledging needs

Feeling "different" can be so painful that, if you have diabetes, you may find yourself minimizing your need and desire for emotional support. You may feel stronger and more in control if you tell yourself that nothing is changed and you don't need any help. You may even be a little frightened of being "needy"; what if others feel overburdened? What if they don't come through for you?

It is important to acknowledge that we all have emotional needs, regardless of our circumstances. And whether or not illness enters the picture, all relationships require these elements to thrive:

- Give and take,
- Mutual respect,
- Honest communication,
- Genuine listening, and
- Knowing when to back off or let something go.

A medical and emotional condition

Remember that having diabetes can generate strong emotions, especially at first. Dealing with these feelings is a central part of managing your illness. Painful feelings aren't going to go away just because you deny or minimize them. Instead, they are likely to result in behaviors that can jeopardize self-care.

It's not that different

We all depend on one another. You need to be heard and to be helped; you also need to hold up your end, to hear and to help. So having diabetes doesn't make you that different after all. You're ahead of the coping game if you can acknowledge your need for social support. And your relationships needn't change greatly if you do your part and keep applying the necessary elements.

Good relationships are based on mutual affection, but they also rely on the effort and skills of the people involved. Let's take a look at some ways to help keep relationships strong when diabetes hits home.

Coping skills for couples

Chronic illness can really test the depth and maturity of the bond between life partners; it can also enhance that depth and maturity. A "committed relationship" is truly that when a couple successfully face the challenge of long-term illness.

But what is the best way to pull together instead of pulling apart?

Honest communication

This is the most important task for couples facing difficult issues. The easier (though not always easy) part of it is to communicate to each other your love, support, and your promise to be there for the long haul. The harder part, with the biggest payoff in terms of safeguarding the relationship, is to communicate honestly about tough feelings like

- Anger,
- Blame,
- Fear,
- Loss or grief, and
- Guilt.

It is hard for people who care deeply about one another to express these feelings. But the fact is that

I don't need more advice than most people, and I don't need a 'policeman' telling me what to do. Hey, I know what I'm supposed to do! I just need you to listen for a while. That's what really helps.
—Angela, age forty-six, with type 2 diabetes

they will come up between partners when one has a
chronic illness. This is natural and unavoidable. You
may become angry if your partner develops diabetes, especially if your partner has not been taking
good care of him- or herself. At the same time, you
may blame yourself for not doing more to encourage healthy behavior in your partner. You may fear
what the future will bring, and you may feel grief at
the loss of your partner's former health. With these
feelings can come guilt.

If you have diabetes, you may feel angry at the
world, especially with people who don't have diabetes, like your partner. You may feel shame or guilt
about being sick, and you may blame yourself. You
may have fears about the future and feel guilty at the
thought of burdening your mate. You may even feel
guilty about mentioning your fears.

No wonder it can seem easier, even wiser, to tuck
these unpleasant feelings away. But, as discussed
above, hidden feelings do not disappear; in fact,
they tend to become more powerful precisely
because they've gone underground. A hidden force
is more dangerous than one that is out in the open.
Suppressed problems can't be worked on and
resolved. What's more, they can cause stress, which
can elevate blood sugar and blood pressure.

The real risk in not acknowledging painful feelings, however, is not that the emotions will run
amuck; it's that you and your partner can slowly
become emotionally estranged from each other.
Often what happens is that negative or hurtful
behaviors begin taking over the function of expressing emotions that are better expressed through
talking.

Behaviors like the silent treatment, "forgetting"
to do the things you've promised to do, avoiding or

Timesaver
If your partner
has just been
diagnosed with
diabetes, ask the
doctor or dia-
betes educator
for a referral to
an education and
support group for
partners.
Anticipate that
you will need
information and
support.

withholding sex, and sniping at each other in front of friends are hardly a healthy alternatives to taking the leap and talking honestly to each other.

Get an education

It is very important for partners of people with diabetes to educate themselves about the disease and its management. The point is not that you should direct your partner's self-care, but that accurate, up-to-date knowledge is a powerful weapon against fear and helplessness. And in order to empathize with your partner's situation, you need to understand the basics of what he or she is coping with. Finally, you need to know how to recognize and react to the signs of diabetic emergencies like hypoglycemia and ketoacidosis.

Getting your "diabetes degree" can have the added benefit of putting you in touch with other people who have experienced what you're going through. This can provide invaluable emotional support, as well as information about community and other resources for people with diabetes.

Keep your roles clear

If you are the partner of a person with diabetes, it is not your job to make sure that your partner is managing the diabetes properly. It can take a while for this to sink in. After all, you love your mate and want the best for him or her. You've taken the time to learn about blood-sugar control, the importance of monitoring, the way to count carbohydrates, and what to do if severe hypoglycemia occurs. So reminding your loved one to check blood glucose levels, to take a pill, or to go easy on the chocolate cake seems to come naturally. You only want to help!

But "policing" people with diabetes—or most people, for that matter—doesn't help. The bottom line is that your partner's diabetes is just that: your partner's diabetes. It is up to the person who has diabetes to manage the illness. And let's face it: He or she knows full well what to do. Your reminders, or worse, your criticisms aren't adding to your partner's store of knowledge, only to a store of resentment.

Your role is not to nag, even when (and this is a tough one) you are worried. If you are truly worried, state this in a non-judgmental way that expresses your feelings, not criticism. But if you are constantly worried, always fretting, always trying to control your partner's self-care activities, this is a sign that you are taking on the responsibility for your mate's health, which is both impossible and unfair to your mate. You will have to let that sense of responsibility go.

What, then, is your role? Your role is to take the edge off the anger, fear, and hardship by

- Listening, not advising (unless specifically asked).

- Understanding that diabetes can be scary, frustrating, and demanding, and that the fact that your mate expresses these feelings does not mean he or she is going to give up on self-care.

- Asking if there is anything you can do to make things easier and then following through.

- Providing hugs, humor, praise, and attention.

When you think about it, this is a heck of a lot easier than trying to control something you cannot: another person's behavior.

We want to end this section by pointing out once again that if your partner has diabetes, it is not your

Bright Idea
Ask your partner with diabetes to write down a list of behaviors and phrases that he or she finds truly supportive, encouraging, and helpful. Keep the list in a special place where you can refer to it often.

role to be in charge of his or her health. Just as important, it is not fair for the person with diabetes to expect anyone else to do it. Keep in mind that if you have diabetes, taking care of your health is a part of taking care of your relationship. Your partner can't be blamed for worrying over and being angry about serious or chronic negligence on your part. And he or she will naturally be less willing to listen to your worries and frustrations if you are not doing all that you can to preserve your health.

Deal with sexual problems

A happy sex life is an important part of a lasting relationship. When a person's body is affected by illness, however, it's easy for problems in a couple's sex life to develop. In Chapter 12, we describe some of the sexual difficulties that can trouble people with diabetes. We give treatment options, and we strongly encourage patients to discuss sexual concerns with their health-care practitioners.

Our message here is that you must not neglect or avoid dealing with sexual problems. Make a commitment to keep your sex life healthy. If problems arise, discuss them openly and promptly and seek medical help.

Don't let your sex life go by the wayside. If it has been an important part of your relationship, it should stay that way. Protect your bond by taking care of this special, most intimate part of it.

Hold on to your dreams

When you first fell in love with your partner, it seemed that he or she hung the moon and stars. Your perception changes with time, of course. You're less starry-eyed now, but the qualities you fell in love with are still there.

Bright Idea
Rather than telling your partner what to do, why not show him or her? Stopping smoking, following an exercise program, and eating healthy foods are actions that speak louder than words. They are also things that you and your partner can do together.

When one person in a couple develops an illness, it's easy to lose sight of romance, hopes, and dreams. Your partner with diabetes can suddenly seem fragile and weak.

You may both feel overwhelmed by the physical changes, and changes in routine, that come with diabetes. There is a great deal of emphasis on the health status of the person with diabetes. This is understandable and appropriate. But try not to let it become the only perspective on the partner and your relationship. You both are still fundamentally the same people you were when you met and fell in love.

Make an effort to treat each other as you did in the beginning, to spend time together, to date, and to make plans. This is something that all couples must work on over time, and so should you.

Seek additional support

Even when both partners are healthy, it's not wise to try to be each other's only source of emotional support. This is especially true when one partner has a chronic illness. To avoid overburdening your relationship and disappointing each other, it's necessary to turn to outside sources of support—to friends, relatives, and support groups.

Don't hesitate to ask your medical team for referrals to support groups for each of you. One or both of you may seek out individual counseling, as well. The goal is to have one or more safe places where you can voice your personal concerns.

Coping skills for parents

There may be nothing harder in life than wanting the best for your children and feeling that there is nothing you wouldn't do to protect them. It's both a source of great joy and, at times, of heartache.

Watch Out!
You need a place to vent your anger or frustration with your partner or your role in the relationship. If this anger builds up, it can be poisonous. Protect your relationship by staying connected to a support system outside it.

Parents of children with chronic illnesses have an acute awareness of this joy and heartache. It's devastating to learn that your child has a serious illness, even if it is a manageable one. The wish to take away your child's hardship is very strong and often accompanied by irrational but powerful feelings of guilt: "Did I cause this? Have I failed my child?" And self-doubt: "Am I a good enough parent to help my child with this?"

Unofficially...
"It could be worse" is one of the least helpful things you can say to someone struggling to cope.

Your role in helping your child manage diabetes will change as your child changes. There are, however, some guidelines you can follow that apply to all stages of your child's development.

Keep your marriage strong

It's easy to lose sight of the importance of this when you are worried about a child. But your own emotional health and well-being are essential to the development of your child's. You and your mate have the responsibility, and also the right, to do what it takes to keep your relationship on solid ground.

Don't ignore your own needs! It's a recipe for falling apart.

Don't blame yourself

Blaming yourself for your child's diabetes is medically unfounded, helps no one, and is a waste of your emotional energy. Your child is likely to pick up on it, causing guilt in him or her. More important, blaming yourself can lead you to make parental choices out of guilt, rather than from the perspective of what is best for your child. It may cause you to be overprotective, or even to distance yourself, in an effort to ease your painful self-blame.

Be informed

Make sure that your knowledge of diabetes and diabetes management is accurate and up-to-date. Go to healthcare appointments prepared to ask questions. Utilize printed and online material to keep abreast of information relating to children and diabetes. (See the Resource Guide in Appendix B for sources of information for parents.)

Seek the advice and support of other parents

This is one of the most practical, sustaining, and reassuring things you can do. Ask your child's doctor, diabetes educator, or your local American Diabetes Association for help in linking up with a parents' support group. Don't try to go it alone.

Consider modifying the family diet

If your family has long enjoyed snacks high in sugar and fat that a child with diabetes should not eat, think about upgrading everyone's menu to healthier foods. You can't eliminate sweets from your children's life, but you can take steps to provide a better diet for all your children while lessening your diabetic child's sense of being deprived. This can cut down on unhappiness and conflict. You'll be a good role model, and your own health will probably improve.

Children shouldn't be denied treats just because a brother or sister has diabetes. But the overall amount of sweets available can be changed and healthier choices introduced. In the meantime, be sure to learn how to make food and insulin adjustments that will allow your child with diabetes to "eat like a kid" on special occasions.

Talk to a diabetes educator or nutritionist about healthy substitutes for your family's favorite dishes and snacks.

Listen to your child

All children need their parents to listen to their feelings and concerns. When your child has an illness, this can be especially challenging because you are worried, and you want so much for the child to be as well as possible. When your child complains about having to cope with diabetes, it can be difficult to listen without reminding him or her of the importance of doing all the self-care chores.

But remember that your child will always have diabetes. He or she will have to learn to cope with feelings about it as part of living successfully with the disease. Your child needs to learn to recognize and express these feelings in safe and appropriate ways. This will help to identify problems, both medical and social, which in turn will help to pinpoint solutions.

Remember also that your child will someday have to be his or her own medical advocate. If you react to negative feelings by telling the child that "it's not so bad," you are sending the message that the child's problems aren't real or important. This can lead to unassertiveness down the road.

When negative feelings come up, listen for a while and acknowledge how difficult coping with diabetes can be. This may be enough. But you may also need to engage your child in problem solving. Ask him or her what might be done to make things better.

Avoid overprotecting your child

Naturally, your instinct as a parent is to do all that you can to protect your child from emergencies, worsening diabetes, or complications. But your real task as a parent is to find the balance between being involved in your child's diabetes control and fostering the child's independence.

Bright Idea
Diabetes camps provide tremendous social support and peer interaction for children with diabetes, which is good for the entire family. For information on diabetes camps, call the American Diabetes Association at (800) 342-2383, or visit this Web site: www. childrenwithdiabetes.com.

This is where guidance and reassurance from your child's health-care team, and from other parents of children with diabetes, can really help you get some perspective. These people can help you determine the appropriate degree of self-care responsibility for your child at a given stage of development.

As we've said above, your child will need to handle diabetes for his or her entire life. It is crucial that the child learn step by step that ultimately he or she is in charge of meeting diabetes management goals.

Overprotecting your child, excusing lapses in self-care, or constantly trying to do everything for your child can cause him or her to feel incapable or inadequate. That's not good training for someone who will need to deal capably with diabetes. It can result in your child's needing to prove his or her own capability, sometimes by ignoring or sabotaging treatment.

Give yourself some credit!

You're hanging in there with your child. Some days are better than others, and some days your child's glucose control is better than others. But you should think of him or her always as a child first and a child with diabetes second. You must accept, love, and guide your child without regard to diabetes.

Don't forget to give yourself a pat on the back for all that you are providing as a parent. Perfection isn't the goal; being there is. Good for you!

Friends and co-workers: diabetes etiquette

It can be a touchy issue: How can you be supportive of a friend or colleague with diabetes without being nosy, bossy, or otherwise unhelpful?

Watch Out!
Overprotecting or overcontrolling your child is an exhausting effort, and therefore not a good coping response for parents who are already under stress. Get help in learning the difference between loving involvement and taking over.

To begin with, there is, of course, no specific etiquette for acknowledging diabetes. Common sense
and basic good manners should tell you not to stare
at the person who happens to have diabetes: He or
she is not an exotic zoo inhabitant or a tourist
attraction. Diabetes is a personal matter. If you have
questions or comments, it's best to keep them to
yourself (and educate yourself) unless you are very
friendly with your colleague who has diabetes or he
or she brings up the topic and seems comfortable
taking an educational role.

If you are a friend of someone with diabetes,
what is your role?

Don't play doctor

Who was it who said, "Everybody's an expert?" Like
pregnant women who have to endure tummy touch-
ing and advice giving from total strangers, people
with diabetes are often subjected to advice and
prognostications from those around them.
Everybody, it seems, has had an aunt or uncle or
cousin with diabetes and therefore knows all about
it and how to control it.

Unless you have diabetes or are an endocrinologist or a certified diabetes educator, it is extremely
doubtful that you are qualified to tell your acquain-
tance who has diabetes what he or she should or
should not eat, do, or expect in the way of complications. Resist the urge, however well intentioned,
to make suggestions or control behavior.

If you are truly worried about a friend's health,
let the person know in a noncritical way. But examine your motives first: Is your worry genuine and
well-founded, or do you enjoy taking on the role of
advisor?

> **"**
> Parents of chil-
> dren with dia-
> betes often use
> negative words
> such as 'cheat-
> ing,' 'bad,' and
> 'unreliable' when
> dealing with dia-
> betes manage-
> ment issues. The
> resulting guilt or
> resentment can
> virtually shut
> down communi-
> cation.
> —Melissa
> Strugger, social
> worker and dia-
> betes educator,
> in *Diabetes Self
> Management*,
> January/February
> 1997
> **"**

Don't dwell on complications

People who don't have diabetes tend to associate it only with dire complications, like blindness and amputation. This is understandable, and it is true that serious complications can occur.

People who have diabetes, however, do not need to be reminded of this threat. You can be sure that your friend or associate with diabetes is perfectly aware of the complications that can develop, and why. He or she does not need warnings, or the sad story of what happened to Great Aunt Hattie. Trust that your friend is fully informed and managing diabetes as he or she deems best.

You can listen

The onus is off you to provide your friend with diabetes advice or warnings. What can you offer?

We believe that parents and partners of people with diabetes provide a real service when they simply listen to that person's feelings about having diabetes.

This is certainly true of good friendships. If your friend with diabetes is down in the dumps, frustrated, or angry, you can offer a sympathetic ear. You can ask if there is anything you can do to help. You needn't come up with brilliant suggestions. Just listen.

You have limits

There may come a time when you feel overburdened by a friend's problems. This can be very difficult to deal with. If you're feeling used or sense that your relationship is becoming one-sided (focusing solely on your friend with diabetes), you owe it to yourself and the friendship to let your friend know.

You may also feel that your friend is not doing enough to help him- or herself. For example, does your friend

- Keep appointments with health-care professionals?
- Engage in positive activities, like exercise, hobbies, and education?
- Have other friends?
- Make use of support groups or counseling?

If not, you may have reason to feel unfairly burdened with your friend's problems.

If this is a friendship you value, you owe it to yourself and to the relationship to speak honestly to your friend. You do have limits, and you have a right to abide by them. Indeed, you can't really do otherwise. The friendship will be destroyed if limits aren't respected.

The good host

There are a few questions you might ask your friend with diabetes when inviting him or her to a dinner or party, such as:

- Do you need to eat at a specific time?
- Do you have any food or beverage needs I should know about?

Don't expect to get one sort of answer. Treatment plans and personal choices vary widely.

Think about including some healthy, low-fat and low-sugar foods along with more sumptuous party fare. These days, many of your guests will be grateful, not just those who have diabetes.

Two final pointers

- Never push food on anyone who politely declines it. It's not good hosting to insist that "a

Bright Idea
Planning a party? Ask your friend(s) with diabetes to suggest some healthy, fun things to eat. Borrow a favorite recipe!

Watch Out!
If you know a
dinner guest has
diabetes, don't
subject him or
her to a lengthy,
undernourished
cocktail hour.
The same goes
for planning an
evening on the
town.

little bit won't hurt" or to take offense if food is declined.

- Never draw attention to a guest's individual food needs or choices.

Extra support: consulting a mental health professional

Sometimes emotional problems can make you feel like a small boat on a storm-tossed sea. You keep heading for the shoreline, but somehow it never appears. Despite your best efforts, and encouragement from family and friends, you just can't make it to solid ground.

Many problems in life resolve themselves. When problems repeat or persist, however, and when they begin to interfere with meeting the demands of daily life, then it may be time to consider professional counseling.

Do I need help?

Even if you are feeling bad, it can be hard to know when to seek professional help. Begin by asking yourself a few questions:

- How long have I had this painful feeling, or struggled with this particular problem? Days? Weeks? Months? Do I remember feeling this way in the past? Have I had the same problem before?

- Is this feeling or problem interfering with my ability to care for myself, meet daily responsibilities, or enjoy life?

- Am I out of ideas for ways to feel better or resolve the problem on my own?

- Have other people expressed concern about how I'm doing, such as friends, family, or a member of my health-care team?

Identifying serious depression and anxiety

Many emotional problems involve feeling depressed, anxious, or both. Since life can and does throw us curve balls that cause sadness or worry, you might not know whether your particular case of "nerves" or the blues is worthy of professional attention.

Depression

Often, feeling depressed can be linked to a specific, saddening event that has recently occurred in one's life. Such reactive depression tends to lift with time and adjustment. Sometimes, though, the trigger is not clear or the depression lingers. Mental health professionals refer to serious or prolonged depression as major, or *clinical*, depression. According to the American Psychiatric Association, the diagnosis of clinical depression is made when at least five of the following symptoms are present:

- Depressed, irritable, or anxious mood
- Markedly diminished interest or pleasure in usual activities
- Significant weight loss or gain
- Insomnia or hypersomnia (sleeping more than normal)
- Agitation or slow responses to those around you
- Fatigue or loss of energy
- Feelings of worthlessness or guilt
- Impaired concentration or indecisiveness
- Recurrent thoughts about death or suicide

In some people, clinical depression is caused by chemical imbalances in the brain. This is referred to as biological, or *endogenous* ("internally caused") depression. It may also be that prolonged

Watch Out!
Some recent research suggests that clinical depression is about three times more prevalent in people with diabetes than in the general population.

psychological depression interferes with normal brain chemistry in some people.

Treating depression

Today, clinical depression is usually treated with a combination of psychotherapy and antidepressant medications. We describe different types of psychotherapy below. The antidepressant medications most often prescribed today are

- **Selective serotonin reuptake inhibitors (SSRIs).** These newer medications help to maintain adequate levels of serotonin in the brain. Serotonin is a naturally present neurotransmitter that can positively affect mood. (Neurotransmitters are substances in the brain that allow messages to pass between brain cells.) Examples of SSRIs are Prozac (*fluoxetine*), Paxil (*paroxetine*), Effexor (*venlafaxine*), Wellbutrin (bupropion), and Zoloft (*sertraline*). In some people, SSRIs can cause nervousness, insomnia, decreased appetite, and reduced sexual drive and response.

- **Tricyclics.** Today, these are less commonly prescribed than SSRIs. They have been in use since the 1950s, and it is believed they work by increasing the amount of neurotransmitter chemicals in the brain. Examples are Elavil (*amitriptyline*), Sinequan (*doxepin*), Desyrel (*trazodone*), and Trofanil (*imipramine*). Side effects can include dry mouth, sedation, increased appetite, and reduced sexual drive or response.

Antidepressant medications usually take anywhere from two to eight weeks to begin taking effect. Keep in mind that each person reacts somewhat differently to these medications. It may take some experimentation to find the most effective medication for you.

Additional measures

Besides professional counseling and antidepressants, there are some self-care steps you can take on your own to help relieve depression, such as:

- Exercising regularly
- Staying socially active
- Avoiding alcohol, which has been shown to aggravate depression and makes blood-sugar control more difficult
- Sticking to normal activities and routines
- Sticking to your normal sleep schedule
- Learning and practicing a relaxation technique
- Changing your thoughts by practicing positive thinking

Anxiety

We all have worries, especially if we are coping with a chronic disease that can cause serious complications. But just as there is a difference between "having the blues" and clinical depression, there is a difference between being worried and having a clinical anxiety disorder.

A clinical anxiety disorder involves unrelieved, fearful worrying that has lasted for at least six months and that interferes with normal functioning or enjoyment of life. It also includes the frequent occurrence of at least three of the following symptoms:

- Restlessness or feeling on edge
- Easily growing tired
- Difficulty concentrating or mind going blank

Unofficially...
Fifty to 65 percent of depressed people begin to feel better within six to eight weeks of treatment combining psychotherapy with antidepressant medication.

- Irritability

- Muscle tension

- Sleep disturbance (difficulty falling or staying asleep; restless or unsatisfying sleep)

Treating anxiety

The first course of action is to identify clearly the rational sources of worry, and to see if changes or improvements can be made in areas of life that are causing anxiety. Counseling may be necessary to get at the root of persistent or irrational anxiety, to address fears, or to suggest new ways to cope with anxiety-provoking situations.

There are some medications that are prescribed for anxiety:

- Ativan (*lorazepam*)

- BuSpar (*buspirone*)

- Serax (*oxazepam*)

- Tranxene (*clorazepate*)

- Xanax (*alprazolam*)

Be aware that some of these medications, like Ativan and Xanax, can be addictive. Be sure to follow your doctor's recommendations for use.

Because the symptoms of depression and anxiety overlap, anti-depressant drugs may also be prescribed to treat anxiety.

Relaxation techniques, like breathing exercises, guided imagery, muscle relaxation, and massage, can be very helpful in relieving anxiety. If phobias (fears that disrupt daily functioning) are a part of the anxiety disorder, behavior modification treatment may be necessary. This usually involves gradual desensitization to the feared object or situation by slowly increasing exposure to it.

Eating disorders

One form of emotional and behavioral problem that requires professional help is an eating disorder. Since eating disorders are about ten times more common in women than in men, we cover them in Chapter 13 in the discussion of women and diabetes. But we draw attention to them here, as well, because they are serious, potentially life-threatening psychiatric disorders. Symptoms include

- Having an intense fear of gaining weight and of eating.

- Seeing yourself as fat despite being very underweight.

- Binge eating, forced vomiting after eating, or manipulating insulin doses to lose weight.

If you have any of these symptoms, or feel that preoccupation with calories and body image are interfering with your life, you should seek help from a mental health professional.

Seeking help for children and teens

Children and teens, especially those who are coping with diabetes, may develop clinical depression and anxiety. Symptoms can be identical to those described above, but they can also take slightly different forms.

"Acting out" behaviors

Children and teens may express depression or anxiety by engaging in rebellious, aggressive, or behaviors that are essentially cries for help. These actions provide a release for painful emotions, and also tend to draw the attention of adults.

Because young people are in a dependent, relatively powerless position, they are more likely to be frightened by symptoms of depression and anxiety. They may cope with this by desperately seeking the help of adults. At the same time they may feel angry at the powerful adults in their lives and hold them responsible for this depression and anxiety. The result can be tantrums, fighting, skipping school, smoking, drug and alcohol abuse, refusal to follow a diabetes treatment plan, or other angry, negative behaviors that "act out" (express through actions) the emotional state of the child or teen.

All children defy their parents or rebel at times. It is a normal part of growing up. But repeated, prolonged, uncontrollable negative or dangerous actions signal a need for professional evaluation and care. The cause could be underlying depression, anxiety, or both.

Other warning signs for children with diabetes and their families

In its guidelines for doctors who treat diabetes, the American Diabetes Association identifies certain exceptionally stressful situations and problems involving children with diabetes and their families that may call for help from a mental health professional. These may occur

- At the time of a child's initial diagnosis.

- When a child is diagnosed in a single-parent family.

- When an infant or toddler is diagnosed.

- When the family is already coping with another serious illness or disorder.

- When the child cannot or will not perform age-appropriate diabetes management tasks.

- If the child has had more than one diabetes-related hospitalization for unexplained reasons within one year.

- When there is weight loss and chronically high blood-sugar levels, especially in teenage girls.

- When there is repeated conflict between parent and child over diabetes care tasks.

The mental health professions

There are a number of different credentials that indicate a qualified mental health professional. The three largest mental health professions are

- **Psychiatry.** The psychiatrist is a medical doctor (M.D.) who has received special training in the treatment of psychological and neuropsychological disorders. Look for a doctor who is board certified in psychiatry. The psychiatrist can provide psychotherapy and diagnostic evaluations, and can prescribe medications. Psychiatrists are expensive, typically charging $80 to $200 per hour.

- **Psychology.** The psychologist holds a Ph.D. or master's degree in psychology, usually clinical or counseling psychology for psychologists who perform psychotherapy. The psychologist can provide psychotherapy and can perform psychological testing, but cannot prescribe medication. A Ph.D.-level psychologist may charge close to what a psychiatrist charges. Master's level psychologists are often less expensive, generally charging from $50 to $90 per hour.

- **Social work.** The social worker holds a bachelor's degree or, preferably, a master's degree from an accredited school of social work. Look for the credentials M.S.W., C.S.W., and L.C.S.W. The social worker can provide psychotherapy and, often, is skilled in assisting clients in dealing with larger systems, like Social Security,

Bright Idea
Did you know that keeping a journal or writing unsent letters can help relieve stress and depression? Writing down your feelings in an unedited fashion can be a remarkably effective way to feel better.

schools, hospitals, or insurance companies. Hourly fees for most social workers range from $50 to $100, depending upon the social worker's degree of experience.

Other professionals who may provide mental health counseling are those holding various master's degrees in counseling, such as marriage and family counselors, pastoral counselors, ministers, rabbis, and persons holding advanced degrees in divinity (M.Div.)or in education (Ed.D. or M.Ed.).

Types of psychotherapy

We can't give a detailed description of the many schools of psychotherapy here, but we can summarize the most common types of therapy available today.

By the way, the type of psychotherapy that a professional practices does not depend upon his or her credentials. A psychiatrist and a social worker, for example, may both practice the same type of therapy. It depends upon the individual's personal preference and beliefs. Qualified professionals have received additional training in the type of psychotherapy they practice.

Psychodynamic psychotherapy

This type of therapy has its origins in psychoanalysis, invented in Germany by Sigmund Freud. It is psychoanalysis that utilizes the famous couch and free-association techniques.

Psychodynamic therapy involves exploring one's childhood, especially the relationship with the parents. The goal is to recognize the way in which perceptions and emotional experiences from childhood shape your adult life.

Cognitive-behavioral therapy

Cognitive refers to the thought processes. A cognitive-behavioral therapist does not focus on childhood or the past. Instead, this therapist believes that current thoughts and behaviors influence feelings, and that changing your thoughts and behaviors can change your feelings. The cognitive-behavioral therapist will help you to identify and challenge negative, distorted thinking.

Systemic therapy

This therapy involves focusing on the system of relationships among people. The goal is to identify and change negative patterns of relating to one another. The emphasis is on the here-and-now and on changing behaviors within relationships.

Choosing a therapy

Choosing what type of therapy to pursue depends upon your personal feelings about what is troubling you, as well as what type of therapy sounds most comfortable to you.

Another consideration is what type of therapy, if any, your health insurance will cover, and how many sessions per year. Some forms of therapy, like psychoanalysis and some psychodynamic therapies, take a long time to complete and can cost thousands of dollars a year. Others focus on shorter-term results. Today, the majority of insurance companies will not pay for long-term psychotherapies. Most will cover only a limited number of mental health appointments a year, for example, six to twelve. Some policies will fully reimburse for a limited number of appointments, after which they will reimburse for a part of the fee. Know your insurance coverage, and keep it in mind when selecting

Moneysaver
Many universities or university-affiliated hospitals run mental health clinics staffed by qualified, closely supervised professionals-in-training. Such clinics often have lower fees.

Bright Idea
The American
Psychiatric
Association
offers a free
brochure on
"Managed Care
and Your Mental
Health," a guide
to getting the
most out of your
insurance plan.
Write to the
American
Psychiatric
Association,
Division of Public
Affairs,
Department HE,
1400 K Street
NW, Washington,
DC 20005.

a type of therapy. (See Chapter 7 for more information on selecting a mental health professional.)

Finding a therapist

This, too, may be affected by your insurance coverage, especially if you are required to stick to a list of practitioners.

If you are searching for referrals or trying to choose a name from a list of providers, think about

- Asking your doctor or diabetes educator for a referral.

- Asking your clergyman or clergywoman for a referral.

- Asking a friend or relative who has had a positive experience with psychotherapy to suggest someone he or she has worked with or known.

Other sources for referrals include

- Your employer, if you have an Employee Assistance Program.

- The department of psychiatry or psychology at a respected local hospital.

- Your community mental health center or organization.

- Your local Social Services office.

- Your local American Diabetes Association chapter.

- A university or university-affiliated hospital that runs a mental health clinic as a professional training unit. Such an institution may offer services for lower fees.

Just the facts

- Acknowledging emotional needs is an important part of diabetes self-care.

- Couples and families coping with diabetes need to communicate honestly about the feelings it brings up.

- Trying to "police" or control someone with diabetes does not lead to better self-care, only to resentment.

- Support groups or counseling can take the pressure off marriage and family relationships.

- If emotional or behavioral problems recur or persist, or if they interfere with daily functioning, consider professional mental health counseling.

PART VI

Past and Present

GET THE SCOOP ON...
Ancient descriptions of diabetes ▪ Medieval
treatments ▪ The starvation diet ▪ Banting and
Best ▪ The first insulin patient ▪ Other advances
in diabetes treatment

Since Antiquity: A Brief History of Diabetes and Medicine

Chapter 15

D iabetes has been recognized since ancient times. The unique symptoms and deadly effects of untreated diabetes attracted medical attention thousands of years ago, when Hindu healers noticed that ants and flies were attracted to the urine of people suffering intense thirst, huge urine output, and wasting of the body. This was recorded in 1500 BC. The ancient Egyptians also recorded their observations of diabetes, in the *Papyrus Ebers*, a medical text dating back to 1550 BC.

It wasn't until 1921, when Canadian physician Frederick Banting discovered insulin, that diabetes ceased to be rapidly and inevitably fatal. It is little wonder that Banting was awarded the Nobel Prize for taming the disease that had fascinated, mystified, and tragically frustrated physicians for millennia.

The siphon: earliest medical references

The Greek Apollonius of Memphis is thought to have given diabetes its name sometime around

250 to 230 BC. *Diabetes* translates literally as "to go through," or to siphon. This refers to early observations that people with this disease take in huge amounts of water that seems to pass right through their bodies and out again as large amounts of urine.

In 150 BC, the Greek Aretaeus of Cappodocia described diabetes as "a melting down of the flesh into urine."

Eventually, the Greeks added to diabetes the Latin word for honey, *mellitus*, and the modern term *diabetes mellitus* was coined. *Mellitus* refers to the sweetness of the diabetic's urine.

Wine and roses

Ancient healers tried various remedies to control diabetes. *Venesection* (the cutting of veins) was employed, as were herbal concoctions including endive, lettuce, dates, myrtle, and juices of knotgrass. Red wine, sometimes diluted with water, was mixed with herbs. Poultices of vinegar, rose oil, and navel-wort were applied to the back in order to strengthen the kidneys, which were thought for centuries to be the source of diabetes.

Along with bloodletting, various purging methods were tried. Vomiting and sweating were induced, although diuretics (promoting water loss and urination) were prohibited.

For the latter stages of diabetes, some healers prescribed opiate drugs; others recommended lukewarm baths and wine.

During the latter half of the 1600s, Western physicians rediscovered the ancient Hindu writings on diabetes. These were interpreted in light of the prevailing medical theory of the time, which held that the illness is caused by imbalances in the body's "humors," or essential fluids. Emphasis shifted away from the kidneys; diabetes was now thought to be a disorder of the blood. Astringents were prescribed—agents thought to have a binding effect on the blood.

Progress in understanding diabetes

In 1798, a man named John Rollo documented for the first time that the blood of people with diabetes, not just their urine, contains excess sugar.

Timesaver
For a good synopsis of the history of insulin, visit the Web site of the world's oldest manufacturer of insulin, Eli Lilly and Company, at www.lilly.com.

In 1813, French researcher Claude Bernard theorized that this excess blood sugar is caused by the conversion of glycogen, stored in the liver, into glucose (blood sugar).

Scientific understanding of diabetes slowly advanced, but treatment remained medieval. Physicians continued to employ bloodletting and the use of narcotics as treatments for diabetes into the mid-1800s, when a German medical scientist named Ludwig Traube noted the connection between eating carbohydrates and the presence of sugar in the urine. Eliminating carbohydrates from the diet, he noted, eliminated most of the sugar in the urine.

Perhaps as a result of Traube's discoveries, one treatment that emerged in the late 1800s was the starvation diet. It is most closely associated with Frederick Allen, the leading American diabetologist at the turn of the century.

Allen surmised that since the diabetic's body could not absorb all the food eaten, then perhaps limiting the amount of food would keep the diet within a range that the person with diabetes could handle.

The starvation approach was a difficult, even cruel treatment to undergo. It meant living on about 500 to 800 calories a day, eating mostly fats and proteins, and strictly avoiding nearly all sugars and starches. For many it was a nightmare of deprivation and fatigue, but it accomplished what bloodletting and opium had not: It kept some people alive for a few years longer than they would otherwise have lived.

As the discovery of insulin approached, Allen's treatment served the purpose of keeping some people with diabetes alive long enough to begin insulin treatment.

The twentieth century: closing in on insulin

As the 1800s came to a close, the importance of the pancreas in diabetes began to be recognized. In 1869, a German medical student named Paul Langerhans discovered the tiny multicellular structures in the pancreas that we now know as the *islets of Langerhans*. The islets contain the beta cells that produce insulin. Langerhans was unable to discover the function of the islets.

A turning point in the understanding of diabetes came in 1889, when two German physiologists, Oskar Minkowski and Joseph von Mehring, accidentally produced diabetes in a laboratory dog. While studying carbohydrate metabolism, the two researchers surgically removed the dog's pancreas, looking for evidence for their theory that the pancreas secretes a substance that controls the conversion of foods to energy. To their surprise, the dog began urinating frequently and was very thirsty. Recognizing the classic symptoms of diabetes, Minkowski and von Mehring checked the dog's blood-sugar level and discovered that it was excessively high.

Unofficially...
Elizabeth Evans Hughes developed diabetes in 1918. She was the daughter of Charles Evans Hughes, governor of New York and later Chief Justice of the United States Supreme Court. Dr. Allen's starvation diet kept Elizabeth alive until she began insulin treatment in 1922. Her recovery from near death was reported worldwide. Elizabeth lived into her seventies.

Then, in 1901, a Baltimore pathologist named
Eugene Opie observed that the islets of Langerhans
in a young woman who had died of diabetes were
unaccountably small and withered.

Pancreatic extracts

The link between diabetes and the pancreas was
now established. No one was aware, as yet, of the
hormone insulin and its critical role. During the
early 1900s, researchers began focusing on the way
to use preparations, or *extracts*, of the pancreas to
treat diabetes.

Much of what follows is based on the information provided in Michael Bliss's definitive book, *The
Discovery of Insulin* (University of Chicago Press,
1982).

One well-known early researcher was young
Georg Ludwig Zeulzer, an internist in Berlin.
Zeulzer eagerly pursued a pancreatic solution that
would control diabetes. He used pancreas tissues to
make ingestable compounds. He developed an
injectable pancreatic compound that he called *acomatrol*. A patient of Zeulzer who was dying of diabetes received injections of acomatrol and actually
improved for awhile. Unfortunately, the patient
died when the supply of acomatrol ran out.

In 1911, Zeulzer took out an American patent
on one of his solutions, called a "Pancreas Preparation Suitable for the Treatment of Diabetes." He saw
little success, however, and lost his laboratory during World War I.

Frederick Banting and Charles Best

The war ended in 1919, and the world had but a
short time to wait before the first effective treatment
for diabetes, insulin, would be found.

> 66
> If you were
> transported back
> to the world of
> 1920, you'd
> probably be
> impressed by all
> the technology
> you saw: Early
> versions of the
> automobile. The
> radio. Movies,
> telephones, heli-
> copters, air con-
> ditioners. But if
> you had dia-
> betes? You'd be
> undergoing
> treatment that
> seemed rooted in
> the dark ages.
> —Eli Lilly and
> Company, cele-
> brating "75 Years
> of Insulin"
> 99

Frederick Banting was a young veteran of World War I, a Canadian who had graduated with a degree in medicine in 1916. His own life had been marked by diabetes: his childhood sweetheart had died of the disease when Banting was a teenager. Since that time he had dreamed of finding a cure.

Banting was an orthopedic surgeon who taught physiology at the University of Western Ontario after the war. In his free time he studied all the research available on diabetes. He was familiar with the work of Minkowski and von Mehring, and eager to do his own research, which he was certain would expand upon earlier findings.

Lacking the funds and the equipment for his research, Banting approached Professor J. J. R. Macleod of the University of Toronto, a famous authority on carbohydrate metabolism, for help in establishing a laboratory. At first, Macleod turned down the young, inexperienced orthopedist. When Banting would not take no for an answer, however, Macleod finally relented and gave him the use of a lab, ten laboratory dogs, and the help of an unpaid assistant, a recent biochemistry graduate named Charles Best, who had lost an aunt to diabetes. Banting and Best began their work in the spring of 1921.

Banting had long suspected that only a portion of the pancreas secreted a substance that had to do with diabetes. He focused on the islets of Langerhans, theorizing that these cells secrete something directly into the bloodstream that affects blood-sugar levels.

Banting and Best tested this theory by surgically tying off the duct leading from the dogs' pancreases to their intestines. This caused the digestive enzymes produced by the pancreas to accumulate, killing the enzyme-producing pancreatic tissue in about six weeks. Banting's objective was to target only the enzyme-producing tissue, thus isolating and identifying the pancreatic cells that do not produce digestive enzymes.

Sure enough, when Banting and Best removed the pancreases, they found that only the islets of Langerhans were still alive and functioning. This finding confirmed that these cells were producing a substance that does not enter the digestive system, but the blood instead.

Isolating insulin

Having confirmed that the islets of Langerhans have a different function from that of the rest of the pancreas, Banting and Best went about the task of isolating the special substance produced by the islets. They were able to harvest this substance, which they immediately tested by injecting it into one of their lab dogs, which was dying of diabetes. The dog revived within hours, and its urine became free of sugar. Sadly, without another injection, it died the next day.

Banting and Best then knew that the special pancreatic substance needed to be supplied on a daily basis. They began the laborious process of traveling by streetcar to the Toronto stockyards to purchase quantities of fresh beef pancreases. (Banting had sold his car to help pay for the research.) Their efforts proved worthwhile, as the two young men were able to extract the "isletin," as they first called insulin, from the beef pancreases.

From the laboratory to the world

Banting and Best were satisfied that they had found a treatment for diabetes. As a precautionary measure, they injected the newfound substance into one

Unofficially...
The first insulin used to treat Leonard Thompson looked like "thick brown muck," according to colleagues of Banting and Macleod. Today, insulin is clear or slightly cloudy.

another, and found that neither of them suffered any ill effects.

At this point, Macleod stepped in and asked Banting and Best to repeat their experiments. When the success was replicated, Macleod assigned a bio-chemist named John Collip to the task of purifying isletin, which Macleod suggested be called *insulin*. Within six months, Macleod had approved the first use of insulin in a human with diabetes.

The first person to receive insulin was Leonard Thompson, a fourteen-year-old boy who lay emaci-ated and dying in a Toronto hospital. The boy did not improve immediately, and Collip worked on fur-ther purifying the insulin solution. About six weeks after Leonard's treatment began, the newly refined insulin began to take effect. Leonard Thompson revived and began to gain weight. His glucose level dropped from 520 to 120 mg/dl. He lived for the next thirteen years, receiving regular insulin injec-tions along with the rapidly growing numbers of Banting's other diabetes patients. Thompson died of pneumonia at age twenty-seven.

Recognition and discord

In 1923, just two years after Banting and Best began their research, Banting and Macleod were awarded the Nobel Prize for medical research. Banting, furi-ous that Charles Best had not been recognized, shared half of the award money with Best. Macleod split his award with James Collip.

Rivalry and anger had flared among the researchers following the success with Leonard Thompson. In particular, Collip initially refused to tell Banting and Best how he had purified the insulin, going back on an earlier agreement to share all his information. Collip may have been hoping to patent the refined insulin. It is reported that Collip and Banting actually came to blows over this conflict. A cartoon was published depicting Banting sitting on Collip and choking him, a scene captioned "The Discovery of Insulin."

Insulin develops

Somehow the conflicts were resolved well enough to allow the men to continue their research for the next twenty years. By 1923, insulin was available to doctors and patients all over the world. Macleod died in 1935; Banting died in a plane crash in Newfoundland in 1941. Best lived until 1978 and enjoyed a distinguished career at the University of Toronto, during the course of which he succeeded Professor Macleod and became Banting's superior.

Eli Lilly and Company was the first company to receive a license to manufacture insulin, not long after its discovery. Demand for insulin was so high that a large pharmaceutical company was needed to take over production. Lilly entered into a formal agreement with the University of Toronto, giving Lilly manufacturing rights in exchange for payment of royalties to the University. These funds were used to support insulin research and development.

During the 1930s and 1940s, insulin was further refined, and long-acting and intermediate types were developed. *NPH* insulin was developed in the 1940s and the *lente* insulins in the 1950s.

Throughout this time and into the 1970s, insulin was derived from animal pancreases. A big breakthrough for manufacturers came in September of 1978, when synthesis of "human type" insulin through recombinant DNA engineering began. The newest synthetic human insulin, the rapid-acting *lispro* (Humalog), was approved for use in

66
Doctors interested in history know that it helps provide perspective and humility in daily practice. It teaches us that today's 'correct' therapy may be viewed as wrong-headed nonsense by future generations, much as we view primitive therapies of the nineteenth century and earlier.
—Lawrence Martin, M.D., author of *We Can't Kill Your Mother and Other Stories of Intensive Care* (Lakeside Press, 1991)
99

Bright Idea
Dr. Elliott Joslin, who founded the world-renowned Joslin Diabetes Center in 1898, was one of the first diabetes experts to emphasize that nutrition, exercise, and lifestyle were as important as insulin in managing diabetes.

1996. Today, ultra-long-acting insulins are in development.

Beyond insulin

The majority of people with diabetes have type 2 diabetes, and many of these people do not use pharmaceutical insulin. Oral medications for type 2 diabetes—the class of medications called *sulfonylureas*—were introduced in the 1950s. These stimulate the pancreas to produce more insulin. Phenformin, a precursor of today's metformin, became available in the 1960s.

In the 1960s, technology called *radioimmunoassay* made possible the measurement of insulin levels in people and refined our understanding of the distinctions between the two types of diabetes. Since then, more oral medications specifically for treating type 2 diabetes have been produced, including metformin, acarbose, repaglinide, and troglitazone. These medications work in different ways to combat high blood sugar and insulin resistance, a major problem for people with type 2 diabetes.

Besides the development of insulin and oral medications, progress has been made in other areas of diabetes treatment.

For example, prior to the 1960s, sugar levels were tested using urine. The earliest urine test, called the *Benedict test*, required that the urine sample be boiled in a test tube with "Benedict solution," which would change color if sugar were present. Eventually, the boiling method was replaced by tablets that could be placed in the sample, indicating the approximate sugar level by changing color.

By the 1960s, a far simpler urine test was available: the strip test. Strips of chemically treated paper were exposed to urine; their color indicated an approximate sugar level, which one found by matching the strip color to a color chart.

However, urine can give only a rough idea of the status of blood sugar; only blood testing can give accurate glucose levels. It was a big step forward for diabetes management when home blood glucose testing was introduced in the 1970s.

The first home glucose tests also employed chemically treated paper strips, which were matched to a color chart once a drop of blood was applied to the strip. The strips were accurate within about 60 mg/dl of the actual glucose level.

In the mid-1980s, the glucose meter was introduced. Today most people with diabetes use one of these small, sophisticated tools to monitor blood-sugar levels. A drop of blood is placed on a strip of paper and inserted into the meter. Within minutes, the meter provides a highly accurate digital reading of the glucose level.

Changes in insulin regimens

With the development of intermediate- and short-acting insulin came insulin injection regimens based on more frequent injections. This emerged along with growing insight into the workings of the healthy pancreas, and with the spread of glucose self-monitoring tests.

The healthy pancreas is exquisitely attuned to rises and falls in blood glucose, and secretes just the right amounts of insulin to keep glucose within a normal range at all times. With advances in insulin preparations and glucose testing, people with diabetes can now follow insulin injection programs that more closely mimic the action of the normal pancreas. More frequent, rapidly effective shots allow people with diabetes greater freedom in the timing of meals and in food choices.

Unofficially...
In 1897, the average life expectancy for a ten-year-old diagnosed with diabetes was 1.3 years. By 1945, that child had a life expectancy of forty-five years.

Tight blood-sugar control

Through the years, researchers have gained new understanding into the devastating long-term complications of diabetes. While it has long been known that, over time, high blood-sugar levels lead to complications, medical researchers debated the question of how much glucose control was enough to prevent or delay these complications. Should people with diabetes strive to keep their blood-sugar levels as close to normal as possible, or was that asking too much for too little gain?

The debate continued, but meanwhile it was becoming easier for people with diabetes to coordinate their insulin, food intake, medication use, and exercise with their blood-sugar levels. There were more tools available—new insulins, and convenient and accurate glucose tests—to help people with diabetes keep glucose levels within normal ranges.

Finally, in 1993, the results of the Diabetes Control and Complications Trial ended the debate about the importance of maintaining near-normal glucose levels. This landmark ten-year study of 1,400 people with type 1 diabetes showed that those who kept tight glucose control, through frequent blood testing and multiple daily insulin injections (or use of an insulin pump), dramatically reduced their risks for serious complications. Recent studies, including the United Kingdom Diabetes Prospective Study, show that people with type 2 diabetes who maintain good blood-sugar control also have a reduced risk for eye, kidney, and cardiovascular complications.

Since its introduction in the early 1980s, the insulin pump has taken intensive insulin therapy to new heights. Although the insulin pump is far from perfect and is not for everyone, it illustrates medical science's resolve to find newer and better ways to compensate for the unhealthy pancreas.

As we enter the twenty-first century, science shows no sign of slowing down when it comes to diabetes research. Read on for a glimpse into current research and what the future holds for the treatment of diabetes.

Just the facts

- Diabetes has been recognized since at least 1500 BC.

- Bloodletting and the use of opium were common treatments for diabetes from ancient times through the mid-1800s.

- Prior to the discovery of insulin, the only treatment that had any beneficial effect whatsoever was the starvation diet.

- Insulin was discovered by Frederick Banting and Charles Best in their laboratory in Toronto, Canada, in 1921.

- The first successful treatment with insulin occurred in 1922.

- Improved home glucose monitoring methods have been almost as important in the treatment of diabetes as the discovery of insulin.

- Recent research shows that "tight" glucose control decreases the risk of diabetic complications for people with both type 1 and type 2 diabetes.

GET THE SCOOP ON...
Progress in genetic research ▪ The difference
between ACEs and AGEs ▪ New forms of insulin ▪
New type 2 medications ▪ Blood tests without
finger sticks

The Cutting Edge: A Look at Current Diabetes Research

A s we've seen, the mysteries of diabetes have captured the attention of healers, medical doctors, and scientists for thousands of years. Today, almost 20 million Americans have diabetes (about half of whom have not been diagnosed), and we spend close to $130 billion dollars annually on treating this disease. The incidence of diabetes has tripled in the last thirty years, and the numbers will swell as the population ages and continues to gain weight, and subtler diagnostic criteria and tests identify more "silent" cases of diabetes.

Unfortunately, the public is not yet fully aware of diabetes's frightening toll. For years, funding for diabetes research has fallen below that of headline-grabbing diseases such as AIDS, breast cancer, and heart disease. But diabetes research received a well-deserved boost in 1998, when President Clinton dedicated $300 million over the next five years to

Chapter 16

this critically important work. And as a larger portion of the population is diagnosed with diabetes, manufacturers of drugs and medical supplies are also putting more money into diabetes research.

The assault on diabetes is taking place on more fronts than ever before. Research into what causes diabetes—and how to improve treatment—is beginning to flourish. No one can say exactly when, where, or how diabetes will be conquered, but today the chances are better than ever that that day will come.

What is being researched?

One of the highlights of diabetes research in recent years has been a growing interest in type 2 diabetes. For years, type 1 diabetes has received the lion's share of scientific scrutiny, and rightly so: it is a very serious disease that affects both children and adults, and its treatment is complicated. Since the discovery of insulin, much work has gone into developing insulin and refining insulin treatment.

With success in that arena and with the graying of the Baby Boomers, science has turned more of its attention to the majority of diabetics, type 2 diabetics. Type 1 diabetes, however, still continues to be a subject of inquiry. Below, we provide an overview of some of the major questions being asked in diabetes research today, and we report on new advances in treating diabetes. In the next chapter, we'll take a look at research into diabetes prevention and the prospects for a cure.

Understanding insulin resistance and how insulin works

Insulin was discovered over seventy years ago, but scientists still do not completely understand how it

Bright Idea
For reliable information on diabetes research, try these Web sites: www.jdfcure.org (Juvenile Diabetes Foundation); www.diabetes. com (Diabetes.Com); www.niddk.nih. gov (National Institute of Diabetes and Digestive and Kidney Diseases); and www. diabetes.org (American Diabetes Association).

does what it does. How, exactly, does insulin make cells receptive to glucose? How do insulin receptors work or fail to work? What is the true cause of insulin resistance, and why is it linked to obesity? We don't yet know the answers to these and many other questions about the way insulin interacts with the body's cells.

The better we understand the workings of insulin, the better our treatments based on insulin therapy will be. And the more we understand insulin resistance, the more effective our treatments for type 2 diabetes will be. For these reasons, the study of insulin is a perennially active and important area of diabetes research.

Genetic causes of diabetes

This very important topic has long been and continues to be of interest to diabetes researchers. Unfortunately, the genetics of diabetes is highly complex, and our understanding of how to identify and manipulate genetic factors is far from complete.

Ideally, researchers would like to identify a single "diabetes gene," or a single genetic defect, that could be detected and altered. So far, however, research does not indicate that one gene or defect is responsible for causing diabetes.

Instead, scientists are making progress in identifying genetically influenced characteristics that appear to be related to the development of diabetes.

The PC-1 protein

Researchers have discovered that a protein called *PC-1* is more prevalent in people with type 2 diabetes than in nondiabetics. The overproduction of PC-1 is a genetically determined trait. It is

Unofficially... Among pairs of genetically identical twins in which one twin has type 1 diabetes, 50 to 75 percent of the remaining twins never develop diabetes.

significant because PC-1 interferes with the normal functioning of insulin receptors. In people who produce too much of this protein, insulin resistance can occur.

The "obesity gene"

Another area of interest to genetic researchers studying type 2 diabetes is the so-called "obesity gene." Obesity is highly correlated with type 2 diabetes, although the majority of obese people do not develop diabetes. But research begun in 1994 on obese laboratory mice (a breed called *ObOb*) showed first, that the mice's obesity is inherited and second, that the ObOb mice develop a disease very much like type 2 diabetes.

The gene controlling obesity identified in the ObOb mouse was discovered to have problems producing a protein called *leptin*. Human beings have the same leptin-producing gene.

In humans, however, there are many factors contributing to the development of obesity, and researchers cannot point to a single-gene origin for obesity or obesity-related diabetes. But the research into the genetic underpinnings of many traits associated with diabetes continues.

The GENNID study

In 1993, the American Diabetes Association initiated a nationwide effort to gather and coordinate information about the genetic causes of type 2 diabetes. *GENNID* stands for "Genetics of Non–Insulin Dependent Diabetes," as type 2 diabetes was formerly called.

The GENNID Study will amass a database of blood samples, glucose tolerance test results, and other diagnostic measures taken from volunteers whose family and ethnic backgrounds put them at

Bright Idea
Pimigadine is an experimental drug that may inhibit the development of AGEs. Its ability to slow the progression of diabetic complications is being tested in clinical trials in more than 100 centers across America. For more information on these trials, call (800) 41-ENROLL.

risk for developing type 2 diabetes. Family members of volunteers will also provide samples. Working from the premise that a number of genes, not just one or two, predispose people to diabetes, the GENNID Study hopes its database will help researchers to identify relevant genes and eliminate others.

Type 1 diabetes and the HLA and tap genes

In the area of type 1 diabetes, in recent years researchers have begun studying a set of genes called *human leukocyte antigens,* or *HLAs.* Each of us has many HLA genes; we inherit a set from each parent.

HLA genes are significant in type 1 research because these genes govern the antigen molecules on the surface of our body's cells. The antigen molecules are what makes our cells familiar to our immune systems, preventing the immune system from destroying them. In people with type 1 diabetes, it may be that the genes controlling the antigens present on the pancreatic beta cells cause those antigens to appear as "foreign invaders" to the immune system, triggering the autoimmune destruction of beta cells.

Scientists are researching a form of the HLA gene called the *HLA-DR,* which seems to be linked to the development of type 1 diabetes. 95 percent of people who have type 1 diabetes have the DR3 form of the HLA gene, the DR4 form, or both. And most people with type 1 diabetes also have another type of HLA gene, the *HLA-DQ,* as DQw2, DQw8, or both. So there is evidence that these HLA-DR and HLA-DQ gene types may predispose people who have them to type 1 diabetes. But the picture is complicated by the fact that many people who have these HLA gene types do not develop diabetes.

Researchers at Harvard Medical School and Massachusetts General Hospital have recently implicated two more genes in the development of type 1 diabetes. These are called *Tap-1* and *Tap-2,* and like the HLA gene types, they appear to influence the interaction between cell antigens and the immune system. When healthy Tap genes were inserted into diabetic cells, 40 percent of the cells became recognizable as familiar to the immune system.

Research into the genetics of diabetes is advancing at a rapid pace, but it still has far to go. Both type 1 and type 2 diabetes are emerging as diseases caused by multiple genes working in combination with a number of environmental factors.

Immunology: understanding the immune system's attack on beta cells

The fundamental physiological cause of type 1 diabetes is the destruction of insulin-producing beta cells in the pancreas, brought about by an attack by the immune system on the body's own cells. One active area of diabetes research is the study of what causes this autoimmune attack within the body.

We've hinted at some of the factors in the preceding section on genetic research. Medical scientists are looking into the destructive interaction between the immune system's white blood cells, or *T cells,* and the beta cells of the pancreas. Why do the T cells in people with type 1 diabetes perceive the body's pancreatic beta cells as foreigners that must be destroyed? How are autoimmune attacks activated?

Researchers are working on identifying the molecular factors, like antigens on cell surfaces, that interact or communicate with molecules on the surfaces of T cells. The goal is to discover what goes wrong with the signaling between cells in type 1 bodies and their T cells.

Normally, the T cells fight off foreign invaders such as viruses and bacteria. T cells are helped in this fight by the B cells, which produce proteins called *antibodies.* Antibodies recognize invading cells.

But some B cells produce antibodies, called *autoantibodies,* that perceive body cells as invaders. Three of these autoantibodies are especially common in people with type 1 diabetes. They target and destroy

- Islet cells in the pancreas;

- Insulin;

- GAD, or *glutamic acid decarboxylase,* a protein made by pancreatic beta cells.

Scientists have long known that type 1 diabetes can be prevented or delayed if drugs that suppress the immune system are given during the disease's early stages. But these powerful immunosuppressive drugs are highly toxic and cause the person treated to become very vulnerable to infections and tumors. Today, researchers are looking into safer, nontoxic ways to prevent the immune system from attacking beta cells.

Because autoimmune destruction of pancreatic cells is at the bottom of type 1 diabetes, study of the immune system may ultimately lead to a means for preventing type 1 diabetes. But at present, the immune system and its relationship to diabetes is only poorly understood. Like genetic medicine, immunological research is still in its early stages. But it holds promise for greater understanding, control, and possible prevention of diabetes.

Unofficially...
In people newly diagnosed with type 1 diabetes, 70 to 80 percent have autoantibodies to islet cells, 30 to 50 percent have autoantibodies to insulin, and 80 to 95 percent have autoantibodies to GAD.

Diabetes complications

Medical scientists continue actively to pursue the mystery of how high blood sugar causes the serious complications of diabetes—kidney, eye, and heart disease, and nerve damage that can occur throughout the body.

AGEs

One area of research on diabetes complications is the study of AGEs, or *advanced glycosylation endproducts*. AGEs are created when blood glucose binds with proteins in the body. AGEs slowly accumulate in all people as they grow older. In people with diabetes, however, they accumulate much more quickly, forming a kind of biological "glue" that adversely affects the body's cells, tissues, and blood vessels, causing them to become stiff and clogged. (This is one reason why it is important to get regular glycosylated hemoglobin tests.) Some liken the process to the toughness that occurs in meat that has been overcooked. A browning effect of glycosylation can actually be seen in body tissues affected by AGEs.

Accumulation of AGEs can affect the body at both the micro- and macrovascular level, and it is implicated (although its role is not fully understood) in all of the major complications of diabetes. For this reason, AGEs are a hot topic in diabetes research.

ACE inhibitors

Research on diabetes complications is also focusing on the use of a type of drug called *angiotensin-converting enzyme inhibitor*, or *ACE inhibitor*, in preventing or delaying microvascular kidney and eye disease.

ACE inhibitors (like *captopril, lisinopril,* and *enalapril*) are primarily used to treat hypertension, or high blood pressure. Research has already demonstrated that diabetics with high blood pressure who have proteinuria (the presence of protein in the urine, a marker of kidney disease) have a reduction in their proteinuria when using ACE inhibitors. Research is now being conducted to test the effectiveness of ACE inhibitors in delaying or preventing retinopathy, which is damage to the small blood vessels in the retina.

C-peptide

Scientists at Washington University in St. Louis, working with Eli Lilly and Co., have discovered evidence that a protein called *C-peptide* may not only prevent some complications of diabetes but also reverse them.

C-peptide is made by the body, and it aids the production of insulin in the pancreas. (The islet cells in the pancreas make insulin in to chains of amino acids, called the alpha and beta chains, which are connected by C-peptide.) Scientists have long wondered if C-peptide has any other uses. Recent experiments using diabetic rats have shown that injecting larger-than-normal amounts of C-peptide with insulin reduced leakage of blood from arteries by as much as 70 percent. In rats with early diabetes, C-peptide prevented arteries from leaking and also prevented nerve damage over time.

Weak, leaking blood vessels are a major vascular complication in people with diabetes. Further research may mean that C-peptide could one day be added to pharmaceutical insulin preparations.

Other research related to complications

There is new interest in the effects of antioxidants on preventing the complications of diabetes. Antioxidants are natural substances that help to destroy the harmful byproducts of certain biochemical reactions in the body. Examples of antioxidants are vitamins E and C, and beta-carotene. The effects of these substances on the accumulation of AGEs is being studied.

Foot ulcers that resist healing, sometimes leading to amputations, are another diabetes complication that is the subject of research. New grafting materials to cover wounds are being developed. Treatments that promote wound healing using recombinant human-growth factor derived from blood cells called platelets (such as the topical gel Regranex), electrical, and even magnetic stimulation are under research. Kosta Mumcuoglu, a research associate at Hadassah-Hebrew University School of Medicine, has had significant success using maggot therapy (yes, fly larvae—laboratory-bred and germ-free) to heal seriously infected ulcers: maggots placed in the wound feed on the infected tissue. This is unpleasant to think about, perhaps, but it is painless and effective. Footwear manufacturers are working on unique shoe designs and technology that may help prevent ulcers from occurring.

Researchers will also continue to seek improvements in methods used to maintain tight glucose control, which is the best means we now have for preventing complications.

Research related to diabetes treatment and tools

So-called "pure" science seeks to understand the underlying causes of things, while "plied" science looks for practical ways to control or treat them. Both types of science are alive and well in diabetes research today.

Unofficially...
Scientists are studying a human growth factor known as *Veg-F,* which has been implicated in the overgrowth of blood vessels that occurs in advanced diabetic eye disease. Researchers want to discover how to turn the growth factor on and off. Veg-F may have positive uses in the treatment of heart disease.

We've just taken a look at some of the areas of diabetes research that delve into causes. Now let's look at some current areas of research involving diabetes treatments and its tools.

Inhaled insulin

People with diabetes who inject insulin have long awaited the development of insulin that can be administered without needles. Today researchers are coming closer to meeting this goal.

Pfizer Inc., a major pharmaceutical manufacturer, is working with the company Inhaled Therapeutic Systems (ITS) on insulin that is not injected, but inhaled. ITS (based in Palo Alto, California) is developing a portable insulin delivery device that disperses tiny particles of crystallized insulin through a plastic tube. The person using it inhales the insulin crystals from the tube. Insulin enters the lungs and is absorbed rapidly into the bloodstream.

Inhaled insulin is now undergoing trials with the Food and Drug Administration. If all goes well and FDA approval is granted, inhaled insulin could be available in one to two years.

Insulin pills

Insulin in pill form would be a marvel of ease and convenience. So far, this has been an impossibility because insulin is broken down by contact with digestive juices in the stomach. But researchers are working hard on ways to get around this difficulty.

One study, funded by the National Institutes of Health and conducted at Brown University, used insulin delivered in very tiny plastic beads. When the beads were ingested by mice, the insulin remained intact throughout the digestive process.

Bright Idea
The results of the United Kingdom Prospective Diabetes Study (UKPDS), the largest diabetes study ever conducted, show that better glucose control significantly reduces the risks for diabetes complications. What's more, the UKPDS showed that controlling high blood pressure is even more important in reducing risks for complications.

When the beads entered the bloodstream, the plastic disintegrated and the insulin went to work.

In another NIH-sponsored study, conducted at the University of Maryland School of Medicine, a substance called *zonula occluding toxin,* or *ZOT,* was used to allow insulin to pass intact through the walls of the small intestine. Researchers plan to test ZOT on diabetic monkeys and then, perhaps, on humans.

More choices in insulin action times

Advances in techniques for genetically altering bacteria allow scientists to make new kinds of insulin. Bacteria can be altered to make insulin with different absorption times. A recent example is the development of lispro insulin, which is genetically similar to human insulin (it differs only by the arrangement of two amino acids, lysine and proline) and has a rapid onset of action.

Insulin can be produced that has very specific and predictable action times, allowing for ever-greater flexibility in glucose control regimens.

Oral medications for type 2 diabetes: new and improved

Major advances in oral medications for type 2 diabetes were made in the 1990s, which saw the introduction of four new classes of drugs: *acarbose* (Precose) and miglitol (Glyset), *metformin* (Glucophage), *troglitazone* (Rezulin), and *repaglinide* (Prandin). These drugs work in an entirely different way from that of the older oral medications, the sulfonylureas.

More advances are on the horizon for those who take oral diabetes drugs. Researchers are focusing on drugs that increase the type 2 diabetic's sensitivity to insulin.

Rosiglitazone

This drug, currently in the final stages of pre-approval, is a close chemical cousin of troglitazone. Like troglitazone, rosiglitazone helps to make body tissues more sensitive to insulin, apparently not causing the rare but serious liver problems that troglitazone can. It also appears to be more potent than troglitazone, so that smaller doses can be used.

Dopamine agonists

These drugs are designed to improve insulin sensitivity by affecting levels of certain chemicals (called *dopamines*) in the brain that regulate blood-sugar metabolism. Early tests of dopamine agonists show that they improve glucose control and also reduce post-meal levels of triglycerides and fatty acids, perhaps protecting against heart disease.

Targretin

This drug was developed as a treatment for cancer, but it seems also to lower insulin resistance. It is being tested as an oral medication for type 2 diabetes in Belgium and the Netherlands, by Ergo Science Corporation.

Pramlintide

Pramlintide is a drug that works similarly to the hormone *amylin,* a natural substance that is produced by the pancreatic islet cells. Like insulin, amylin plays a role in regulating blood glucose levels. Providing pramlintide to people with type 2 diabetes, who are deficient in amylin and insulin, may improve glucose control. Pramlintide is being tested by Amylin Pharmaceuticals as an adjunct to insulin treatment, and as a single-drug treatment for people with type 2 diabetes not using insulin. It may also have a role in treating type 1 diabetes.

"

The future of people with diabetes will be no needles. I am confident that somebody will do it [develop oral insulin].
—Alessio Fasano, M.D., University of Maryland School of Medicine

"

New methods for monitoring blood sugar

One area of research and product development that is booming and very competitive is that of improvements in the accuracy, rapidity, and convenience of blood-sugar monitoring.

Glucose monitoring is one of the most important, and least pleasant, parts of diabetes management. We can put a man on the moon, as the saying goes, but we can't seem to come up with a painless way to collect blood samples.

But lancet-free blood testing may be just around the corner. Some of the new methods for blood testing that may be available soon include

- Glucose enzyme sensors using catheters, not needles.

- Low-level, painless electrical currents that measure blood glucose.

- Skin patches that collect fluid from the skin's surface from which blood glucose levels can be measured.

- Infrared light that measures blood glucose levels within the finger.

- Implantable glucose sensors.

- Painless laser beams that withdraw fluid from the skin's surface from which blood glucose levels can be measured.

- Flexible, "microfine" blood glucose sensors that can be inserted just under the skin.

- A vacuum device that permits blood glucose testing in parts of the body other than the sensitive fingertips.

Between insulin injections and finger sticks, people with diabetes can sometimes feel like human pincushions. Happily, those days may soon be over.

Implantable insulin pumps

Within several years, implantable insulin pumps may be approved for marketing. Surgeons insert these pumps, each about the size of a hockey puck, under the skin of the abdomen. The pump automatically delivers a basal dosage of insulin; before meals, the pump user tests his or her glucose levels and signals the pump (using a remote control device) to dispense the appropriate burst of additional insulin.

The pump is filled with insulin every few months by a needle inserted through the skin and into the pump. This brief procedure sounds painful, but it is not.

Automatic glucose monitors

Researchers are also working on a related technological product that will take longer to develop: a device that can automatically and continuously measure blood glucose levels. Ideally, such a device could be linked to an implanted insulin pump, and would signal the pump to release the right amounts of insulin based upon current glucose levels. This technological feat would represent the nearest approximation yet to a mechanical replacement for the normal pancreas, sometimes referred to as a *virtual pancreas.*

Diabetes research is wide-ranging, vital, and critical to the advancement of treatment techniques and healthier lives for diabetics. We encourage you to keep informed about progress in diabetes research and to support research in any way you can.

Bright Idea
You can help support diabetes research by participating in the American Diabetes Association's campaigns or the Juvenile Diabetes Foundation's campaigns. You can make financial contributions to diabetes organizations or research centers. You can even volunteer to be a subject in a research study. Call the ADA or JDF, or check your local newspaper.

Just the facts

- Diabetes research is active and growing.

- There is new research interest in type 2 diabetes.

- Medical research has not identified a "diabetes gene," but is studying a number of genetic characteristics that may be related to diabetes.

- The immune system's attack upon the pancreas in type 1 diabetes remains a vital area of diabetes research.

- Scientists are making progress in understanding how high blood sugar causes the complications of diabetes.

- Researchers and manufacturers are actively developing needle-free insulin delivery systems and lancet-free blood glucose monitoring.

Looking Ahead

GET THE SCOOP ON...
How insulin shots may prevent diabetes ▫
Teaching T cells ▫ A historic study on
preventing type 2 diabetes ▫ Progress in
pancreas transplants ▫ Whether the end of the
century will bring an end to diabetes

PART VII

New Hope for Prevention and Cure

Most of us would agree that the best medical treatment is prevention. Isn't it better to prevent disease in the first place, instead of becoming ill and having to undergo treatment?

But treatments and, ultimately, cures for disease are extremely important nonetheless. Today, diabetes research is making strides toward discovering ways to prevent diabetes, and to cure it as well.

As our understanding of the causes of diabetes grows, so does insight into possible means for preventing the disease in people who are predisposed to it. For both type 1 and type 2 diabetes, researchers are looking into genetic and antibody screening and early treatment interventions that might protect vulnerable individuals from developing diabetes. Keep in mind that even delaying the onset of diabetes is a significant advance, as it reduces the risks for serious complications of diabetes, which usually take ten or more years to develop.

435

Preventing type 1 diabetes

In 1994, the National Institutes of Health launched the Diabetes Prevention Trial-Type 1 (DPT-1), a nationwide, two-phase study that is investigating whether diabetes can be prevented if at-risk individuals take insulin.

The diabetes prevention trial-type 1

The DPT-1 is the first of its kind. It is looking at people between ages three and forty-five who are related to someone with type 1 diabetes. Persons chosen as DPT-1 subjects are those for whom blood tests indicate an intermediate to high risk for developing type 1 diabetes within the next five years.

Since DPT-1 began, over 50,000 potential subjects have been screened nationwide. Since only 3.6 percent of all people screened will be appropriate for the trial, DPT-1's organizers plan to screen up to 80,000 people, with the goal of finally enrolling 830 volunteer research subjects.

Phase One of DPT-1 began in early 1994. This phase is exploring whether insulin injection treatment will delay or prevent diabetes in high-risk individuals.

Phase Two began late in 1997. It will look at whether crystallized insulin, taken orally in capsules, will delay or prevent diabetes in intermediate-risk individuals.

It is too soon to tell what the results of DPT-1 will be. In its 1998 Research Progress Report, however, the Juvenile Diabetes Foundation (in an article written by A.T. McPhee) reports on the status of one of the first participants in the trial. Sean Finley was "on the verge of becoming diabetic" at age fourteen. He began taking low-dose insulin shots twice daily and at age twenty-two remains free of diabetes.

Identifying who will develop diabetes

If we could know in advance which individuals will develop type 1 diabetes, we would have a jumpstart on applying preventive measures.

While we have developed the technology to identify those who are genetically susceptible, we are not yet able to predict who will actually develop diabetes; not all genetically susceptible individuals do.

One significant clue to this is the presence of certain autoantibodies in people who are genetically at risk for diabetes. Autoantibodies are proteins that react destructively toward other cells or proteins in the body. Research done by George Eisenbarth, M.D., and epidemiologist Marian Rewers at the Barbara Davis Center in Denver, Colorado, is shining a light on which autoantibodies are associated with diabetes, and at what point they develop in children with and without a family history of the disease.

Dr. Eisenbarth's work so far suggests that, among children at highest genetic risk for developing diabetes, about 40 percent develop specific autoantibodies related to diabetes by age two.

It may be possible someday to identify and treat children before the destructive autoantibodies develop.

Changing the immune system's response to beta cells

Type 1 diabetes is caused by the destruction of insulin-producing beta cells in the pancreas when the body's immune system mounts an autoimmune attack on those cells.

Researchers are exploring ways to block or deter this autoimmune attack in people predisposed to

Bright Idea
Think you might make a good DPT-1 volunteer subject? Or just want more information? Call (800) HALT-DTM1 ([800] 425-8361).

type 1 diabetes. One method may be to remove the immune system's T cells from a person in the beginning stages of diabetes and "teach" them, through exposure to the proteins found on that person's beta cells, to recognize the beta cells as "self." This would stop the T cells from attacking the beta cells, thereby halting the progression of diabetes. (T cells normally fight off viruses and bacteria.)

An alternative to removing T cells would be to make them tolerant by giving oral preparations of the proteins the T cells are mistakenly attacking. This process, called *oral tolerization,* is thought to "re-educate" the immune system. For example, researchers know that the protein glutamic acid decarboxylase (or GAD), found on the surface of beta cells, is one of the first targets of the immune system in the early stages of diabetes. If diabetes-prone individuals could take GAD orally, it might prevent this autoimmune response. Since GAD is not readily available for this purpose, some researchers are developing ways to produce it outside the body.

Another approach is to alter the genetic or molecular structure of the beta cells themselves to change or hide whatever is triggering T cells to attack them. Altering the structures on the T cells that respond to these triggers is also a future possibility. The goal is to stop the mistaken signaling that occurs between T cells and pancreatic cells.

For example, Michael Clare-Salzler, M.D., a researcher at the University of Florida in Gainesville, has found evidence that one type of prostaglandin, which is naturally produced by the body, may somehow spark T cells to attack islet cells in people who are predisposed to develop type 1 diabetes. If scientists can discover which genes are responsible for prostaglandin production, this may lead the way to blocking this problem in people at risk for diabetes.

Preventing type 2 diabetes

Interest in preventing and treating type 2 diabetes is at an all-time high, as facts and figures increasingly demonstrate the enormous impact of this disease. This new commitment on the part of medical science is made clear by the National Institutes of Health's recent announcement of a large-scale study on preventing type 2 diabetes.

The diabetes prevention program

In June of 1996, the NIH launched the first nationwide study to determine whether type 2 diabetes can be prevented or delayed in people susceptible to the disease.

NIH researchers set a goal of recruiting 4,000 volunteer research subjects, half of whom will be African Americans, Latinos, Native Americans, and Asian and Pacific Island Americans. These ethnic groups have disproportionately high rates of type 2 diabetes. Twenty percent of the research subjects will be people age sixty-five or older, and 20 percent will be women who have had gestational diabetes (drawn from the same ethnically diverse subject pool).

All research subjects for the Diabetes Prevention Program will have a condition called *impaired glucose tolerance*, or *IGT*. In IGT, blood-sugar levels are higher than normal, but not as high as those in diabetics. IGT is considered to be a precursor of type 2 diabetes.

Once the volunteer subjects have been selected, they will be placed in one of three research groups, each looking at different preventive treatments:

> **66**
> In years to come, it is likely that DPT-1 will be remembered as a truly historic, landmark trial. It will provide us with our first answers to questions about whether it is possible to alter one's biological destiny, to prevent or delay the onset of type 1 diabetes. Jay S. Skyler, M.D., DPT-1 Study Chair and Professor of Medicine at the University of Miami
>

Watch Out!
Approximately
21 million
Americans have
higher-than-
normal blood-
sugar levels, or
impaired glucose
tolerance. Most
are unaware of
this and the fact
that it puts them
at greater risk
for developing
type 2 diabetes
at some point in
their lives.

n Intensive lifestyle changes resulting in a 7 percent weight loss.

n Treatment with the oral medication metformin.

n "Treatment" with placebo pills and information on diet and exercise.

The study originally included a fourth research group to examine the effectiveness of the oral medication troglitazone in preventing or delaying type 2 diabetes. Concerns about the risk for liver damage caused by troglitazone (a statistically rare occurrence) prompted program officials to discontinue this part of the study.

As of this writing, the NIH reports that volunteer recruitment for the Diabetes Prevention Program is about 50 percent complete. It is likely that we won't see results from the Program before the year 2002. Like the DPT-1, the Diabetes Prevention Program is a landmark study that is sure to offer new insights into preventing diabetes. If you would like to be a volunteer subject, call (888)DPP-JOIN ([888] 377-5646).

Corporate-funded research on prevention

As type 2 diabetes is increasingly recognized as a disorder affecting millions of Americans, American medical technology and biotechnology businesses are stepping up their efforts to find preventive treatments and diagnostic tests for this potentially lucrative disease.

There are many examples of this heightened activity, and we can't cite all of them here. But the following may illustrate the growing involvement of American businesses in diabetes research:

In September of 1998, the United States Patent and Trademark Office awarded Millennium

Pharmaceuticals, Inc., a Cambridge, Massachusetts–based company, a patent for a test that determines whether a person has, or is at risk for developing, "certain forms of type 2 diabetes."

The test works by detecting specific mutations in a gene called *hepatic nuclear factor 1*, or *HNF1*. This gene regulates some of the characteristics that ultimately show up in the liver and pancreas. Millennium's test looks for a specific mutation in the HNF1 gene that increases the risk for developing liver and pancreatic problems that, in turn, lead to type 2 diabetes.

If doctors can pinpoint who is at risk for diabetes, they can recommend early interventions, such as those being tested in the Diabetes Prevention Program, that may prevent diabetes from developing.

A cure?

At present, the only treatment available to people with diabetes that offers the hope of giving them normal pancreatic functioning and normal blood-sugar levels is the pancreas transplant.

Unfortunately, those contemplating this procedure must weigh freedom from diabetes and its complications against the lifelong need to take powerful drugs following transplant surgery, drugs that suppress the immune system in order to stop it from rejecting the foreign organ.

For many, the risks posed by taking these drugs, as well as the expense of transplant surgery and the relative scarcity of donor organs, have made the pancreas transplant an impractical choice for diabetes treatment.

But people with diabetes can take heart from the fact that transplants are becoming more common,

> " With current surgical techniques and immunosuppressive regimens, most recipients of a successful pancreas [transplant] can expect to remain insulin-free.
> — David Sutherland, M.D., Ph.D., transplant surgeon at the University of Minnesota "

success rates are rising, and advances are being made in transplantation techniques and in the immunosuppressive drugs used after transplantation.

Much of the following information on progress in transplantation technology is based on the excellent "1998 Research Progress Report" written by Michael Burton for the Juvenile Diabetes Foundation. (JDF Research Progress Reports are available on the JDF Web site, www.jdfcure.org.)

The pancreas transplant

Unofficially...
Each year, about 100 more pancreas transplants are performed than in the previous year.

Pancreas transplants have usually been done in tandem with kidney transplants. Traditionally, it has been people with diabetes who are facing kidney failure, and who have to undergo immunosuppressive drug treatment following a kidney transplant, who have been selected as appropriate pancreas transplant recipients. Another procedure is to have a pancreas transplant at some point following a kidney transplant.

These procedures have mixed success rates. In about 80 percent of people who have kidney-pancreas transplants, independence from insulin is achieved after one year. The rate is about 70 percent in those who receive a pancreas after receiving a kidney. However, the American Diabetes Association reports that about 15 percent of pancreas recipients die within five years of surgery due to the severe diabetes that is typically present prior to the operation, as well as post-operative stress on the body.

The organ rejection rate for people who receive both organs simultaneously is about 3 percent at one year. For pancreas-only recipients, it is about 9 percent at one year.

Some transplant centers are encouraging wider use of pancreas-only transplants. So far, most transplants are done in people whose diabetes is advanced and who are suffering severe complications. As transplant technology and post-transplant drug therapy improves, pancreas-only transplants may become more common. This could lead to the preemptive use of pancreas transplants in people at high risk for developing complications. Eventually, pancreas transplants could be used in people who are genetically at high risk for developing diabetes.

Islet cell transplants

The islet cells are the cells in the pancreas that produce insulin. (Beta cells are one type of islet cell.)

Researchers are working on techniques for transplanting healthy islet cells into the pancreases of people with diabetes. Their hope is that this procedure will provide the benefits of whole-organ pancreas transplants while eliminating the need for whole-organ donors and major surgery. The problem of potential rejection of the transplanted tissue remains, however.

Experimentation with islet cell transplant in humans is still relatively rare. In the last decade, more than 200 islet cell transplants have been performed in humans, but only 10 percent of recipients have achieved insulin independence. However, many islet cell recipients have been able to lower their insulin doses and have found it easier to achieve stable glucose levels.

Researchers are still trying to figure out exactly how much islet cell tissue must be transplanted in order to produce adequate amounts of insulin. Another problem hampering progress is the need to use steroid drugs as part of the post-transplant immunosuppressive regimen. Steroids are known to cause diabetes, and they place great stress upon the islet cells.

Research is underway to find new, safer anti-rejection drugs, with the goal of eliminating steroids from post-transplant drug therapies.

Some other areas of islet cell research are

- Animal sources of transplantable islet cells. For example, pig insulin differs from human insulin by only one amino acid.

- Implantation of insulin-producing genes into other body cells to create surrogate islet cells.

- Genetic modification of diabetic islet cells that will stop the immune system from attacking them.

- Implantation of transplantable human or animal islet cells inside protective gel microcapsules, which may block the immune system's rejection response.

Islet cell transplant holds great promise for one day providing a cure for diabetes. But throughout its twenty-five-year experimental history, progress has been frustratingly slow. Much has been learned, but much remains to be understood and resolved before this potentially glorious diabetes treatment becomes reliably successful and widely available.

By the year 2000?

Lois Jovanovic-Peterson is a medical doctor specializing in diabetes who was diagnosed with type 1 diabetes while just beginning her medical career. Dr. Jovanovic-Peterson was no stranger to diabetes; her father had died of the disease at age fifty. Upon his death, Lois Jovanovic-Peterson vowed to devote her life to finding a cure for diabetes.

Today, Dr. Jovanovic-Peterson (who uses an insulin pump) is the medical director and chief executive officer of the Sansum Medical Research

Foundation in Santa Barbara, California. In February of 1997, Sansum announced the Santa Barbara Diabetes Project, a worldwide collaborative effort to discover a cure for type 1 diabetes by the end of the century. The project will seek to establish working relationships among international diabetes experts with the object of accelerating progress in diabetes research.

An unusual feature of the project is its bringing together of academic and industrial researchers. In the past, diabetes research has suffered from competition and lack of communication among non-profit and business institutions.

The project is headquartered at the Sansum Medical Research Foundation, but research is taking place in individual laboratories around the world. The laboratories communicate through a "virtual laboratory" on the Internet. Progress will also be shared once or twice each year in meetings held in Santa Barbara.

The Santa Barbara Diabetes Project hopes that this collaborative approach will speed up progress in the three areas of research it deems most promising:

- Creation of a "virtual pancreas," or a glucose sensor-insulin pump system that replicates pancreatic functioning.

- Genetic engineering of body cells to create surrogate insulin-producing cells.

- Pancreas transplant technology.

Time will tell whether the Santa Barbara Diabetes Project will achieve its goal by the end of the century. Whether it succeeds or not, it stands as an example of the new energy, scope, and

> **"**
> Our recently launched Santa Barbara Diabetes Project is aiming for a cure by the end of the century. We're going to bring together the 'brightest lights' in science, medicine, and engineering to solve this problem. The time is right.
> —Lois Jovanovic-Peterson, M.D., director of diabetes research at the Sansum Medical Research Foundation in Santa Barbara, California, and a person with type 1 diabetes.
> **"**

Bright Idea
Walk for the cure! The Juvenile Diabetes Foundation conducts walkathons benefiting its research for a cure. Walkathons are held at 160 locations throughout the United States. For information on one near you, call (800) WALK-JDF ([800] 925-5533).

sophistication of diabetes research that keeps hope alive in this century and leads the way into the next.

Just the facts

- New understanding of what causes diabetes is generating methods for preventing it.

- Progress is being made in the effort to identify who is most likely to develop diabetes.

- Researchers are experimenting with ways to stop the immune system from attacking insulin-producing cells, which could prevent or help treat type 1 diabetes.

- Scientific interest in treating and preventing type 2 diabetes is at an all-time high.

- Progress is being made in improving pancreas transplants and related procedures.

- Technological advances are moving closer to the development of a "virtual pancreas": a combined glucose sensor and insulin pump that will automatically release appropriate amounts of insulin in response to blood-sugar levels.

Glossary

Acarbose Brand name Precose. An oral medication for treatment of type 2 diabetes. Acarbose helps to control rises in blood sugar after meals by slowing down the absorption of some carbohydrates in the intestinal tract.

ACE inhibitors Angio-tensin converting enzyme inhibitors. These are medications used to treat high blood pressure. ACE inhibitors may be used in people with kidney disease or who are at risk for kidney disease to help prevent or control kidney problems.

Acute diabetic ketoacidosis Also called DKA, diabetic ketoacidosis, ketoacidosis, and diabetic coma. This is a severe condition occurring almost exclusively as a result of *type 1 diabetes* that is caused by insufficient insulin. Symptoms are very high blood glucose levels (over 240 mg/dl); *ketones* in the urine; a sweet, fruity odor on the breath; shortness of breath (air hunger); nausea; and possibly coma.

Adult-onset diabetes Former term for *type 2 diabetes.*

447

AGEs (advanced glycosylation endproducts) The by-products of chronic high blood-sugar levels that accumulate in cells throughout the body. AGE accumulation may cause toughening or stiffening of tissues, contributing to *microvascular* and *macrovascular* complications such as eye, kidney, nerve, and heart disease.

Air hunger A symptom of *acute diabetic ketoacidosis*; refers to panting or shortness of breath in the absence of physical exertion. It is caused by the body's attempt to rid itself of excess ketones through oxygen leaving the lungs.

Americans with Disabilities Act of 1990 Federal legislation that protects the rights and interests of people with disabilities in the workplace and public places.

Antihyperglycemic: oral medications Oral drugs for treatment of type 2 diabetes, for example, *repaglinide, acarbose, miglitol, meformin,* and *troglitazone.* (*Sulfonylureas* are sometimes called *oral hypoglycemics.*) All of these medications help to keep blood sugar at lower levels.

Antioxidants Natural substances that block the generation of harmful free radicals, which are the by-products of many chemical reactions in the body. Free radicals may contribute to *AGE* development, and thus to complications of diabetes. Examples of antioxidants are vitamin C, vitamin E, and beta-carotene.

Atherosclerosis Narrowing and hardening of the artery walls; the presence of raised areas or "plaques" on the inner linings of arteries. Atherosclerosis reduces or blocks blood circulation and increases the risk for heart disease and stroke.

Autoimmune disorder A disease or condition in which damage to the body is caused by the body's own immune system, which mistakenly attacks body cells as "foreign invaders." *Type 1 diabetes* begins as an autoimmune disorder in which insulin-producing cells in the pancreas are destroyed by the immune system.

Basal insulin Slowly absorbed, intermediate- or long-acting insulin that supplies the body with a steady, low, "background" level of insulin (mimicking the natural action of the pancreas). Also applies to the small, steady release of fast-acting insulin from an *insulin pump*. Contrast with *bolus insulin*.

Beta cell A specialized type of cell found in the islets of Langerhans in the *pancreas*, the area that produces and secretes *insulin*. In people with *type 1 diabetes*, the beta cells have been destroyed by autoimmune attack. In people with *type 2 diabetes*, beta cells may produce too little insulin.

BIDS Stands for "bedtime *insulin,* daytime *sulfonylurea,*" a mixed insulin/oral medication treatment regimen for people with *type 2 diabetes* for whom oral medications alone are not effective in controlling blood sugar.

Blood sugar Also called *glucose.* A simple form of sugar that is produced by the breakdown of foods, especially carbohydrates, during digestion. Blood sugar travels through the blood to all the body's cells; it is the body's source of energy. The amount of sugar in the blood is called the blood-sugar level.

Body Mass Index (BMI) A ratio of weight to height that, when calculated, may more accurately determine whether a person is obese than does that person's weight on a scale. The BMI is found by multiplying your weight in pounds by 703, multiplying your height in inches by itself, then dividing the first number by the second. BMIs from nineteen to twenty-five indicate a healthy weight. See Appendix D for more information on using the BMI.

Bolus insulin Rapid- or short-acting *insulin* injected before meals to provide a quick rise in insulin levels, mimicking the pancreas's natural release of insulin following meals. This prevents postmeal blood-sugar levels from rising too high. Contrast with *basal insulin.* Basal and bolus insulin combine throughout the twenty-four-hour cycle to keep blood-sugar levels under control.

"Borderline" diabetes An incorrect term, sometimes used for *impaired glucose tolerance* (IGT). There is no such condition as borderline diabetes; a person either has diabetes or does not. Having impaired glucose tolerance is a risk factor for developing *type 2 diabetes.*

Carbohydrate One of the three major sources of calories (energy) in the diet. (The other two are fats and protein.) Carbohydrate is supplied by sugars (the simple carbohydrates, like fruits, syrups, and sweets) and starches (the complex carbohydrates, like bread, potatoes, pasta, and rice). Carbohydrate broken down during digestion has the greatest impact on blood-sugar levels.

Carbohydrate counting A type of meal plan for people with *diabetes* that helps to control blood-sugar levels by limiting the amount of carbohydrates eaten each day. People using carbohydrate counting meal plans learn to count the number of carbohydrate grams in each serving.

Certified Diabetes Educator (C.D.E.) A health-care professional, often a registered nurse,

nurse-practitioner, or registered dietitian, who has completed a course of training that meets American Diabetes Association standards. The C.D.E. helps people with diabetes learn the basics of diabetes self-care, for example, preparing and administering *insulin* injections or proper use of oral medications.

Charcot's foot   Deformity of the bones in the feet caused by diabetic nerve damage. Numbness in the feet leads to unevenly balanced pressure on the feet. Charcot's foot can cause foot ulcers from pressure spots caused by deformities.

Cholesterol   A waxy substance produced by the liver, used by the body to build cell walls and to make certain hormones. It also is found in meat and dairy foods. Too much cholesterol and saturated fat in the diet, a genetic predisposition for high cholesterol levels, or both can cause cholesterol to accumulate along the inside lining of blood vessels. This increases the risk for heart attack and stroke.

Claudication   Muscle pain in the calf of the leg or buttock during exercise that usually disappears when exercise is stopped. It can be a symptom of blocked or narrowed arteries (*atherosclerosis*) in the legs.

Creatinine clearance   A test of kidney function, used to detect kidney disease.

CSII (continuous subcutaneous insulin infusion)   Another term for insulin treatment with the *insulin pump*.

Dawn phenomenon   In the hours just before awakening (typically 4 to 8 a.m.), the daily release of cortisol and growth hormones may oppose the action of insulin. Blood-sugar levels may be elevated upon rising. Changes in the bedtime treatment plan can help to correct this problem.

Diabetes   A disease in which the insulin-producing organ, the *pancreas*, does not produce enough *insulin*, or in which the body cannot use insulin properly (a condition called *insulin resistance*). The hallmark of diabetes is abnormally high blood-sugar levels.

Diabetes Control and Complications Trial (DCCT) A ten-year study sponsored by the National Institutes of Health, ending in 1993. The DCCT studied over 1,400 people with *type 1 diabetes*, who were divided into two study groups: those who followed *"tight"* glucose control and aimed for near-normal blood glucose levels and those who aimed for standard glucose levels. The DCCT proved that tight glucose control reduces the risk of diabetic complications.

Diabetes Prevention Trial (DPT)   The first nationwide study to look at whether *type 2 diabetes* can be prevented or delayed in people at risk for the disease. Sponsored by the National Institutes of Health, the DPP was launched in 1996 and will study 4,000 Americans. Results are expected by about 2002.

Diabetic ketoacidosis   See *Acute diabetic ketoacidosis.*

Diabetologist   A medical doctor who specializes in treating diabetes. Most diabetologists are *endocrinologists*, but internists and family medicine doctors may also be diabetologists.

Dialysis   Medical treatment for people whose kidneys have failed or are only partially functioning. Dialysis is a process that substitutes for the kidneys by filtering toxic substances from the blood and maintaining blood pressure and blood chemical balances.

Endocrinologist   A medical doctor who specializes in diagnosing and treating disorders of the glands and hormones. *Insulin* is a hormone made by the *pancreas,* which is a gland. Many diabetes doctors are endocrinologists.

Exchange plan　A meal plan that helps regulate the amount of calories and fat, protein, and carbohydrate eaten in one day. Servings of different foods within these three groups are designated, each of which is equivalent in calories and fat, carbohydrate, or protein grams (depending upon the group). Within each group, any serving is exchangeable with any other, allowing for variety while caloric and nutritional goals are met.

Family and Medical Leave Act of 1993 (FMLA) Federal legislation that allows for up to twelve weeks per year of unpaid leave from work for employees who are coping with chronic illness or who have a family member coping with illness or disability.

Fasting glucose　The amount of glucose, or blood sugar, present in the blood after no food has been eaten for eight hours or more. In people with uncontrolled diabetes, fasting glucose levels are 126 *mg/dl* or higher. In people without diabetes, the fasting glucose level is about 70 to 115 *mg/dl.*

Fats　The most concentrated source of calories in the diet. Fats may be saturated (found primarily in meat and dairy products and in foods containing hydrogenated vegetable oils), monounsaturated (olive and canola oils), or polyunsaturated (corn and other vegetable oils). Too much fat in the diet, especially saturated fat, can cause obesity and high blood fat levels, increasing the risk for heart disease and stroke.

Foot ulcer　A wound or sore on the foot that is slow to heal or will not heal. People with diabetes are vulnerable to foot ulcers, which can become infected and lead to amputation.

Gastroparesis   A form of diabetic *neuropathy* that slows down the contractions of the stomach that move food into the intestines. Delays in food digestion can make blood-sugar control more difficult for people with diabetes.

Gestational diabetes mellitus (GDM)   A temporary form of diabetes that occurs in about 2 to 5 percent of nondiabetic women during the later stages of pregnancy. GDM disappears following delivery, but women who have GDM are at increased risk for developing GPM in their future pregnancies and for developing *type 2 diabetes* within 5 to 10 years.

Glucocorticoids   Steroid medications, such as cortisone, that can interfere with *insulin* action.

Glucagon   A hormone produced by the *pancreas* that stimulates the liver to secrete stored glucose, raising blood-sugar levels when necessary.

Glucagon emergency injection kit   A kit containing a prepared injection of *glucagon*, to be administered to people with severe *hypoglycemia* who are too impaired to eat carbohydrates.

Glucophage   See *metformin.*

Glucose   See *blood sugar.*

Glucose meter   A palm-sized, computerized device that reads the amount of *glucose* in blood samples inserted into the meter on blood test strips. The glucose level appears within minutes as a digitally displayed number (some meters "speak" the result for visually impaired users).

Glycemic index   A list of the effect of different foods on blood sugar, as compared to the effect of a slice of bread. Some people with diabetes find the

glycemic index helpful in making food choices for better glucose control.

Glycogen   Glucose that has been stored in the liver or muscles. If the blood-sugar level drops too low, glycogen can be converted back into glucose and released into the bloodstream.

Glycosylated hemoglobin; glycated hemoglobin; glycohemoglobin (also called hemoglobin A1c)   The term for the attachment of *glucose* to the hemoglobin protein in red blood cells and the medical test for this process. The percentage of glucose attached to hemoglobin increases when blood glucose levels are chronically high. The glycosylated hemoglobin test evaluates average blood glucose control over the preceding two to three months.

Glyset   See *miglitol.*

Health Insurance Portability and Accountability Act of 1996 (HIPAA)   Federal legislation that allows people to maintain health insurance coverage through job changes, including people who have "preexisting" medical conditions.

Hemoglobin A1c   See *glycosylated hemoglobin.*

Honeymoon phase   A period during which some people who are newly diagnosed with *type 1 diabetes* may need little or no pharmaceutical *insulin* because their own *beta cells* have temporarily begun producing more insulin (perhaps because insulin treatment has given the cells a rest or a boost). The honeymoon phase can last from a few weeks to a year or so.

Hormone   A chemical substance, produced by a gland, that is released into the bloodstream and influences other organs or functions in the body. *Insulin* is a hormone.

Humalog   See *lispro*.

Hyperglycemia   The condition of higher-than-normal blood-sugar levels (generally 140 *mg/dl* and above). Symptoms of hyperglycemia include increased thirst, frequent urination, and weight loss.

Hyperglycemic hyperosmolar nonketonic syndrome (HHNS)   A condition most often seen in people with *type 2 diabetes* in which blood-sugar levels become grossly elevated (600–2,000 *mg/dl*). Dehydration sets in as the body attempts to rid itself of excess sugar through increased urination. *Ketoacidosis* does not occur. Hyperosmolar syndrome can lead to coma if untreated.

Hypoglycemia   The condition of lower-than-normal blood-sugar levels (60 *mg/dl* or lower). Symp-toms include shakiness, perspiration, rapid heartbeat, hunger, mood changes, and eventual seizures or loss of consciousness if not treated.

Hypoglycemia unawareness   In some people, symptoms of hypoglycemia may be muted or imperceptible. Hypoglycemia unawareness may be caused by diabetic *neuropathy* or by repeated episodes of hypoglycemia.

Immunosuppressive drugs   Drugs given to people who have had kidney, *pancreas*, or other organ transplants that prevent the immune system from attacking the transplanted organ. Transplant recipients must take these medications for life. Immuno-suppressive drugs increase the risk for infections and tumors.

Impaired glucose tolerance (IGT)   A condition in which blood tests reveal that a person's blood glucose level is between normal and diabetic levels. People with impaired glucose tolerance do not have

diabetes or "borderline" diabetes, but they have an increased risk for developing diabetes.

Insulin   A *hormone* produced by the *pancreas.* Insulin helps the body to make use of glucose in the bloodstream by "unlocking" cell walls and allowing glucose to enter them. This is how body cells receive energy. Pharmaceutical insulin is made by drug manufacturers for use by diabetics who do not produce their own insulin.

Insulin-dependent diabetes   Former term for *type 1 diabetes.*

Insulin pump   A small, computerized device that delivers insulin through a tube and needle inserted just under the skin, usually on the abdomen. The pump is worn outside the body and is programmed to deliver continuous *basal insulin* throughout the day and *bolus insulin* with meals or snacks.

Insulin reaction   *Hypoglycemia* caused by too much insulin relative to food or glucose.

Insulin resistance   A condition in which the body does not respond properly or efficiently to *insulin,* leading to high blood-sugar levels. Insulin resistance is a primary cause of *type 2 diabetes.*

Intensive diabetes treatment   Also called *"tight"* diabetes treatment, a treatment approach that has the goal of attaining near-normal blood-sugar levels. Intensive treatment includes frequent daily blood-sugar monitoring, three or more insulin shots a day (or use of the *insulin pump*), and adherence to meal and exercise plans. The *DCCT* study showed that intensive treatment lowers the risk for *diabetes* complications.

Islet cells   Cells in the *pancreas* that form the islets of Langerhans, which contain the insulin-producing *beta cells.*

Juvenile diabetes   Former term for *type 1 diabetes*, which begins mostly (but not exclusively) in people under age thirty.

Ketoacidosis   See *acute diabetic ketoacidosis.*

Ketone strips   Chemically treated paper strips used to check urine samples for the presence of *ketones.*

Ketones   Ketones are a by-product of the burning of fat for energy. Normally, the body burns glucose for energy. Without sufficient *insulin*, glucose can't enter body cells, and the body begins burning fat instead (while blood sugar rises). If ketones accumulate, *ketoacidosis* occurs.

Lente   A form of pharmaceutical *insulin* that is intermediate acting. Lente insulin is active about one hour after injection, peaks at six to eight hours, and lasts twelve to eighteen hours.

Lipoatrophy   A condition that can occur at *insulin* injection sites. A dent appears at the site due to the breakdown of fatty tissue underneath the skin. Lipoatrophy is more common in people who use animal-derived insulins, which may trigger an immune response.

Lipohypertrophy   A skin condition that can occur at overused *insulin* injection sites. The skin appears lumpy or like scar tissue due to an overgrowth of cells there. See also *lipoatrophy.*

Lispro   A newer form of pharmaceutical *insulin* that is rapid acting. Lispro insulin is active within about fifteen minutes of injection, peaks in about one-and-a-half hours, and lasts about three hours. (Brand name *Humalog.*)

Macrosomia   Oversized newborn babies, generally weighing ten pounds or more. Macrosomia often occurs if the mother's *diabetes* or *gestational diabetes* is poorly controlled during pregnancy. Macrosomia increases the risk for premature and complicated deliveries.

Macrovascular complications Complications of diabetes that affect the heart, arteries, and circulation in the body and brain.

Metformin Brand name Glucophage. An oral medication for treatment of *type 2 diabetes.* Metformin works by preventing the liver from releasing too much stored glucose into the blood, helping to keep blood-sugar levels normal.

Mg/dl Milligrams per deciliter. This indicates the milligrams of glucose per deciliter of blood. It is used to describe blood-sugar levels.

Microalbumin test; microalbuminuria A test for tiny particles of protein in the urine (a condition called microalbuminuria). Particles may indicate the beginning of kidney disease.

Microvascular complications Complications of diabetes that affect the internal structures and veins of the eyes and kidneys, as well as the nervous system.

Miglitol Brand name *Glyset.* An oral medication for treatment of type 2 diabetes. It works very similarly to *acarbose (frecose).*

NPH insulin A form of pharmaceutical *insulin* that is intermediate-acting. NPH is active about one hour after injection, peaks at six to eight hours, and lasts about twelve to eighteen hours.

Nephropathy Kidney disease. It can be one of the complications of diabetes.

Neuropathy Nerve damage. It can be one of the complications of diabetes. It can cause numbness, pain, or strange sensations in the hands and feet, as well as impaired digestive, cardiac, urinary tract, and sexual functioning.

Non–insulin dependent diabetes Former term for *type 2 diabetes*.

Opthalmologist A medical doctor who specializes in diagnosing and treating diseases of the eye.

Oral hypoglycemics See *sulfonylureas*.

Pancreas A banana-shaped gland located under and behind the stomach. It produces hormones and enzymes that help regulate digestion and the body's use of energy from food. The healthy pancreas produces *insulin,* which regulates the entry of glucose into body cells.

Podiatrist A doctor (not an M.D.; but a D.P.M., doctor of podiatric medicine) who specializes in preventing and treating foot disorders, including *foot ulcers* and infections.

Prandin See *repaglinide*.

Precose See *acarbose*.

Protein One of the three primary sources of calories in the diet. It is found in meats, eggs, and milk, many beans and legumes, and to a lesser extent in grains and some vegetables. Protein is used by the body to build and repair muscle, body tissue, blood cells, *hormones,* and other important substances.

Proteinuria The presence of protein in the urine. This may indicate kidney damage or kidney disease.

Receptors (insulin receptors) The molecular "locks" or sites on cell walls that react to *insulin,* allowing the cell to open up and let glucose enter. One cause of *type 2 diabetes* is an insufficient number of insulin receptors.

Registered dietitian (R.D.) A person who has training and expertise in diet and nutrition.

The registered dietitian has passed a national examination, and is an important part of the diabetes health-care team.

Regular insulin   A form of pharmaceutical *insulin* that is short acting. Regular insulin is active within about forty-five minutes after injection, peaks in about two hours, and lasts for four to six hours.

Repaglinide   Brand name Prandin. One of the newest oral medications for treatment of *type 2 diabetes*. Repaglinide works by stimulating the pancreas to release more *insulin* after meals.

Retinopathy   Damage to the small blood vessels in the eye. It can be a complication of diabetes. In earlier stages, retinopathy is called nonproliferative or background retinopathy and may cause blurred vision. More advanced retinopathy is called proliferative retinopathy; it can lead to detached retina or blindness if untreated. Retinopathy may be treated with laser surgery techniques.

Rezulin   See *troglitazone.*

"Silent" disease   A disease that can be present without symptoms that are noticeable to the person who has it. *Type 2 diabetes* can be present for years before symptoms become obvious.

SMBG (self-monitoring of blood glucose)   The taking of a small drop of blood from one's finger in order to test one's blood-sugar level. The drop of blood is placed on a paper strip that is inserted into a *glucose meter* (or is matched against a blood glucose color chart). SMBG is an essential part of diabetes self-care, and is typically performed four to eight times a day (more frequently during pregnancy).

Somogyi Effect   A reaction of the liver to a period of hypoglycemia. The liver "overcorrects" by releasing too much glucose, causing the blood-sugar level to rise too high.

Sulfonylureas   A class of oral medications for treatment of *type 2 diabetes* that work by stimulating the *pancreas* to release more *insulin*. The sulfonylureas are the oldest oral diabetes medications. They were discovered in the 1940s and are still an important part of type 2 diabetes treatment.

TIA (transient ischemic attack)   Temporary neurological problems, such as slurred speech or numbness of the arm, caused by partial blockage of an artery or arteries in the brain.

"Tight" insulin control   See *intensive diabetes treatment.*

Triglycerides   The fats found in our diets and also in our bodies and bloodstream. Dietary triglycerides come from both animal and vegetable sources and are saturated, unsaturated, or monounsaturated. Doctors check the triglyceride levels in the blood when they check cholesterol levels. There is some evidence that high levels of triglycerides in the blood increase the risk for heart disease in people with diabetes.

Troglitazone   Brand name Rezulin. An oral medication for treatment of *type 2 diabetes.* Troglitazone works by increasing fat and muscle cell receptivity to insulin.

Type 1 diabetes (formerly called juvenile diabetes and insulin-dependent diabetes)   A form of diabetes that usually appears in people age thirty or under but may occur at any age. It usually is caused by the attack of the immune system on the cells in the *pancreas* that produce *insulin.* People who have type 1 diabetes cannot produce their own insulin and must take insulin injections to survive.

Type 2 diabetes (formerly known as adult-onset diabetes and non–insulin dependent diabetes) A form of diabetes that usually, but not always, occurs in people over the age of forty. Type 2 diabetes is caused by *insulin resistance* and, in some cases, insufficient insulin production. Type 2 diabetes can sometimes be treated with diet and exercise alone, but often oral medications or insulin injections are necessary.

Ultralente insulin A pharmaceutical form of *insulin* that is long-acting. Ultralente insulin is active within about two to four hours after injection, peaks at about eight to twelve hours, and lasts for about thirty-six hours.

Velosulin A buffered form of regular insulin that is often used in *insulin pumps*.

Virtual pancreas Scientists are working to create this innovation in diabetes treatment, which would be a combination glucose sensor and automatic *insulin pump*. It would mimic the functioning of a healthy *pancreas*. The glucose sensor would continuously monitor blood-sugar levels, and would trigger the pump to release the right amount of insulin. The device would be implanted.

Resource Guide

Note: Web site addresses (URLs) are included throughout the Resource Guide following addresses and telephone numbers. The separate section for Internet resources provides Web site addresses only for selected diabetes-related sites.

Diabetes organizations

American Diabetes Association
1660 Duke Street
Alexandria, VA 22314
Phone: (800) 342-2383
Web: www.diabetes.org

Association Latinoamericana de Diabetes
Av. Potosi No. 425
San Luis Potosi
Mexico
Fax: (52481) 330-050
Web: www.info.pitt.edu/~imdl1/diabetes/
ALAD.html

Canadian Diabetes Association
15 Toronto Street, Suite 1001
Toronto, Ontario M5C 2E3
Canada
Phone (416) 363-3373
Web: www.diabetes.ca

Central Diabetes Program
U.S. Indian Health Services
Indian Health Services Headquarters West
5300 Homestead Road NE
Albuquerque, NM 87110
Phone: (505) 248-4182
Web: www.tucson.his.gov
From the home page, go to "Site Map." Scroll down
to "Health Care and Administrative Resources,"
then down to "IHS Diabetes Program."

Diabetes Division
Centers for Disease Control and Prevention
National Center for Chronic Disease Prevention and
Health Promotion
TISB Mail Stop K-13
4770 Buford Highway NE
Atlanta, GA 30341-3724
Phone: (770) 488-5080

Juvenile Diabetes Foundation
120 Wall Street
New York, NY 10005
Phone: (800) 533-2873
Web: www.jdfcure.com

Diabetes advocacy

Taking Control of Your Diabetes
149 7th Street
Del Mar, CA 92014
Phone (619) 755-5683
Web: www.tcoyd.com

A nonprofit organization dedicated to educating people with diabetes about how to live longer and to be self-advocates within their health-care programs.

Health-care professional organizations

American Academy of Opthalmology
Customer Service Department
PO Box 7424
San Francisco, CA 94120-7424
Phone: (415) 561-8500
Web: www.eyenet.org

American Association for Marriage and Family Therapy
1133 15th Street NW, Suite 300
Washington, DC 20036
Phone: (202) 452-0109
Web: www.aamft.org

American Association of Clinical Endocrinologists
1000 Riverside Avenue, Suite 205
Jacksonville, FL 32204
Phone: (904) 353-7878
Web: www.aace.com

American Association of Diabetes Educators
444 North Michigan Avenue, Suite 1240
Chicago, IL 60611
Phone: (800) 338-3633
Web: www.diabetesnet.com/aade.html

American Board of Medical Specialties
47 Perimeter Center East, Suite 500
Atlanta, GA 30346
Phone: (800) 776-2378
Web: www.abms.org; www.certifieddoctor.org

American Board of Podiatric Surgery
1601 Dolores Street
San Francisco, CA 94110
Phone: (415) 826-3200
Web: www.abps.org

American Dietetic Association
216 West Jackson Boulevard, Suite 800
Chicago, IL 60606
Phone (312) 899-0040; (800) 366-1655
Web: www.eatright.org

American Medical Association
515 North State Street
Chicago, IL 60610
Phone: (312) 464-4818
Web: www.ama-assn.org

American Psychiatric Association
1400 K Street, NW
Washington, DC 20005
Phone: (202) 682-6000
Web: www.psych.org

The Endocrine Society
4350 East West Highway, Suite 500
Bethesda, MD 20814-4410
Phone: (301) 941-0200
Web: www.endo-society.org

National Association of Social Workers
750 First Street, NE, Suite 700
Washington, DC 20002
Phone: (800) 638-8799
Web: www.socialworkers.org

Pedorthic Footwear Association
9861 Broken Land Parkway, Suite 255
Columbia, MD 21046-1151
Phone: (800) 673-8447
Web: www.pedorthics.org

Medical organizations and foundations

American Amputee Foundation
PO Box 250218
Little Rock, AR 72225
Phone: (501) 666-2523
(Web site under construction)

American Association of Kidney Patients
3926 Granger Drive
Chamblee, GA 30341
Phone: (770) 451-4579
Web: www.aakp.org

American Council of the Blind
1155 15th Street, NW, Suite 720
Washington, DC 20005
Phone: (800) 424-8666
Web: www.acb.org

American Heart Association
7272 Greenville Avenue
Dallas, TX 75231
Phone: (800) 242-8721
Web: www.americanheart.org

Diabetic Retinopathy Foundation
350 North LaSalle, Suite 800
Chicago, IL 60610
(Telephone number not available)
Web: www.retinopathy.org

Impotence Institute of America
10400 Little Patuxent Parkway, Suite 485
Columbia, MD 21044
Phone: (800) 669-1603
(No Web site available)

Medic Alert Foundation
PO Box 1009
Turlock, CA 95381-5378
Phone: (800) 432-5378
Web: www.medicalert.org
Note: The Medic Alert Foundation provides medical
ID bracelets (for a fee) and other emergency med-
ical assistance services with membership.

National Amputation Foundation
73 Church Street
Malverne, NY 11565
Phone: (516) 887-3600
(No Web site available)

National Federation for the Blind
1800 Johnson Street
Baltimore, MD 21230
Phone: (410) 659-9314
Web: www.nfb.org/diabetes.htm

National Kidney Foundation
30 E. 33rd Street
New York, NY 10016
Phone: (800) 622-9010
Web: www.kidney.org

National Osteoporosis Foundation
1150 17th Street NW, Suite 500
Washington, DC 20036
Phone: (202) 223-2226
Web: www.nof.org

Wound Care Institute, Inc.
1541 NE 167th Street
North Miami Beach, FL 33162
Phone: (305) 919-9192
Web: www.woundcare.org

Diabetes journals and magazines

Diabetes Advocate
American Diabetes Association
Government Relations Department
1660 Duke Street
Alexandria, VA 22314
Phone: (800) 342-2383
E-mail: advocate@diabetes.org
To preview online: www.diabetes.org, click on "Legislation Info."
The *Diabetes Advocate* newsletter, published ten times per year, reports on current legislation and public policy affecting diabetes treatment, research, and people with diabetes. It is a rallying cry for the diabetes community.

Diabetes Forecast
American Diabetes Association
1660 Duke Street
Alexandria, VA 22314
Phone: (800) 342-2383; (800) 806-7801
E-mail: customerservice@diabetes.org
To preview online: www.diabetes.org, click on "Read Our Magazine."
The official magazine of the ADA, "America's leading diabetes magazine" began publication in 1948. You must be a member of the ADA to subscribe. Published monthly.

Diabetes Interview
Kings Publishing, Inc.
3715 Balboa Street
San Francisco, CA 94121
Phone: (800) 234-1218
E-mail: diabetes@best.com
To preview online: www:diabetesworld.com/
index2.html
Diabetes Interview is a monthly newspaper-style publication serving the diabetes community that provides in-depth coverage of all aspects of living with diabetes. Lots of reader input is included.

Diabetes Is Not a Piece of Cake Newsletter
Lincoln Publishing, Inc.
PO Box 1499
Lake Oswego, OR 97035-0499
Phone: (800) 266-5748
Written by certified diabetes educator Janet Meirelles, author of the funny, information-packed book *Diabetes Is Not a Piece of Cake,* this newsletter covers nutrition, research, recipes, and much more. It is published eleven times yearly.

Diabetic Reader
Prana Publications
5623 Matilija Avenue
Van Nuys, CA 91401
Phone: (800) 735-7726
E-mail: prana2@aol.com
To preview online: http://members.aol.com/
prana2
The *Diabetic Reader* is published twice a year, in Spring/Summer and Fall/Winter. It is a warm, personal conversation between readers and two former librarians—one with diabetes—who research all topics relating to diabetes and solicit information from readers and health-care professionals.

Diabetes Self-Management
R.A. Rapaport Publishing, Inc.
150 West 22nd Street
New York, NY 100ll
Phone: (800) 234-0923
E-mail: staff@diabetes-self-mgmt.com
To preview online: www.diabetes-self-mgmt.com
Published six times yearly, *Diabetes Self-Management* magazine offers expert, accessible information on all aspects of diabetes self-care in articles written by experienced diabetes professionals.

Scientific journals

For help in researching and evaluating new and alternative medical treatments:

British Medical Journal
BMJ Publishing Group
PO Box 590A
Kennebunkport, ME 04046
Phone: (800) 236-6265
Web: www.bmj.com/bmj

Harvard Health Letter
Harvard University Publications
164 Longwood Avenue
Boston, MA 02115
Phone: (617) 432-1485
Web: www:countwaymed.harvard.edu/
publications/Health

Integrative Medicine
Elsevier Science
PO Box 945
New York, NY
10159-0945
Phone: (888) 437-4636
Web: www.elsevier.com

Journal of the American Medical Association
Subscriber Services Center
PO Box 10945
Chicago, IL 60610
Phone: (312) 670-7827
Web: www.ama-assn.org/
publications/journals/jama/jamahome/html

The Lancet
655 Avenue of the Americas, 5th Floor
New York, NY 10010
Phone: (212) 633-3800
Web: www.theLancet.com

New England Journal of Medicine
10 Shattuck Street
Boston, MA 02115-6094
Phone: (617) 734-9800
Web: www.nejm.org

Prevention
Customer Service
PO Box 7319
Red Oak, IA 51591-0319
Phone: (800) 813-8070
Web: www.healthyideas.com

Science
PO Box 1811
Danbury, CT 06813
Phone: (800) 731-4939
Web: www.sciencemag.org

The Internet

For general information on diabetes

American Diabetes Association
Web: www.diabetes.org
A bright, well-designed, comprehensive Web site. It includes basic diabetes facts, information on research and legislation, ADA membership, and previews of *Diabetes Forecast* and *Diabetes Advocate*. This should be your first stop on the "diabetes Web."

Children With Diabetes
Web: www.childrenwithdiabetes
Do *not* miss this wonderfully comprehensive Web site! *Children With Diabetes* provides information and resources for all people with diabetes, but especially for parents and children. It includes a unique Q-and-A forum with diabetes health-care professionals, a great online links directory, and much more. (The "One-Page Care Guide for Children in School" and "Before School Starts Checklist for Parents" documents in Appendix D of this book are from this site. Take a look.)

Diabetes.Com
Web: www.diabetes.com
Another strong site for up-to-date information on all aspects of diabetes. Special sections on tight diabetes control, complications, and sexual concerns, plus a community message board.

Diabetes Webring
Web: www.webring.org/cgi-bin/
webring?ring=diabetes&list
This terrific site links you to thirty-five diabetes-related Internet sites! For example, link up with *Big Men Who Have Diabetes*, or *Diabetes and Sports* (about

a South American man who competed in the Ironman triathlete event). This site is a must for Internet surfers seeking diabetes information.

It's Spelled D-I-A-B-E-T-E-S

An excellent, down-to-earth source of general diabetes information. To visit, log on to *Diabetes Webring*, discussed above, and then click on "It's Spelled D-I-A-B-E-T-E-S."

Informacion para personas con Diabetes

Web: www.cica.es/~samfyc/informhtm

A Spanish-language Web site containing lots of general diabetes information, as well as links to other Spanish-language sites.

Juvenile Diabetes Foundation

Web: www.jdfcure.org

Answers to all your basic questions about type 1 diabetes, and excellent information on diabetes research.

Rick Mendosa: A Writer on the Web

Web: www.mendosa.com

Rick Mendosa is a well-traveled, interesting health and business writer and poet who happens to have type 2 diabetes. He has compiled an incredibly comprehensive list of Internet diabetes resources, including detailed reviews of each site. Visit his home page and click on "directory." A rich resource!

ScienceWeb

Web: http://diabetes.sciweb.com

Be sure to visit this Center for Diabetes Education. Includes information on books, medication, research, diabetes news, and online links.

Sharing the World of Diabetes
Web: www3.edgenet.net/dare/
This Web site seeks to take "an active role in uniting the world of people with diabetes." Great, first-person profiles, general information, recipes, a message board, and more.

For information on foot care and foot ulcers
Amputation Prevention Global Research Center
Web: www.diabetesresource.com
This center is a collaborative effort between the Boehringer-Mannheim and Eli Lilly companies, and is "dedicated to a global effort to prevent amputations in persons with diabetes."

Woundcare
Web: www.woundcare.org
Dedicated to the advancement of wound healing and the treatment and prevention of diabetic foot pathology.

Online chats, support groups, message and bulletin boards
America On-Line Diabetes Bulletin Board
From AOL, go to "Channels." Then click on "Health." Click on "Illnesses and Treatments," then "Diabetes," and then "Thrive: Diabetes." Look for the "Support Groups and Message Board."

Diabetes Mailing List Home Page
Web: www.cde.com/diabetes.world/
Communicate via e-mail with other people living with diabetes. A mix of personal experience, medical information, scientific news, and support.

Diabetes Support Board
Web: www.nucleus.com/~munro/bbs/
diabetes.html

This message board strives to educate people about diabetes and hopes that participants "perhaps make a difference in their own, or someone else's lives."

Support Diabetes Kids
From www.childrenwithdiabetes.com, click on "On-Line Links," then on "General On-Line Sources," then on "alt.support.diabetes.kids."
Parents trade stories, advice, questions, and problems about the challenges of parenting children with diabetes. Lots of real life information!

Information for parents
Children With Diabetes
www.childrenwithdiabetes
See entry above, under general information sites. This is a wonderful resource for parents and children created and managed by the father of an eleven-year-old girl with type 1 diabetes, who was diagnosed at age two.

Diabetes Life Network (Boehring-Mannheim)
www.roche.com/diagnostics/
This corporate-sponsored Web site has good general diabetes information, and also a nice section on "Kids and Parents." From the home page, click on "Diabetes Care," then on "Kids and Parents."

Family's Guide to Diabetes
Web: www.diabetes.cbyc.com
Help for parents and families. Contains sections on school and diabetes, diabetes in young children, and the "DiabetiChat" message board.

Juvenile Diabetes Foundation
Web: www.jdfcure.org
See entry above, under general information. From the home page, click on "Diabetes Information and

Publications." Look for FAQs about "Diabetes" and "Children with Diabetes"; also, check out JDF's publication for children, *Countdown for Kids.*

For information on diabetes research

American Association of Clinical Endocrinologists
Web: www.aace.com
Updates on endocrinology research and patient advocacy initiatives.

American Diabetes Association
Web: www.diabetes.org
From the home page, click on "Research Update."

Diabetes Wellness and Research Foundation
Web: www.charities.org/dirs/health/
drwf/index.html
This foundation provides support for scientific research into diabetes treatments and a cure; diabetes screenings, evaluations, and education; and the prevention of complications.

Juvenile Diabetes Foundation
Web: www.jdfcure.org
From the home page, click on "Research."

National Institutes of Health/National Institute of Diabetes and Digestive and Kidney Diseases
Web: www.niddk.nih.gov
From the NIDDK home page, click on "Research Funding and Programs."

For information on diabetes supplies

American Diabetes Association
Web: www.diabetes.org
From the home page, click on "Read Our Magazine," then on "Buyer's Guide to Diabetes Products" (published each fall).

Children With Diabetes
Web: www.childrenwithdiabetes.com
From the home page, go to "On-Line Links," then to "Mail Order Supplies." CWD has compiled a fantastic listing of mail-order diabetes supplies companies, with telephone numbers and other information.

Resources for travelers

Centers for Disease Control
Twenty-four-hour International Travelers Hotline
Phone: (404) 332-4559

Diabetes Traveling and Living Well (on the Internet)
Web: www.ishops.com/diabetes/
Information on managing diabetes during intercontinental travel. Includes *Diabetes Traveler,* a quarterly newsletter.

International Association for Medical Assistance to Travelers
417 Center Street
Lewiston, NY 14092
Phone: (716) 754-4883
www.sentex.net/~iamat/
Can provide a list of doctors in foreign countries who speak English and who received postgraduate medical training in North America or Great Britain.

International Diabetes Federation
1 rue Defacqz
B-1000 Brussels
Belgium
Fax: +32-2-538-5114
Web: www.idf.org
Since 1950, the IDF's mission has been to enhance the lives of people with diabetes throughout the world. It has associations in 122 countries, including

in Africa, South America, Europe, and Southeast Asia. It can offer assistance when you're traveling.

Resources for exercisers

International Diabetic Athletes Association
1647 Bethany Home Road, #B
Phoenix, AZ 85015
Phone: (800) 898-4322
Web: www.diabetes-exercise.org

Employment discrimination resources

American Bar Association
Commission on Mental and Physical Disability Law
740 15th Street NW
Washington, DC 20005-1009
Phone: (202) 662-1570
Web: www.abanet.org
From the home page, click on "Public Information," then look under "Additional Resources for the Mental and Physical Disability Law."

Americans with Disabilities Act Document Center (on the Internet)
Web: http://janweb.icdi.wvu.edu/kinder/
From the home page, click on "Employment Considerations for People with Diabetes".

Americans with Disabilities Act Information Line
Phone: (800) 514-0383

Disability Rights Education and Defense Fund, Inc.
2212 6th Street
Berkeley, CA 94710
Phone: (510) 644-2555
Web: www.dredf.org

Equal Employment Opportunity Commission
1801 L Street NW
Washington, DC 10507
For help in filing a charge:
Phone: (800) 669-4000 (connects to your local EEOC office)

For publications on the Americans with Disabilities Act:
Phone: (800) 669-3362
Web: www.eeoc.gov

National Information Center for Children and Youth with Disabilities
P.O Box 1492
Washington, DC 20013-1492
Phone: (202) 884-8200
Web: www.nichy.org
Provides up-to-date information on disability topics.

National Institute on Disability and Rehabilitation Research
U.S. Department of Education
Washington, DC 20202
Phone: (800) 949-4232
Web: http://janweb.icdi.wvu.edu/kinder/nidrr.html
With ten regional offices, the NIDRR provides information, referrals, and technical assistance on all aspects of the American with Disabilities Act.

Legislation

Americans with Disabilities Act
On the Internet: http://janweb.icdi.wvu.edu/kinder/
For the text of the ADA, click on "Public Law 101:336—The ADA Itself."

Also try the ADA home page:

Web: www.usdoj.gov/crt/ada/

A copy of the fifty-one-page ADA can be ordered from the Government Printing Office for $1.50. Call (202) 512-1800 or 1808, or look in your telephone book lue ages under "US Government, Government Printing Office Bookstore." Or order a copy online: At http://thomas.loc.gov, look for "Congressional Internet Services" (left margin). Click on "GPO," then on "Sales Product Catalogue." In the search box, type the name of the act or legislation you wish to order, and follow directions from there.

Family and Medical Leave Act

On the Internet: http://thomas.loc.gov

(Congress on the Internet). On the home page, go to "Public Laws by Law Number." Click on "Previous Congresses," then "103 (1993-94)," then on "103-1 to 103-50." Scroll down to #3, HR 1. Click on this and then on "Text of Legislation."

A copy of the FMLA can be ordered from the Government Printing Office. See instructions, above, under American With Disabilities Act.

Health Insurance Portability and Accountability Act of 1996

On the Internet: http://thomas.loc.gov

(Congress on the Internet). On the home page, go to "Public Laws by Law Number." Click on "Previous Congresses," then "104 (1995-96)," then "104-151 to 104-200." Scroll down to "#191, HR 3103." Click on this and then on "Text of Legislation."

A copy of the HIPAA can be ordered from the Government Printing Office. See instructions, above, under American with Disabilities Act.

Recommended Reading List

General books on diabetes

American Diabetes Association. *Complete Guide to Diabetes.* Alexandria, VA: American Diabetes Association, 1996.

Beasor, Richard S. *The Joslin Guide to Diabetes.* New York: Fireside, 1995.

Meirelles, Janet. *Diabetes Is Not a Piece of Cake,* 3rd Edition. Lake Oswego, OR: Lincoln Publishing, 1997.

Saudek, Christopher D. *The Johns Hopkins Guide to Diabetes.* Baltimore: The Johns Hopkins University Press, 1997.

Books on type 1 diabetes

American Diabetes Association. *The Take-Charge Guide to Type 1 Diabetes.* Alexandria, VA: American Diabetes Association, 1994.

Dominick, Andie. *Needles*. New York: Scribner, 1998.

Walsh, John, Ruth Roberts, and Lois Jovanovic-Peterson. *Stop the Rollercoaster*. San Diego, CA: Torrey Pines Press, 1995.

Books on type 2 diabetes

American Diabetes Association. *Type 2 Diabetes: Your Healthy Living Guide*. Alexandria, VA: American Diabetes Association, 1997.

Edelman, Steven V. and Robert R. Henry. *Diagnosis and Management of Type II Diabetes*. Caddo, OK: Professional Communications, Inc., 1997.

Monk, Arlene. *Managing Type II Diabetes*. Minnetonka, MN: ChroniMed Publications, 1996.

Books for parents

Brackenridge, Betty and Richard R. Rubin. *Sweet Kids*. Alexandria, VA: American Diabetes Association, 1996.

Johnson, Robert W. *Managing Your Child's Diabetes*. Sandy, OR: Mastermedia Publications, 1996.

Books for children and teens

Betschart, Jean and Susan Thom. *In Control*. Minnetonka, MN: ChroniMed Publications, 1995. (A self-help guide for teenagers with diabetes.)

Betschart, Jean. *It's Time to Learn About Diabetes*. Minnetonka, MN: ChroniMed Publications, 1995. (For children age eight to ten.)

Peacock, Carol and Adair Gregory. *Sugar Was My Best Food: Diabetes and Me*. Mortongrove, IL: Albert Whitman and Co., 1998.

Other special interest diabetes books

Henry, Walter and Kirk Johnson. *Black Health Library Guide to Diabetes.* New York: Henry Holt and Co., Inc., 1993.

Hirsch, Irl B. *How to Get Great Diabetes Care.* Alexandria, VA: American Diabetes Association, 1996.

Lois Jovanovic-Peterson, June Biermann, and Barbara Toohey. *The Diabetic Woman,* revised edition. New York: Putnam Publishing Group, 1996.

Lodewick, Peter A., June Biermann, and Barbara Toohey. *The Diabetic Man.* Los Angeles: Lowell House, 1996.

Insulin pumps

Frederickson, Linda, ed. *The Insulin Pump Therapy Book.* Hawthorne, NY: Walter DeGruder, Inc., 1995.

Walsh, John. *Pumping Insulin.* San Diego, CA: Torrey Pines Press, 1994.

Exercise and diabetes

Gordon, Neil F. *Diabetes: Your Complete Exercise Guide.* Champaign, IL: Human Kinetics, 1993.

Diabetes and your emotions

Rubin, Richard. *Psyching Out Diabetes.* Los Angeles: Lowell House, 1997.

Important Documents

This appendix contains the following documents:

- Calculating your Body Mass Index
- The Glucagon Emergency Kit
- Instructions for Using the Glucagon Emergency Kit
- To Inject Glucagon
- Sample Blood-Sugar Log
- Daily Treatment Log
- Instructions for Mixing Insulins
- How to Prepare a Single Dose of Insulin
- How to Inject Insulin
- Instructions for Safe Sharps Disposal
- Carbohydrate Gram and Calories Counting Guide
- One-Page Care Guide for Children in School
- Before School Starts Checklist for Parents

The authors gratefully acknowledge Mr. Gilbert Jibaja for permission to reprint the Daily Treatment Log, and Mr. Jeff Hitchcock and www. childrenwithdiabetes.com for permission to reprint the One-Page Care Guide for Children in School and the Before School Starts Checklist for Parents.

Calculating your body mass index

Are you overweight?

Obesity is a known risk factor for type 2 diabetes. How do you know if you are overweight? Medical experts now say that your Body Mass Index (BMI) is a better indicator of obesity and associated health risks than the numbers on your scale.

Use this three-step method to calculate your BMI. A calculator will help.

Step 1: Multiply your weight in pounds by 703.

Step 2: Multiply your height in inches by itself.

Step 3: Divide the first number by the second.

Round to the nearest whole number for your Body Mass Index.

Interpreting your BMI
BMI under 19: Underweight
BMI 19 to 25: Healthy weight
BMI 26 to 30: Overweight
BMI 31 to 39: Very overweight
BMI 40 and above: Extremely overweight

For help in calculating and interpreting your BMI, visit the Web site of Shape Up, America!, a national program promoting healthy weight and increased exercise. The Web address is www.shapeup.org.

The glucagon emergency kit

How it works

Glucagon is a medicine given by injection that raises blood sugar very rapidly, in case of a low blood-sugar (hypoglycemia) emergency. If your blood-sugar level gets so low that you pass out or can't swallow, you will need glucagon.

Is it safe?

Glucagon is a safe drug, and there is no danger of overdosing or taking too much. However, it should be taken only during an emergency and should be used only under your doctor's direction.

What the kit contains

A Glucagon Emergency Kit includes all the supplies needed to administer the injection. Each emergency kit contains one bottle of glucagon in dry powder form and one syringe filled with a specially prepared liquid. Ask your doctor for a prescription.

How others can help

If you use insulin, you should always have an Emergency Glucagon Kit nearby. Your family, friends, co-workers, and even your exercise partners should learn how to give glucagon *before* you need it—because in an emergency you won't be able to give it to yourself. Most people find it extremely difficult to give an injection, especially in an emergency, so make sure your friends and family get plenty of opportunities to practice by giving you regular insulin injections.

If you pass out at home, at work, in the gym, or at a friend's house, the people around you should always be prepared to give you glucagon, even if they don't know exactly how low your blood sugar is.

Instructions for using the glucagon emergency kit

Note: Do not mix glucagon until you are ready to inject it.

To prepare glucagon for injection

1.
Remove the flip-off seal from the bottle of glucagon. Wipe the rubber stopper on top of the bottle with an alcohol swab.

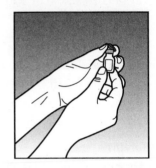

2.
Remove the needle protector from the syringe. Inject the entire contents of the syringe into the bottle of glucagon.

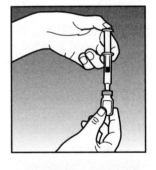

3.
Remove the syringe. Shake the bottle gently until the glucagon powder dissolves and the solution becomes clear. **Glucagon should not be used unless the solution is clear and waterlike.** Inject the glucagon immediately after mixing.

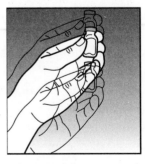

To inject glucagon

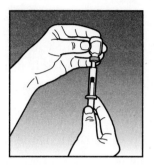

1.
Using the same syringe, withdraw all of the solution (1 mg mark on syringe) from the bottle. (If the shot is being given to a small child, and if a doctor recommends it, withdraw ½ of the solution from the bottle [0.5 mg mark on the syringe].)

2.
Cleanse an injection site on the buttocks, arm, or thigh with an alcohol swab.

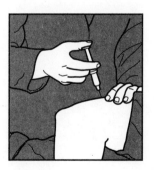

3.
Insert the needle into the subcutaneous fat at the clean injection site. Inject all of the glucagon solution. **There is no danger of overdose.** Apply light pressure at the injection site and withdraw the needle.

Turn the unconscious person on his or her side, in order to prevent choking when he or she awakens.

As soon as the person awakens and is able to swallow, give him or her a fast-acting source of sugar, such as a regular (nondiet) soft drink or orange juice, and a longer-acting source of sugar, such as crackers and milk or cheese.

Warning: The patient may be in a coma from severe hyperglycemia (high blood sugar) rather than hypoglycemia. In such a case, the patient will NOT respond to glucagon and will require immediate medical attention.

Once the person revives, his or her doctor should be notified immediately.

Note: Make sure your family and friends always have emergency phone numbers for your doctor and the nearest emergency room on hand.

Sample blood-sugar log

Sample Blood-Sugar Log

	BLOOD-SUGAR TEST RESULTS AND INSULIN DOSAGE								
DAY/DATE	BREAKFAST		LUNCH		DINNER		BEDTIME		COMMENTS
	Blood Sugar-Value	Insulin	Blood Sugar-Value	Insulin	Blood Sugar-Value	Insulin	Blood Sugar-Value	Insulin	Diet, exercise, ketones, stress, feelings, general health

← Note!
You can make your own blood-sugar log by making copies of this sample and keeping them in a ring binder. Simply enlarge the copies to the desired size and punch the necessary number of holes. The diagonal line under Blood-Sugar Value allows you to record mg/dls before and after each meal.

Daily treatment log

DAILY TREATMENT LOG

	ARISE	BKFST	LUNCH	SUPPER	BEDTIME
Glucose/Ketones in Urine:	_____	_____	_____	_____	_____
Blood Glucose*:	_____	___/___	___/___	___/___	_____
Insulin Type/Dose:	_____	_____	_____	_____	_____
Other Medications:	_____	_____	_____	_____	_____
Vitamins/ Supplements:	_____	_____	_____	_____	_____

Weight: _____   Blood Pressure: _____   Pulse: _____   Exercise Type: _____   Minutes: _____

Food Intake in Grams

NOTES _____

	CALS	SOD (mg)	Carbs	Fat	Chol.	Protein
DAY TOTALS						

*The diagonal line allows you to record mg/dl values before and after meals.
Copyright 1998 Gilbert Jibaja. Reprinted with permission.

Instructions for mixing insulins

Some people take more than one type of insulin at the same time. For example, you may need a mixture of short-acting insulin and intermediate-acting insulin to keep your blood sugar under control over time. You might use premixed insulin, such as 70/30 or 50/50. But you might need a ration of short-acting to intermediate-acting insulin that does not come premixed. If so, you will need to mix the insulins yourself.

Both insulins can go into the same syringe, so that only one shot is needed. This is called a *mixed dose* of insulin. Mixing should be done just before you inject the insulin. Don't try to mix insulin if you don't know how to handle syringes and insulin. Your doctor or diabetes educator will teach you how to prepare your first mixed dose of insulin. The following instructions are for use as a reminder only.

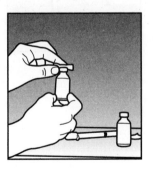

1.
Clean the tops of both insulin bottles with an alcohol swab.

2.
Inject ___ [B] units of air into the **longer-acting** insulin bottle (B = your dose of intermediate- or long-acting insulin). Do NOT pull insulin into the syringe. Take the needle out of the bottle.

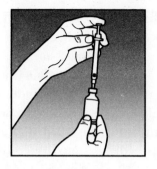

3.
Inject ___ [A] units of air into the **short-acting** insulin bottle (A = your dose of short-acting insulin). Turn the bottle and syringe upside down. Hold the bottle with one hand. Use the other hand to pull back on the plunger until you have ___[A] units of short-acting insulin in the syringe. Be sure to remove any large air bubbles (see How to Prepare a Single Dose of Insulin in this appendix). Take the needle out of the bottle.

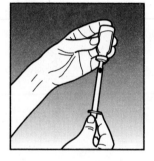

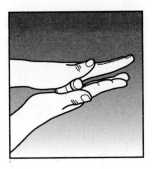

4.
Gently roll or swirl the longer-acting insulin bottle until it is mixed.

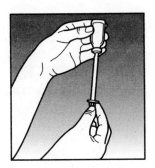

5.
Insert the needle into the bottle of longer-acting insulin. Turn the bottle and syringe upside down. Hold the bottle with one hand. Use the other hand to pull back on the plunger. Pull the plunger back until you have the total of ____(A+B) units in the syringe. Be sure you do not push any of the shorter-acting insulin into the longer-acting insulin bottle.

6.
Remove the needle from the bottle. Give yourself your injection as described in Administering an Insulin Injection, in this appendix.

How to prepare a single dose of insulin

Your doctor or diabetes educator will explain how to give yourself insulin injections. Don't try to do it just by following this guide. It is just a reminder.

1.
Gently mix the insulin by:

—Rolling the bottle between the palms of your hands, or

—Turning the bottle over from end to end several times, or

—Swirling the bottle gently.

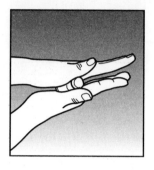

2.
If this is a new bottle of insulin, remove the cap. Do not remove the rubber stopper or the metal band under the cap.

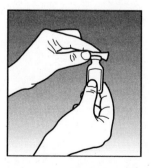

3.
Clean the rubber stopper on the top of the insulin bottle with an alcohol swab.

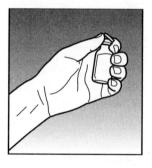

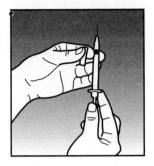

4.
Remove the cover from the needle. Pull the plunger back to bring air into the syringe. Stop pulling the plunger when the tip of the plunger is at the line for ___units (your dose of insulin).

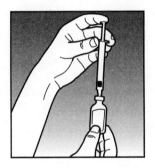

5.
Push the needle through the rubber stopper on the top of the insulin bottle. Push the air from the syringe into the bottle of insulin by pressing on the plunger.

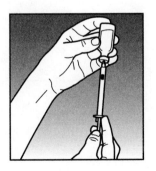

6.
Turn the bottle and syringe upside down. Make sure that the tip of the needle is in the insulin. Hold the bottle with one hand. With the other hand, pull back on the plunger. This will pull insulin from the bottle into the syringe. Stop pulling the plunger back when the tip of the plunger is at the line for ___units (your dose of insulin).

7.
Check the insulin in the syringe. There should be no air bubbles. If you see any air bubbles:

—Use the plunger to push the insulin back into the bottle.

—Slowly pull insulin into the syringe again by pulling back on the plunger.

—Pull the plunger back to the line for your dose of insulin.

—Repeat this until there are no large air bubbles in the syringe.

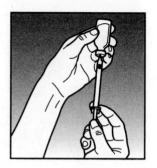

8.
Make sure the tip of the plunger is at the line for ____units (your dose of insulin). Double-check your dose. If you have difficulty seeing the lines on the syringe, magnifiers that connect to the syringe are available.

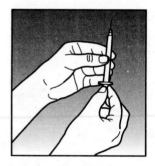

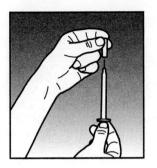

9.
Pull the needle out of the rubber stopper. (Be sure to put the cover back on the needle if you need to lay the syringe down before injecting yourself.)

How to inject insulin

1.
Choose a site for your injection. Clean the skin at the site with a alcohol swab.

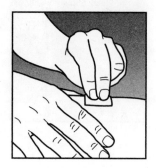

2.
"Pinch up" a large area of skin at the injection site. Push the needle into the skin. Go in at a 90 degree angle, as shown. Make sure that the needle goes all the way in.

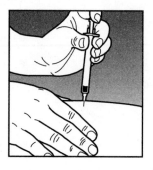

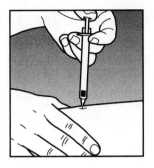

3.
Push the plunger all the way down, so that all of the insulin is pushed from the syringe into your body.

4.
Keeping the needle straight, pull it out of your skin. Do not rub the injection site.

5.
Safely dispose of used needles and syringes. For instructions, see Instructions for Safe Sharps Disposal in this appendix.

Instructions for safe sharps disposal

Follow these guidelines for safe containment and disposal of "sharps"—lancets, needles, and syringes.

- Use a puncture-proof plastic container with a tight-fitting screw top. A plastic soda bottle or bleach bottle is good, or ask your pharmacist about buying containers made specifically for this purpose. Don't use glass; it can break. Coffee cans aren't recommended because the plastic lids come off easily.

- Label the container clearly. Write "Contains Sharps" directly on the container or on masking tape on the container. Use a waterproof marker.

- As soon as you have used a syringe or lancet, immediately place it in the container and screw on the cap. Don't clip or bend needles.

- Keep the container out of the reach of children!

- When the container is full, screw the cap on tightly. Seal the container with heavy-duty tape for extra safety.

- Local laws differ as to how sharps containers may be disposed. Some communities allow full containers to be picked up with household trash; others may have special pickup days or drop-off sites for household medical waste.

- You may be able to drop off sharps containers at a local commercial medical laboratory or hospital laboratory.

- For more information on disposal, call your local public works department or solid waste manager. (Look in the blue pages of your telephone book, under city or county government.)

Or ask your diabetes educator or local American Diabetes Association about sharps disposal programs in your community.

- Do not put the sharps container out with recyclable plastics. Sharps are not recyclable.

Carbohydrate gram and calories counting guide

	Measure	Weight (grams)	Calories	Carbohydrate (grams)
		Dairy Products		
Butter	1/2 cup	113	810	—
	1 tbs	14	100	—
Cheese				
American	1 oz	28	105	—
cheddar	1 oz	28	115	—
cottage	1 cup	210	215	6
cream	1 oz	28	100	1
Swiss	1 oz	28	95	1
Cream				
light	1 cup	240	470	9
	1 tbs	15	30	1
heavy	1 cup	238	820	7
	1 tbs	15	50	1
sour	1 cup	230	495	10
	1 tbs	12	25	1
Eggs	1	50	75	1
yolk only	1	17	60	—
Ice cream	1 cup	133	270	32
Ice milk	1 cup	131	185	29
Milk				
buttermilk	1 cup	120	100	12
chocolate milk 2%	1 cup	250	180	26
evaporated	1 cup	252	340	25
malted milk	1 cup	265	235	29
powdered (skim)	1 cup	246	81	11
skim	1 cup	245	85	12
whole	1 cup	244	150	11

Whipped topping	1 cup	75	240	17
	1 tbs	4	15	1
Yogurt				
plain	8 oz	227	145	16
fruit	8 oz	227	230	43
Combination Foods				
Beef				
potpie	1	210	515	39
stew	1 cup	245	220	15
Chicken potpie	1	232	545	42
Chili con carne				
with beans	1 cup	255	340	31
Franks and beans	1 cup	255	365	32
Macaroni and cheese	1 cup	168	270	32
	3 oz	85	183	17
Pizza	1 piece	120	290	39
Soups, canned (with water)				
bean, bacon	1 cup	253	170	23
beef with vegetables	1 cup	245	80	10
chicken noodle	1 cup	241	75	9
clam chowder, Manhattan	1 cup	245	80	12
consommé, beef	1 cup	240	15	—
consommé, chicken	1 cup	240	12	—
cream of chicken	1 cup	244	115	9
cream of mushroom	1 cup	244	130	9
minestrone	1 cup	241	80	11

continues

	Measure	Weight (grams)	Calories	Carbohydrate (grams)
split pea	1 cup	250	165	27
vegetable with beef	1 cup	244	80	10
Soups, canned (with milk)				
New England clam chowder	1 cup	248	165	17
tomato	1 cup	248	160	22
oyster stew	1 cup	240	200	14
Soups, dry (with water)				
chicken noodle	1 cup	188	40	6
onion	1 cup	184	20	4
tomato	1 cup	189	40	8
Spaghetti with meat sauce	1 cup	248	330	39
Taco	1	81	195	15
Turkey patties	1	64	180	10
Meat & Poultry				
Bacon	3 slices	19	110	—
Beef				
corned	3 oz	85	185	0
hamburger	3 oz	85	245	0
pot roast	3 oz	85	325	0
roast, rib	3 oz	85	315	0
roast, rump	3 oz	85	220	0
steak, porterhouse	3 oz	85	395	0
steak, round	3 oz	85	220	0
steak, sirloin	3 oz	85	240	0
Chicken				
stewed	1 cup	140	250	0

fried	3.5 oz	98	220	1
roasted	3 oz	85	140	0
Duck	1/2	221	445	0
Ham	3 oz	85	250	0
Lamb				
chop, loin	3 oz	80	235	0
leg, roasted	3 oz	85	208	0
rib, roasted	3 oz	85	315	0
Pork				
chop	3 oz	85	275	0
roast	3 oz	85	270	0
Turkey	2 pieces	85	135	0
Veal				
cutlet	3 oz	85	185	0
roast	3 oz	85	230	0
		Seafood		
Bass	3 oz	85	167	5
Bluefish	3 oz	85	135	—
Clams, raw	3 oz	85	65	2
Cod	3 oz	85	144	—
Crabmeat				
canned	1 cup	135	135	1
Fish sticks	4	112	280	16
Flounder	3 oz	85	80	—
Haddock	3 oz	85	140	—
Halibut	3 oz	85	140	0
Herring	3 oz	85	190	0
Lobster	3 oz	85	81	—
Oysters, raw	1 cup	240	160	8
Perch	3 oz	85	185	0
Salmon, canned	3 oz	85	120	0
Sardines, canned	3 oz	85	175	0
Scallops	3 oz	85	95	0

continues

	Measure	Weight (grams)	Calories	Carbohydrate (grams)
Shrimp	3 oz	85	100	1
Swordfish	3 oz	85	150	0
Trout	3 oz	85	175	—
Tuna, canned				
in oil	3 oz	85	165	0
in water	3 oz	85	135	0
		Vegetables		
Artichoke	1	120	55	12
Asparagus	1 cup	180	45	8
Beans				
green	1 cup	125	30	7
lima	1 cup	170	110	32
red kidney	1 cup	255	230	42
yellow	1 cup	125	30	6
Bean sprouts	1 cup	125	25	5
Beets	1 cup	170	55	11
Beet greens	1 cup	145	40	8
Broccoli	1 cup	155	45	9
Brussel sprouts	1 cup	155	55	10
Cabbage	1 cup	150	30	7
raw	1 cup	70	15	4
Carrots	1 cup	156	70	16
cooked	1 cup	156	70	16
raw, strips	18	72	30	7
Cauliflower	1 cup	125	30	6
Celery	1 cup	120	20	4
raw, stalk	1	40	5	1
Collards	1 cup	190	25	5
Corn	1 ear	77	85	19
canned	1 cup	210	165	41
Cucumber	6 slices	28	5	1
Dandelion				
greens	1 cup	105	35	7
Eggplant	1 cup	96	25	6

Endive	1 cup	50	10	2
Kale	1 cup	130	40	7
Kohlrabi	1 cup	165	50	11
Lentils	1 cup	200	212	38
Lettuce				
iceberg	1 cup	55	5	1
loose leaf	1 1/2 cup	56	10	2
Mushrooms	1 cup	156	40	8
Mustard greens	1 cup	140	20	3
Okra, pods	8	85	25	6
Onions				
cooked	1 cup	210	60	13
raw, green	6	30	10	2
Parsnips	1 cup	156	125	30
Peas				
canned	1 cup	170	115	21
fresh	1 cup	160	65	11
frozen	1 cup	160	125	23
Peppers				
green, sweet	1	74	20	4
red, hot	1	45	20	4
Potatoes				
baked	1	101	110	25
boiled	1	136	120	27
French fried	20	100	220	34
fried	1 cup	115	308	37
mashed with milk	1 cup	210	160	37
scalloped	1 cup	245	210	26
Pumpkin	1 cup	228	75	18
Radishes	4	18	5	1
Sauerkraut	1 cup	236	45	10
Soybeans	1 cup	208	270	22
Spinach	1 cup	214	50	7

continues

	Measure	Weight (grams)	Calories	Carbohydrate (grams)
Squash				
summer	1 cup	180	35	8
winter, mashed	1 cup	205	80	18
Sweet potatoes				
baked	1	114	115	28
candied	1	105	145	29
Tomatoes				
canned	1 cup	240	50	10
raw	1	123	25	5
Tomato juice	1 cup	244	40	10
Tomato sauce	1 cup	245	75	18
Turnips	1 cup	156	30	8
Turnip greens	1 cup	144	30	6
Vegetables				
mixed	1 cup	163	75	15
		Fruits		
Apple	1	110	65	16
Applesauce				
no sugar	1 cup	244	105	28
Apricots	3	106	50	12
Avocado	1	173	305	12
Banana	1	114	105	27
Blackberries	1 cup	144	75	18
Blueberries	1 cup	145	80	20
Cantaloupe	1/2	267	95	22
Cherries, canned	1 cup	244	90	22
raw	10	68	50	11
Dates, pitted	1 cup	178	490	131
Figs	1	21	60	15
Grapefruit	1/2	120	40	10
Grapes	10	50	35	9

Lemon	1	58	15	11
Orange	1	131	60	15
Papaya	1 cup	140	65	17
Peach	1	87	35	10
Pear	1	166	100	25
Pineapple	1 cup	155	75	19
Plum	1	66	35	9
Prunes	4	49	115	31
Raisins	1 cup	145	435	115
Raspberries	1 cup	123	60	14
Rhubarb				
with sugar	1 cup	240	280	75
Strawberries	1 cup	149	45	10
Tangerine	1	84	35	9
Watermelon	1 cup	160	50	11
Fruit juices				
apple	1 cup	248	115	29
grapefruit	1 cup	246	95	23
lemon	1 cup	244	60	21
lime	1 cup	246	65	22
orange	1 cup	248	110	26
Grain Products				
Bagel	1	68	200	38
Barley	1 cup	200	700	158
Biscuit	1	28	100	13
Breads				
Boston brown	1 slice	45	95	21
cracked wheat	1 slice	25	65	12
French	1 slice	35	100	18
Italian	1 slice	30	85	17
raisin	1 slice	25	65	13
rye	1 slice	25	65	12
white	1 slice	25	65	12
whole wheat	1 slice	28	70	13

continues

	Measure	Weight (grams)	Calories	Carbohydrate (grams)
Breadcrumbs	1 cup	45	120	22
Cereals				
bran flakes	1 cup	56	180	44
bran flakes w. raisins	1 cup	56	185	42
corn flakes	1 cup	28	110	24
corn, frosted	1 cup	28	110	23
corn, puffed	1 cup	56	220	26
oats, puffed	1 cup	28	110	20
oatmeal	1 cup	234	145	25
rice, puffed	1 cup	28	110	25
wheat flakes	1 cup	28	100	23
wheat, shredded	2/3 cup	28	100	23
Crackers				
graham	2	14	60	11
saltine	4	12	50	9
rye wafers	2	14	55	10
Danish pastry	1	57	220	26
Doughnut	1	60	235	26
Flour				
buckwheat	1 cup	98	340	78
cornmeal	1 cup	138	500	108
enriched white	1 cup	125	455	95
whole wheat	1 cup	120	400	85
Muffin	1	40	120	17
corn	1	45	145	21
English	1	50	140	27
Pancakes				
homemade	1	27	60	9
from mix	1	27	60	8

Pasta

macaroni	1 cup	140	155	32
noodles	1 cup	160	200	32
spaghetti	1 cup	140	155	32

Popcorn

with oil, salt	1 cup	11	55	6

Pretzel	1	16	65	13

Rice

brown	1 cup	195	230	50
enriched	1 cup	205	225	50
instant	1 cup	175	185	41

Rolls

dinner	1	28	85	14
hamburger	1	40	115	20
hard	1	50	155	30

Waffles

homemade	1	75	245	26
from mix	1	75	205	27

Wheat germ	1 oz	28	110	14

Desserts & Sweets

Cake

angel food	1 piece	53	125	29
carrot with frosting	1 piece	96	385	48
cheesecake	1 piece	92	280	26
devils food with frosting	1 piece	69	235	40
fruitcake	1 piece	30	110	18
gingerbread	1 piece	63	175	32
pound	1 piece	43	165	25
sponge	1 piece	30	120	32
yellow with frosting	1 piece	75	275	39

Candy

caramels	1 oz	28	115	22
combination bar	1 oz	28	145	18

continues

	Measure	Weight (grams)	Calories	Carbohydrate (grams)
fudge	1 oz	28	115	21
gum drops	1 oz	28	100	25
hard	1 oz	28	110	28
Chocolate				
milk	1 oz	28	145	16
bitter	1 oz	28	150	16
semi-sweet	1 oz	28	150	16
syrup	1 oz	38	85	22
Cookies				
brownie	1	20	95	11
butter	1	12	61	7
chocolate chip	1	10	45	7
fig bars	1	14	52	11
sugar	1	12	59	7
Cupcakes				
frosted	1	36	129	21
Custard	1 cup	265	305	29
Frosting				
chocolate	1 cup	275	1035	185
coconut	1 cup	166	605	124
white, boiled	1 cup	94	300	76
white, uncooked	1 cup	252	947	206
Gelatin				
made with water	1 cup	240	140	34
Honey	1 tbs	21	65	17
Ice Cream	1 cup	133	270	32
Jams and preserves	1 tbs	20	55	14
Jellies	1 tbs	18	50	13
Marshmallows	1 oz	28	90	23
Molasses	1 tbs	20	43	11

Pie

apple	1 piece	158	405	60
blueberry	1 piece	158	410	55
cherry	1 piece	158	410	61
custard	1 piece	152	330	36
lemon meringue	1 piece	140	355	53
pecan	1 piece	138	575	71
pumpkin	1 piece	152	320	37
Popsicle	1	95	70	18

Puddings

chocolate	1 cup	260	300	50
rice	1 cup	264	310	54
tapioca	1 cup	260	290	50
Sherbet	1 cup	193	270	59

Sugar

brown	1 cup	220	820	212
white, granulated	1 cup	200	770	199
	1 tbs	12	45	12
white, powdered	1 cup	100	385	100

Syrup

corn, maple	1 tbs	21	61	16

Beverages

Alcoholic

beer	12 oz	360	150	13
beer, light	12 oz	355	95	5
wine	3 1/2 oz	102	80	3

Carbonated drinks

artificially sweetened	12 oz	350	0	0
club soda	12 oz	355	0	0
colas, sweetened	12 oz	369	160	41
fruit flavored soda	12 oz	372	170	45

continues

	Measure	Weight (grams)	Calories	Carbohydrate (grams)
ginger ale	12 oz	366	125	32
root beer	12 oz	370	165	42
Miscellaneous				
Barbecue sauce	1 tbs	16	10	2
Bouillon cube	1	4	5	0
Catsup, tomato	1 tbs	15	15	4
Cocoa	1 cup	265	225	30
Coconut, shredded	1 cup	80	285	12
Garlic	1	30	41	9
Mustard	1 tbs	5	5	1
Nuts				
almonds	1 oz	28	795	28
cashews	1 cup	137	785	45
peanuts	1 cup	145	840	27
pecans	1 cup	108	720	20
walnuts	1 cup	125	760	15
Olives				
green	4	13	15	0
ripe	3	9	15	0
Peanut butter	1 tbs	16	95	3
Pickles				
dill	1	65	5	1
relish	1 tbs	15	20	5
sweet gherkin	1	15	20	5

One-Page Care Guide for Children in School

When you send your child to school, you should include some kind of instructions for the teacher that describe what you expect of the teacher. The instructions should include a list of symptoms that your child exhibits when he or she is hypoglycemic, when you expect the child to perform blood glucose tests, and how to respond to episodes of hypoglycemia.

Written instructions are particularly important when your child has a substitute teacher. Make sure that your instructions are prominently posted in the classroom, preferably close to the teacher's desk. You might even want to print it on bright yellow or pink paper so that it stands out.

The following example must be adapted to the needs of your child with the help of your diabetes team.

Remember, this is only an example.

Guidelines for Caring for _____
                                                    [child's name]

When to do a blood-sugar check
She says, "I'm low," especially during or after exercise.
If she has symptoms of low blood sugar, including

- Irritability
- Erratic responses to questions
- Sleepiness

WHAT TO DO BASED ON HER
BLOOD-SUGAR READING

(Remember, this is only an example and must be adapted to your child's specific needs.)

Blood-Sugar Reading	What to Do
Under 60	Give two glucose tablets, followed immediately by food containing 30 grams of carbohydrates. If she doesn't respond within 10 minutes, telephone her mother/ father, [name/name], at [phone number] for further instructions.
61 to 100	Give one glucose tablet. If a meal or snack is within 30 minutes, she can wait; otherwise, give her a snack including carbohydrates and protein, such as cheese crackers with peanut butter or cookies and milk.
101 to 125	She is fine. If exercise is planned before a meal or snack, she must have a snack before participating. This includes recess.
126 to 200	She is fine. She could feel low if she was previously high and is dropping.
201 to 240	She's a bit high, but this is not uncommon for her, especially in the early morning.
Over 240	Her blood sugar is too high. She must be given access to water or other noncaloric fluids. Use of the bathroom must be allowed as needed. She needs to check her urine for ketones. If ketones are present, the parents or the diabetes team should be called for advice. *Note:* She may confuse being this high with being low, since many of the symptoms are similar.

When giving sugar, the following are roughly equivalent:

- Four ounces of fruit juice
- One-half to one cup of milk
- Two glucose tablets (some are different: 10 to 15 grams of sugar are recommended).
- One-half tube of Cake Mate frosting (should be placed between the cheek and gums if unable to swallow)
- One-half can of soda (regular, NOT diet!)

Chocolate candy is not to be used unless there is no other source of sugar available. It is not absorbed quickly enough, due to fats in the candy.

If the blood sugar remains low despite treatment and the student is not thinking clearly, the parent or the diabetes team should be called for advice.

Following an episode of low blood sugar, it can take several hours to fully recover. Hence, the student should not be expected to perform at optimal levels. However, diabetes should never be allowed to become an excuse for school performance.

©1998 Children with Diabetes
Reprinted with permission.

Before School Starts Checklist for Parents

Each school reacts differently to children that need a little extra attention. And children with diabetes do need a little extra attention, especially when they are very young. If you are approaching your first school year with diabetes, here's a list of things you should do *before* school starts:

1. Meet with the school principal and determine the school's specific policies regarding blood testing and access to emergency sugar. Some schools allow the children to test in the classroom, while others require them to test in the clinic.

2. Find out the name of your child's teacher, and make an appointment to see him or her at least one week before school starts. At that meeting, you should

    a. Tell the teacher that your child has diabetes.

    b. Briefly describe what it means to have diabetes. Both the American Diabetes Association and the Juvenile Diabetes Foundation have excellent books and pamphlets to assist you. Particularly good is the ADA publication, *Caring for Children with Diabetes*. It covers the basics about diabetes and, at only 14 pages, is short enough to read in about an hour.

    c. Tell the teacher that your child must eat midmorning and midafternoon snacks, and tell him or her at what time you expect the snacks to be eaten. Regardless of the day's activities, your child must be allowed to eat these snacks. That might mean bringing food to an assembly or field trip.

d. Find out at what time your child will be having lunch so you can plan insulin injections accordingly. Some kids have lunch at 11:00 a.m. while others have lunch at 12:45 p.m. That can make a big difference on morning insulin and snacks.

e. Describe what happens when your child is hypoglycemic. Since every child reacts differently, tell the teacher exactly what to look for and how to respond. You might want to provide the One-Page Care Guide for Children in School (contained in this appendix).

f. Give the teacher a supply of sugar and extra snack foods to keep in her desk in case they are needed. In some schools, you might have to keep these in the clinic.

g. Impress upon the teacher in no uncertain terms that if he or she suspects that your child is experiencing low blood sugar (insulin reaction) that your child is not to be left alone. If your child must go to the clinic to perform a blood test, make sure the teacher understands that someone must go with your child.

3. If you can, obtain a numeric pager. Give your pager number to your child's teacher and the clinic nurse, if there is one. Instruct them to page you with your child's blood-sugar level whenever it is out of the range that you feel is acceptable.

4. Meet with any other teacher that your child will see, including gym teachers, music teachers, art teachers, and the librarian. Let them know that your child has diabetes and ask them to be on the lookout for symptoms of low blood sugar. This is especially important for gym teachers.

5. **An extra note on gym teachers:** Make sure that gym teachers know that your child should *not* exercise with a blood-sugar level of 240 mg/dl or higher, since such a high sugar level can indicate insufficient insulin. In this case, exercise can actually cause the blood-sugar level to rise. One parent reported that her child's gym teacher said that exercise lowers blood sugar, and made a ketonic child run a mile!

References:

1. *Managing Your Child's Diabetes*. Johnson, Robert Wood and Sale Johnson.

2. *A Child with Diabetes in Your Care*, published by the Juvenile Diabetes Foundation.

3. *Caring for Children with Diabetes,* published by the American Diabetes Association.

Important Statistics

- Nearly 20 million people in the United States, or about one in every seventeen people, have diabetes.

- About half of all people who have diabetes do not know that they have the disease and are not receiving medical care.

- Each year, about 650,000 people are diagnosed with diabetes—about 1,800 new cases each day.

- Diabetes is the leading cause of adult blindness, amputation, and end-stage kidney disease in the United States. It also contributes to heart disease, stroke, and nerve damage.

- More women die from diabetes-related complications than from breast cancer.

- Diabetes costs the United States close to $130 billion per year in medical expenses—almost 15 percent of total medical expenditures.

- People who have diabetes are four times more likely to die of heart disease than people who do not.

- Diabetes is one of the most common chronic disorders in children in the United States. Nearly 130,000 children and teens age nineteen and younger have diabetes. That's about eighteen children for every 100,000 people.

- 90 to 95 percent of all diabetes cases are type 2 diabetes.

- Nearly 11 percent of Americans ages sixty-five to seventy-four have type 2 diabetes.

- In Americans ages forty-five to seventy-four, over 14 percent are Mexican Americans and Puerto Rican

Americans who have type 2 diabetes

- Over 10 percent of African Americans have type 2 diabetes.

- About 6 percent of Cuban Americans and Caucasians have type 2 diabetes.

- In some Native American groups, almost half of adults age thirty to sixty-four have type 2 diabetes.

- 75 to 80 percent of all people with type 2 diabetes are or have been obese.

- Each year, about 135,000 pregnant women develop gestational diabetes mellitus.

- Of these women, about 35 to 40 percent will develop type 2 diabetes in the following five to fifteen years.

- About 1,000,000 Americans depend upon insulin injections to live.

The *Unofficial Guide*™ Reader Questionnaire

If you would like to express your opinion about living with diabetes or this guide, please complete this questionnaire and mail it to:

The *Unofficial Guide*™ Reader Questionnaire
Macmillan Lifestyle Group
1633 Broadway, floor 7
New York, NY 10019-6785

Gender: ___ M   ___ F

Age: ___ Under 30   ___ 31–40   ___ 41–50
___ Over 50

Education: ___ High school   ___ College
___ Graduate/Professional

What is your occupation?
_____

How did you hear about this guide?
___ Friend or relative
___ Newspaper, magazine, or Internet
___ Radio or TV
___ Recommended at bookstore
___ Recommended by librarian
___ Picked it up on my own
___ Familiar with the *Unofficial Guide*™ travel series

Did you go to the bookstore specifically for a book on living with diabetes?   Yes ___   No ___

Have you used any other *Unofficial Guides*™?
Yes ___   No ___

If Yes, which ones?
_____
_____
_____

What other book(s) on diabetes have you purchased?

_____

_____

_____

Was this book:
___ more helpful than other(s)
___ less helpful than other(s)

Do you think this book was worth its price?
Yes ___   No ___

Did this book cover all topics related to diabetes adequately?   Yes ___   No ___

Please explain your answer:

_____

_____

_____

Were there any specific sections in this book that were of particular help to you?   Yes ___   No ___

Please explain your answer:

_____

_____

_____

On a scale of 1 to 10, with 10 being the best rating, how would you rate this guide? ___

What other titles would you like to see published in the *Unofficial Guide*™ series?

_____

_____

Are *Unofficial Guides*™ readily available in your area?   Yes ___   No ___

Other comments:

_____

_____

_____

_____

About the Authors

Maria Thomas is a health and mental health writer and a graduate of the University of Michigan, where she received a Bachelor's degree with honors in Psychology and History, and later a Master's Degree in psychiatric Social Work. Before beginning her career as a writer, Maria practiced as a family counselor and mental health therapist for over 13 years. Her background in mental health informs and enriches her reporting on all aspects of living with chronic disease.

Loren Wissner Greene, M.D. graduated from Barnard College cum laude with honors in anthropology and biology. She graduated from New York University School of Medicine where she received the Merck Manual Award in Medicine. She went on to complete a fellowship in Endocrinology and Metabolism at New York University Medical Center. Dr. Greene is board certified in Internal Medicine and in Endocrinology and Metabolism and is a Fellow of the American College of Endocrinology (FACE) and the American College of Physicians (FACP).

She has spoken to professional and patient audiences and written articles for professional and lay journals on diabetes and other areas of endocrinology.

Dr. Greene is a Clinical Associate Professor of Medicine at New York University School of Medicine where she is the co-director of the second year course in Endocrinology, co-director of the Endocrine Clinic at Bellevue Hospital, and a co-director of the Bone Density Unit at New York University Medical Center. She has a private practice in New York City, specializing in Diabetes, Endocrinology, and Metabolism.